CURRENT PRINCIPLES AND PRACTICES OF TELEMEDICINE AND E-HEALTH

Studies in Health Technology and Informatics

This book series was started in 1990 to promote research conducted under the auspices of the EC programmes' Advanced Informatics in Medicine (AIM) and Biomedical and Health Research (BHR) bioengineering branch. A driving aspect of international health informatics is that telecommunication technology, rehabilitative technology, intelligent home technology and many other components are moving together and form one integrated world of information and communication media. The complete series has been accepted in Medline. Volumes from 2005 onwards are available online.

Series Editors:
Dr. J.P. Christensen, Prof. G. de Moor, Prof. A. Famili, Prof. A. Hasman, Prof. L. Hunter, Dr. I. Iakovidis, Dr. Z. Kolitsi, Mr. O. Le Dour, Dr. A. Lymberis, Prof. P.F. Niederer, Prof. A. Pedotti, Prof. O. Rienhoff, Prof. F.H. Roger France, Dr. N. Rossing, Prof. N. Saranummi, Dr. E.R. Siegel, Dr. P. Wilson, Prof. E.J.S. Hovenga, Prof. M.A. Musen and Prof. J. Mantas

Volume 131

Recently published in this series

ISSN 0926-9630

Current Principles and Practices of Telemedicine and e-Health

Edited by

Rifat Latifi

Professor of Clinical Surgery, The University of Arizona, Tucson, Arizona, USA

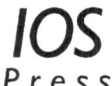

IOS
Press

Amsterdam • Berlin • Oxford • Tokyo • Washington, DC

ISBN 978-1-58603-806-9
Library of Congress Control Number: 2007940963

Publisher
IOS Press
Nieuwe Hemweg 6B
1013 BG Amsterdam
Netherlands
fax: +31 20 687 0019
e-mail: order@iospress.nl

Distributor in the UK and Ireland
Gazelle Books Services Ltd.
White Cross Mills
Hightown
Lancaster LA1 4XS
United Kingdom
fax: +44 1524 63232
e-mail: sales@gazellebooks.co.uk

Distributor in the USA and Canada
IOS Press, Inc.
4502 Rachael Manor Drive
Fairfax, VA 22032
USA
fax: +1 703 323 3668
e-mail: iosbooks@iospress.com

LEGAL NOTICE

The publisher is not responsible for the use which might be made of the following information.

PRINTED IN THE NETHERLANDS

Preface

This book represents the most current developments in the rapidly expanding and changing field of telemedicine and e-health, especially in the developing countries. Much has changed since the publication of the first book in 2004 (Establishing Telemedicine in Developing Countries: From Inception to Implementation). Telemedicine has become more popular, and continues to grow. Over the last three years, I have received many requests for copies of the book from all over the world. While there are many good books and materials on telemedicine, my hope is that this one will become a useful reference for all of those practicing telemedicine and e-health, particularly in developing countries. It is dedicated to all future generations of telemedicine and e-health students, including health care practitioners, administrators, policy makers, technical professionals and others.

Having in mind this vision for the book, I have asked some of the best and the brightest in telemedicine to help me put together this volume, which should be understandable, informative, and un-ambiguous. I am grateful to every one who has contributed to this and to the first edition of this book.

If you want to go anywhere in world, there are maps (although in some parts of the world maps are changing rapidly); if you want to build a motorcycle, a boat or perform a complex surgical procedure, chances are you can find instructions on the internet on how to do it. Well, this is not the case if you require information on how to establish telemedicine and e-health system and programs, not only in the developing countries, but even in your own town, or own country in the developed world.

I hope that this book will be the guide we all wanted to have and will reflect the current status of telemedicine. Perhaps someone else will take over and name this "Telemedicine for Dummies". Maybe we should have called this book exactly that: "Telemedicine and E-Health for Dummies".

Rifat LATIFI, MD, FACS
Professor of Clinical Surgery
Trauma, Surgical Critical Care and Emergency General Surgery
Department of Surgery, The University of Arizona, Tucson, Arizona, USA
Associate Director of Arizona Telemedicine Program, Telesurgery and
International Affairs
President, International Virtual e-Hospital Foundation
Director, Telemedicine Program of Kosova

Contents

V. The Internet and Medicine

VI. New Frontiers of Telemedicine

I. The Development of Telemedicine

Current Principles and Practices of Telemedicine and e-Health
R. Latifi (Ed.)
IOS Press, 2008

3

International Virtual e-Hospital:
The Balkans Journey

Rifat LATIFI, MD, FACS
Professor of Clinical Surgery
Trauma, Surgical Critical Care and Emergency General Surgery
Department of Surgery, The University of Arizona, Tucson, Arizona, USA
Associate Director of Arizona Telemedicine Program, Telesurgery and
International Affairs
President, International Virtual e-Hospital Foundation
Director, Telemedicine Program of Kosova

Abstract. What started in Berlin in May of 2000 as an idea to create the telemedicine program of Kosova in order to help the country rebuild the broken medical system and change the miserable face of medicine, has now spread to other countries in the Balkans. Today, June 29, 2007, as I am rewriting this chapter, ten doctors and engineers from Kosova, Montenegro and Macedonia graduated from a three weeks intensive course on telemedicine, e-health and medical electronic library. This international telemedicine fellowship is organized by the very entity that was created in Berlin 7 years ago: The International Virtual e-Hospital (IVEH). This time, however they are part of a project called "Improving Health Care in the Balkans Using Telemedicine, Advanced Technologies and Cultural Exchange Programs as a Platform" funded by the Bureau of Education and Cultural Exchange of the State department of USA, and is being implemented in collaboration with Arizona Telemedicine Program and University of Arizona Health Science Center Library, as well as Alaska Telemedicine program in Anchorage. The goal of the program is to create the medical and technical leadership that will significantly enhance health care access and quality in the region. This program is creating a powerful international medical education network in the Balkans for further collaboration and development. As part of the project, 48 physicians, nurses and engineers from Kosova, Montenegro, Macedonia and Albania are being trained in telemedicine, e-health, electronic library management, trauma and surgical critical care. A group of experts in these same medical disciplines will conduct workshops, seminars and other cultural and educational activities in the Balkan region. We can say now with certainty that the Telemedicine Program of Kosova is having an impact in the region that goes far beyond telemedicine applications and advanced technologies in the Balkans. It is creating leadership that will take the future in their own hands, as they become the true champions of telemedicine and rebuilding the dream of advancing the health care in their own countries. As we say at IVEH, it is "one country at a time." In October, we will inaugurate the Second Phase of the Telemedicine Program of Kosova. On October 21–23, in Tirana, Albaria, we will organize the Second Intensive Balkan Telemedicine and e-health seminar, a three-day workshop on current principles and practices of telemedicine, e-health, and medical informatics. The journey that started in Berlin is continuing. Soon we will be traveling to Atalaya, Peru and other communities of Amazon River, then Africa. We will not stop. One country at a time!

Introduction

The Telemedicine Program of Kosova has become one of best telemedicine programs in South Eastern Europe and the best in the Balkans, and during this process we have realized, as predicted, that our mission goes far beyond the simple "telemedicine" applications. What started as modern telemedicine center at the University Clinical Center of Kosova in Prishtina, has now has spread to all regional hospitals of Kosova, and as such it has become an inspiration, and above all, the place where hope for change and prosperity meet with the reality. So before you start reading *all you ever wanted to know about establishing telemedicine in developing countries,*" I would like to take you through a personal journey of creating and establishing telemedicine in the Balkans. For me, this has been a great journey filled with joy, excitement, drama, occasional disappointments, and many, many hours traversing the world from one corner to the other. But it was worth it. Every bit of it! The Telemedicine Program of Kosova (TPK) and establishment of telemedicine in other developing countries have become my passion- or more accurately, my obsession, my second professional life, after trauma surgery. But it has been most enriching experience, an experience that I would not trade for anything in the world. It has been a destiny.

1. Journal from my World

1.1. New Haven, Connecticut, 1999

Eight years ago, in June of 1999, I was a surgical chief resident at Yale University in New Haven, CT. The war in Kosova was intensifying and the rivers of refugees, including my family in Shijak, now refugees. Concentrating entirely on working on the surgical oncology service at Yale University was becoming more and more difficult. The day of graduation from my surgical residency on June 19, 1999 was not coming fast enough. I was a trauma surgeon, and it was very difficult to stay on the "sidelines"!

I had purchased a ticket to go to Albania June 21, 1999 a month in advance. Although I wanted peace, and an end to the war. I also was afraid that war would end without my help, before I could get there, somewhere in the mountains of Albania or Kosova.

I had suggested to Dr. Ronald C. Merrell, my chairman, to allow me to go to Albania and bring with me the telemedicine technologies on the ground and support Kosovar wounded and injured. He thought that this was a great idea. He and his team had done something similar to this in Armenia during the catastrophic earthquake. By the time we got to do anything the war ended. I missed an incredibly valuable chance to use telemedicine when it was necessary, and develop a true teletrauma. Reports from refugee camps on the ground were horrifying. The number of wounded, misplaced, and terrorized Kosovars was growing. My parents and sisters family had made it to Albania, but they had traveled through Montenegro. They were somewhere in Shijak, now refugees. Concentrating entirely on working on the surgical oncology service at Yale University was becoming more and more difficult. The day of graduation from my surgical residency on June 19, 1999 was not coming fast enough. I was a trauma surgeon, and it was very difficult to stay on the "sidelines"!

I had purchased a ticket to go to Albania June 21, 1999 a month in advance. Although I wanted peace, and an end to the war, in a way I was afraid that war would end before I could get there, somewhere in the mountains of Albania or Kosova.

I had suggested to Dr. Ronald C. Merrell, my chairman, to allow me to go to Albania and bring with me the telemedicine technologies on the ground and support Kosovar wounded and injured. He thought that this was a great idea. He and his team had done something similar to this in Armenia during the catastrophic earthquake. By the time we got to do anything the war ended. I missed an incredibly valuable chance to use telemedicine when it was necessary, and develop a true teletrauma.

1.2. Tirana, Albania

On June 19th 1999, I graduated from Surgical Residency at Yale University in New Haven, Connecticut, and on June 22, I arrived in Tirana, Albania, but the war had ended ten days earlier. The NATO troops entered Prishtina and liberated Kosova from Serbian forces. Albania had become a large refugee camp from North to South, and East to West. Refugees were in every corner and in every home of Albania. There were numerous wounded Albanians at the Military Hospital in Tirana, but there were no new causalities coming from the Northern front any more. For me, the war had not ended. We had a long way to go. The true war of rebuilding the country, the independence and democratic country has just started. The UN resolution 1244 fell short of all of this. The country was destroyed and it was in total disarray. We were entering a new phase of war. I had to be part of this war now. There were no more excuses.

1.3. Kllodërnicë, Kosova

On July 1, 1999, I returned home to Kosova from Albania with my two brother-in-laws and a river of refugees who were coming back on buses, tractors and all sorts of trucks. Each vehicle held an Albanian and an American flag waving on that warm July night. They were returning to Kosova to find nothing but destruction, death, and misery. Seeing people alive was a real pleasure. No one knew who was dead and who was alive. I felt guilty returning to Kosova with refugees. This was their moment in history. I did not deserve to be with them.

When I arrived in Kllodernice, the village I was born and grew up in, everything was destroyed. I learned that my uncle, aunt, many cousins, neighbors, and friends, had all been killed, all shot at point blank range. I knew our house had been burned also. Our house in Kllodërnicë was burned the same day my wife and I were closing on a new house in Chesterfield County, Virginia. Drita found this ironic. I was hoping that at least some of thousands of books had survived the fire. As I approached the house everything became clear. Everything was gone: the books, the memories. Burned down to ashes. Hope was the only survivor… As I looked over the ravages of my old home, I became numb. There were no tears. There was nothing I could feel or do. I set in the middle of what use to be the guest house or "oda" as we called and asked my brother-in-law to take a picture of me sitting there. This was the last time I sat there. Last time!

"Welcome Home, Sir!"

1.4. Prishtina, July 2 1999

At the gate of University Clinical Center of Kosova in Prishtina, a British soldier stood, with boyish face, a machine gun in his hand, and a frightening look. I pulled out my American passport. Somehow I was able to tell him that I used to work there, pointing at the Surgery Clinic and trying to hide my tears. The soldier stood at attention and saluted me: "*Welcome Home, Sir.*" I fought back my tears again, and saluted him. I have never forgotten his face.

(Eight years later, every time I pass through that gate in my way to the University Clinical Center of Kosova in Prishtina, I see the image of that soldier saluting me, although I never met him again.)

When I entered the emergency room, one of the senior surgeons recognized me and asked if I was on call that night. *"No I am not"*—I replied matter of fact and we hugged each other. *"I do not deserve to be on call now that there is peace. I was not here during the war, thus, I cannot be on call tonight. I just came to find out who is still alive"*—I thought but never said a word. I think he understood me regardless of my lack of words. Since then, I have operated, rounded on many patients, and lectured many times to the students, and doctors and nurses of the University Clinical Center of Kosova. In a way, it feels I never left that day. I think I am on call all the times. Virtually on call.

However, I did leave Kosova that day. As I traveled back, smell of the ashes of the burned homes lingered, although there were no more fires.

For the next twelve hours I traveled back to Shijak, Albania, now home to thousands of refugees placed in the camps and Albanian homes, to tell my parents that everything that they had built during their entire life was gone. My parents and my sisters, Haka and Hava, with their children, remained numb and cried quietly. Fighting the tears from his deep blue eyes and old face, my eighty year old father said *"Selim was my best brother."* His seventy-six year old brother was killed at his doorstep by his Serbian neighbor. For four years after his death, we did not know where the remains of my uncle lay.

1.5. Richmond, Virginia

Later that July of 1999, I moved to Richmond, Virginia to become an assistant professor of surgery and trauma at Virginia Commonwealth University. I joined Dr. Merrell and Dr. Rao R. Ivatury, a mentor and a friend from my surgical critical care and trauma fellowship, Part of my obligations at VCU were to lead the educational programs and distance learning for the Medical Informatics and Technology Applications Consortium (MITAC) that Dr. Merrell had created with a grant from NASA.

After the war was over in Kosova, NATO countries, many NGO's, and other organizations from around the world, poured into Kosova, but concentrated efforts mainly in Prishtina. A British doctor used a laptop computer to send e-mail and jpg pictures of many complicated surgical cases asking for "international" advice. We answered many of these calls from Prishtina and rendered advice for treatment of land mine injuries, burned kids, and those with multiple small bowel fistulae—just to name a few. In a sense, this was the start of the project we should have been doing during the war.

1.6. 2000

Late January 2000, Dr. Merrell, Brett Harnett, and I visited Kosova. During this visit, we operated with Prishtina surgeons, gave ground rounds, signed the MOU with the Medical Faculty in Prishtina, and performed the technical evaluation of telecommunications system at the UCCK. It was clear that the situation was grave in every aspect, and the technical network was almost non-existing and destroyed. The idea of establishing telemedicine program was getting stronger and clear.

Early spring of 2000, Toulouse, France, I participated in a telemedicine conference. This was my first telemedicine conference. I really enjoyed the conference and the City of Toulouse. The delegates certainly knew each other, but I was new to this world.

Dr. Michael Nerlich, a trauma orthopedic surgeon from Regensburg University, Regensburg, Germany, was in charge of organizing part of the program of the final conference of the G-8 meeting in Berlin, to take place on May 3–5, 2000. He invited me to give a talk at that meeting on the health status in Kosova and the possibilities of using telemedicine as a means and way to change and improve healthcare.

That night in Toulouse, I became very anxious about my presentation, which was months away. This was very unusual for me. Actually I asked Dr. Nerlich to invite some one else from Prishtina to do the talk. I offered to help him identify a speaker. Dr. Nerlich insisted that I do it, and I am thankful he did. For the next few months, I worked tirelessly on my presentation. I collected facts, pictures, created and deleted many slides over and over. I titled my talk: *"The Anatomy of Death and Destruction of Kosova: The Alumni's View in Restructuring Healthcare."* [2] Desperately, I asked for help from Prishtina. I needed numbers, real data. Data was hard to come by. Most of it had been destroyed, or frankly never collected.

1.7. Berlin, Germany

When I arrived in Berlin, I was greeted by a beautiful ultra modern city. I stayed at the Madison Hotel. After a short nap that afternoon, I went for a run in a nearby park and was surprised greatly by nude folks enjoying sunbathing in a public park in Berlin. Hotel Madison and Berlin Parliament were few hundred meters away from the (former) Berlin Wall. I do not like walls and borders to begin with, and the Berlin Wall was no exception. The Berlin Wall always reminded me of the border between Albania and Kosova. Once, at age seventeen, October 22, 1972, as a second year high school student, a few friends and I attempted to cross illegally to Albania and break that "wall" that has killed so many Albanians. Instead of getting across the mountain, we ended up in jail for a few days. I never forgot those three days in jail. Although the Berlin Wall was no longer functioning, it has remained bad memory of a human tragedy and a political failure.

On May 3, 2000, my power point presentation was ready but something was unsettling to me. My talk was descriptive, but almost crying. My purpose was to describe the anatomy of the death and destruction of Kosova, and come up with a telemedicine project, but there was something was missing. I did not have a name for it. This was really troubling me. Then, things suddenly changed! As I was sitting with an editor from a major publishing company located in Stuttgart, Germany, listening to one particularly dry presentation, everything came together. It was almost as if someone had delivered a typewritten note to me from the sky that afternoon at the Berlin Parliament. It was as clear as it possibly could be. The telemedicine project of Kosova had a name. The International Virtual e-Hospital—yes, the name International Virtual e-Hospital really sounded great and was quite appropriate for the G-8 conference that I was presenting.

I rushed back to the hotel and picked up my laptop and re-did my entire talk in the next few hours, occasionally paying attention to the speakers of the afternoon plenary session. Putting this together all of a sudden was really easy. The talk was flowing, had a real pulse, and a nice closure. It was dramatic to the point of being bloody, but so what? As a trauma surgeon I function best surrounded by blood. The situation in Kosova was still bloody; the drama was still ongoing and needed to be changed.

I showed the talk that evening to Dr. Michael Nerlich. He thought it was exactly what "*these guys*" needed. "*Let it be real for once,*" he said, almost upset. After the last session was over that afternoon, I went to "East" Berlin and walked for hours around the remains of the wall. On the east side, but now unified Berlin, I asked a bartender to write directly in my lap-top in German, on my last slide: "I love you Berlin."

That night in Berlin was the first time that I had peace of mind with my assignment since it was presented to me at the Toulouse meeting. Everything made sense, my message was becoming clear, and I knew that something big was born that day.

On May 4, 2000, everything was ready. I was the first speaker. The delegates were all in their seats in the modern auditorium at the Berlin Parliament where Bismarck gave his major historical talk and said that politics is not an exact science. This was my first international telemedicine presentation and I was ready. The auditorium was a fantastic place to give this kind of futuristic and promising talk as one needed for the Balkans. I spoke for 30 minutes. When I left the podium of the Berlin Parliament, the slide showed an Albanian flag was waving and on it "I Love You Berlin" in German. Later, I learned there was a spelling error in my phrase, and that the bartender was actually an immigrant from Poland.

Everything and everyone became almost eerily quiet. Speaker after speaker got up to offer me help, but they were unable to talk because they were in tears. It became clear that I had hit a chord, I infused some new blood into this meeting, and I simply challenged the world that if we were serious about offering assistance to developing countries and countries in disarray like Kosova, we should provide real structured help. This was the idea. The message came across clearly to everyone's mind and heart. I felt elated. Immediately after my talk, the organizer of the conference, Dr. Gottfried T.W. Dietzel, invited me to the reception with the Minister of Health of Germany, Mrs. Anne Fisher, at the Building of the German Parliament that was being organized for a select group of people from the conference. During her welcoming speech, she said "*I am very happy that today in Berlin, you have created the International Virtual e-Hospital of Kosova.*" To the rest of the delegates this appeared almost as if it was planned and orchestrated. No one knew that 28 hours ago this concept did not have a name.

I spent a great deal of time with Mrs. Fisher that night, and found her to be a fascinating woman, charismatic and humorous. "*Working with doctors, is a real challenging task*"—she said many times, adding that she did not think that I was a "*real*" doctor! "*You have too much passion, you seem too real,*" she said.

I realized that this was probably the most important talk of my life. I wished someone from Kosova was there, and I wished someone from Kosova had listened to the evening news that night in Germany. The creation of the International Virtual e-Hospital of Kosova became international news on the first day of creation of the concept [3]. As the evening progressed, I became more aware of what really happened that day in Berlin. One thing was for sure: my life changed dramatically and took on a totally new direction.

I am so happy about that! (*Not a day goes by that I do not think of this event. One is really not aware how things can change in your life. It only takes you one event and than things will may never be the same. For good or for bad!*)

From Berlin I went to Munich's outskirts to visit my brother Halil and his family who were refugees. It had been almost four years since we had seen each other. His children had grown up and they had a new son. He had grown older. They were getting ready to be repatriated back to Kosova by German authorities. There was something ironic in all of this. It was in Berlin that the International Virtual e-Hospital concept was created, and it was an official Berlin who was returning all these refugees to Kosova where they had no housing, no jobs, no medical care, and almost no future. Intellectually, it was very disturbing and unsettling, but obviously there is not much intellect in daily political moves.

I returned from Germany ecstatic, and sure that the idea of the International Virtual e-Hospital of Kosova would work. The question was: *"How am I going to make this all happening? I had no money, no script, no support, just a dream!"*

On my way from work, I stopped at Sunday Park, a neighborhood bar and restaurant on the lake and drew on a napkin the three phases of development of the International Virtual e-Hospital network and telemedicine project of Kosova. This drawing is still the main frame of the project.

1.8. Phoenix, Arizona: "You Will Come Back!"

Early June 2000, the Annual Meeting of ATA (American Telemedicine Association) was taking place in Phoenix, Arizona; I gave a short version of "the Berlin talk," in a special session dedicated to international telemedicine. I talked for 10–12 minutes, straight and to the point. I invited people and countries to assist us with the project. Most agreed that this was a great idea for an international collaborative project.

I went out for a run during "high noon," when the temperature was 109 degrees F. I liked Arizona. It was almost that something was telling me, *"You will be back!"*

(*For the last five years I have been in Arizona. I love it here. I call it home for now, but home is where ever you and your family are happy, and you can achieve the intellectual potential and fulfillment. And, the intellectual happiness is the best and most powerful feeling that human can have.*)

1.9. Prishtina, Kosova

In the summer of 2000, I was invited to participate in the International Medical Symposium "Medical Emergencies during the Military Conflicts" that was organized in Prishtina by the Kosova Protection Corps.

This was an important meeting, especially since it was being organized by individuals who were ousted from the University of Prishtina for more than ten years with the last three years at war [4,5].

The last day of the meeting, we were somewhere in Drenica, stalled in a traffic jam, and Shaip and I were discussing the conclusions for the meetings. Everything had gone well during the conference, and we needed good closure. I suggested to have only two conclusions: 1) *creation of a telemedicine program of Kosova*, and 2) *to create a modern trauma system*. This became our purpose and promise for the next few years. So far we have done the first one, and have started on the second one.

1.10. October 2000, Montreal, Canada

At the Montreal meeting I gave my presentation [6] and chaired a session on telemedicine in third world countries [7]. Our group from MITAC had another presentation at this session as well [8]. During my session the room was packed with people who understood the passion and dedication for telemedicine in developing countries. I used Kosova as the example, because I knew the situation there best. Kosova could have been any other country in the world just as well.

1.11. November 2000, Lillie, France

In November 2000, I was invited me to give a talk at the EHTEL meeting in Lillie, France. My presentation was entitled *"Telemedicine in Kosova: Where Do Our Priorities and Responsibilities to our Fellow European Citizens Lie?"* [9,10]. When I finished my talk at this meeting, I thought the audience was numb, as numb as this northern cold French University city was that November. In a way I was afraid I "overdid it" with the bloody slides. I left the podium not disappointed, but still without my usual elation. I still do not know why. It did not feel right.

That evening after the long dinner, I had a dramatic exchange with a French radiologist, who thought that my presentation was very emotional, but said *"we do not like to be told how dirty our garden is,"*! He was considering Kosova a European garden. He was right. I simply asked him to *"clean the garden, and no one will tell him how to clean it."* It was clear that we would be unable to resolve our differences over Kosova that night.

It was meeting that I wish I never attended. The remainder of 2000 I spent in preparation for a trip back to Prishtina and for initiation of the realization of the project.

1.12. 2001 Cairo, Egypt

In January 2001, I was a guest speaker at the 12th Annual Meeting of Egyptian Medical Syndicate in Cairo [11,12]. Both talks were accepted warmly, by all participants. In Cairo, I felt curiously comfortable. Perhaps it is because most of modern Cairo was built by Muhammad Ali Pasha, a creator of modern Egypt, an Albanian.

1.13. Back to Prishtina, Kosova

After the Cairo meeting, Dr. Merrell and I returned to Prishtina, but now with a drafted document for the Memorandum of Understanding between all stake-holders in Kosova including the Ministry of Health, the Medical School, Medical Association of Kosova, and the Kosova Protection Corps (KPC), 40th Medical Battalion, the Department of Surgery of Virginia Commonwealth University, the World Health Organization, and the Kosova Foundation for Medical Development (now the International Virtual e-Hospital Foundation, www.iveh.org), which we had just created in order to help with the realization of this project.

We arrived in Prishtina on January 30, 2001. It was cold day in Prishtina. The next day we made rounds in the hospital, had meetings at the medical school where we met with all the "Who's Who" from the Co-Ministers of Health and downward.

On February 1, 2003, we had a dinner at the NATO restaurant in Prishtina. Before we started dinner, I gave a presentation from my laptop. I insisted it was *"business before pleasure"* and they all agreed. After a few questions, mainly by United Nations Officials that were satisfactorily answered, everyone agreed to sign the MOU the next day. Early that afternoon we visited the hospital at the American base in Kosova, Camp Bondsteel in Ferizaj, and presented our proposed project [13]. As fate would have it, Dr. John Porter, a trauma surgeon with whom I have trained in Bronx New York and had stayed in touch over the years, and I met again unexpectedly, He was an Army reservist and serving at Camp Bondsteel. This led later to my move to Arizona where we now work together.

It was a harsh winter in Prishtina on that day, February 2, 2001. It was snowing heavily, it was cold, and there was no electricity in most of Kosova. The generators were breaking the silence of the falling snow in the city that I grew up in. Early that evening we signed the memorandum of understanding to start the telemedicine project of Kosova in an attempt to change the sad face of medicine in Kosova and in the Balkans. An "official" (not one of the signatories) reminded me that *"This is the Balkans, this is Kosova. All they know is war, suffering, bloodshed, and you want to bring state-of-the-art technology in here... Telemedicine! You must be out of your mind!"* He said that I have become an arrogant American!

We left the ministry of health and walked in silence toward the Grand Hotel Prishtina. As the adrenalin let go, I was numb, tired, feeling miserable. I was unable to understand why I was not exuberant. I knew we had a lot of work ahead of us, but this was not a reason. But despite that fact that we had an MOU signed I was asking myself if this was going to work. Did we take on something that we will not be able to keep the promise? Again, we did not have money all we had was the permission to do it.

We signed the MOU and now officially could to continue our project. It was not an easy task to convince them, although all said yes the night before. The official signed it but it was not pleasant. Not festive. Mother Theresa's picture was on the wall. I felt she was looking at us, she was wondering about our struggle and the officials' hesitation to help their very Ministry that they were managing.

That night I could not fall asleep. I was too disappointed, and too tired. At two in the morning, I called a friend and he invited me to visit him. I took a taxi from the front of the hotel, still debating if this is going to work. It seemed to be all just a far-fetched dream.

As I sat in the back seat of the taxi, the driver greeted me. *"Dr. Latifi, tell me how the project of telemedicine is going? It really sounded great for Kosova, when I heard you the other day on TV. Thank you for doing that..."* I looked at his face in the mirror and said to myself: I will not let this man down... *"We will make it work and we will succeed"*. *"Failure is not an option"*—I thought, remembering a NASA slogan. The rest of the night we never slept. We caught up on things from the past. We had not seen each other in years. In the morning we walked toward the center of the city in the cold and ate "burek" for breakfast. I was as rested as if I had slept all night.

1.14. May 2001, Jeddah, Saudi Arabia

In May 2001, I was the guest speaker at the First International e-Health Association Conference that took place in Jeddah, Kingdom of Saudi Arabia. I presented two talks [14,15]. As during many other meetings, I was desperately looking for funding for our project. Despite great moral support, as at every meeting, the money was difficult to come by. There too many promises never fulfilled or kept.

During the summer of 2001, I flew frequently to Prishtina for many meetings and presentation with the European Agency for Construction and with officials of the Agency and others who were in charge of funding medical development and reconstruction in Kosova. They had accepted the project in principal, but the finalization and realization of the funding was quite slow. We were coming close to get funds from different foundations and governments, but than everything changed in September 11, 2001. The world all of the sudden had a different problem to deal with. My dream of building the International Virtual e-Hospital was not the world's priority.

1.15. October 2001, Kuala Lumpur, Malaysia

On October 15–17, 2001, I participated as a guest speaker at the 2nd International Congress of Emergency Medicine of Malaysia, in Kuala Lumpur [16–18]. I enjoyed Kuala Lumpur tremendously. I have returned there more than once. The best part I like the co-habitation of three nationalities and cultures as one, the kindness of people and the modern city.

I have continued to present the concept of the international virtual e-hospital and our progress on telemedicine in Prishtina at meetings around the world. The meetings our project was presented at, in addition to the ones described include: American Telemedicine Association's meeting of 2001 in Ft. Lauderdale, Florida [19,20], the 42nd Congress of Austrian Surgical Society in June 2001 [21], the Sixth International Telemedicine Conference of International Society for Telemedicine in Upsala, Sweden [22]; the European Society for Telemedicine Scientific Quarterly Meetings, Paris, January 2002 [23]; the 10th European Endoscopic Congress, Lisbon, Portugal June 2002 [24]; the Asia Business Forum, Kuala Lumpur, Malaysia [25], the International Society for Telemedicine in Regensburg, Germany [26,27], the Conference on Curriculum Reform of Medical Faculties of Southeastern Europe Universities in Zagreb, Croatia [28], and the Annual Meeting of Medical Syndicate Cairo, Egypt December 2002 [29–44]. At the 8th International Society for Telemedicine Meeting in Tromsø [30], our project was awarded by Polycom as one of the Best Telemedicine Projects presented at the Conference, out of 32 countries participating at the conference. At the 10th Congress of the International Society for Telemedicine and eHealth and the 2nd Congress of the Brazilian Council of Telemedicine and Telehealth, Sao Paulo, Brazil, our paper Microsoft Scientific Award Recipient, The Role of Disruptive Technology in Redevelopment of Medical Systems: Telemedicine of Kosova as an Example, received the Microsoft Scientific Award Recipient. But the best award of this program will be when we save even a single life, when we reduce the morbidity or prevent the unnecessary transfer of the sick patient.

1.16. Summer, 2002

Let's Stir Things Up: The First Intensive Balkan Telemedicine Seminar

In June 2002, things were still going slowly. I was not happy. I knew we needed to do something to "stir things up." We had accomplished much by now. We had signed an MOU with the University Clinical Center of Kosova, and had the space identified.

Things were moving along, but not quickly enough. Time was running out.

I went on Voice America TV in Albanian and announced that on October 25–27, 2002, we would have the first Intensive Balkan Telemedicine Seminar titled: "Telemedicine and Telehealth in Developing Countries: From Inception to Implementation. The future has just begun." [31] I had created the entire plan and program for the conference and planned to invite the "who's who" in telemedicine around the world to speak. We did not have any money so I asked speakers to pay their own way to Prishtina, and promised them that we would take care of them while in Kosova. No one declined to come. A few of them were able to ensure that someone else would pay their expenses.

This was a risky undertaking by all accounts. We had no money, and the space was not ready.

In September, 2002, I quit my job at Virginia Commonwealth University in Richmond, Virginia and moved to Prishtina to oversee the project. By now, we had a small office at the medical school, two computers and four chairs. The entire team lived in this office for months, working day and night. The building of the center was progressing well. The organization of the conference was going well too. Local support was tremendous; we received a grant from the European Agency for the conference.

1.17. October 25, 2002: "Operation Richmond"

At the opening of the First Intensive Balkan Telemedicine Seminar on October 25, 2002, something almost surreal happened. Everything was coming together as planed. Without a single glitch we brought together 400 people from 21 countries, and started a new chapter in the history of telemedicine and telehealth in the Balkans.

The director of Television of Kosova, Mr. Avni Spahiu, decided to broadcast the opening ceremony live. The prime Minister of Kosova, Dr. Bajram Rexhepi, a surgeon, officially opened the seminar. We arranged to have live wireless connection with Mitrovicë, Peja, Gjakovë and Prizren. We had made plans to broadcast directly live, wireless, a surgical procedure from Operating Room Number Three at the Medical College of Virginia in Richmond to Kosova. This was the first time something of this nature had been attempted in the Balkans. I could not announce publicly just in case things did not go well.

But everything was going well. We linked wirelessly with all four regional hospitals in Kosova, Mitrovicë, Pejë, Gjakovë and Prizren. I looked at Jeton Peja, an intense guy who was in charge of Kujtesa, a local Internet provider. When he gave me the signal to go ahead and announce, that we were "linked" live, with Richmond, I had an indescribable feeling. When we finished "the operation Richmond" I thought we had demonstrated what we were striving to do here in Kosova. It was the best thing that ever happened to me in my career. There was no doubt about it.

At the break, after the opening ceremony, there was hope in the eyes of doctors, students, nurses, and common people. They understood what we were doing.

It was a great event that lasted two and a half days. No participant ever left the "classroom" through out all the entire presentations. The speakers were not used to this undivided attentiveness of the audience.

1.18. The Inauguration of Telemedicine Center of Kosova

On December 10, 2002, we officially inaugurated the Telemedicine Center of Kosova. Once just a dream and an illusion for Kosova, now the Telemedicine Centre of Kosova was a reality.

2. Telemedicine of Kosova 2002–2006

The TCK is located at the UCCK in Prishtina, and is approximately $1,000$ m^2. The center includes a 100-seat electronic auditorium, a computer training room with teaching space for 25, a telemedicine training room, technology support laboratories, a resource room, an electronic library and administrative offices. The center is equipped with computers, fiber connectivity using Integrated services digital network (ISDN), video production equipment, video streaming capability, and computer servers. The TCK operates its own virtual private network (VPN) and a local area network (LAN). This is the highest quality currently available in Kosova. All state-of-the-art equipment has been selected for compatibility, interoperability, and overall effectiveness to ensure sustainability. The electronic library and resource room offers instructional modules with various electronic books and scientific journals through different world-wide programs and other publishing companies and resources. The Learning Center encompasses the latest in image projections systems, interactive capabilities, and diagnostic tools. This center has the capability to effectively encompass, store, and deliver educational content within the UCCK, regional hospitals, and the world. Current systems within the facility allow for acquisition, editing, storage, and streaming of educational modules created by the staff of the TCK and its collaborators. The library has a full range of medical texts online, search capacity, and printers. The faculty and the students of UCCK have direct and unrestricted access to more than 2,100 electronic journals, through the WHO Health InterNetwork Access to Research Initiative (HINARI) program, which provides online access to the major journals in biomedical and related social sciences, the latest medical publications and books (in English). The TCK works closely with publishers to obtain unrestrictive access to publications from companies such as Landes Bioscience (Austin, TX) [6]. The Learning Center is open 24 hours a day/365 days a year, and is widely used by physicians, medical students, nurses and other healthcare professionals. The Center is managed by a team of Kosovar medical personnel and engineers. It serves as an integral part of the UCCK and is closely affiliated with the medical school, which is on the same campus as the hospital.

Personnel were trained at collaborative laboratories in the United States and collaborators from the United States and Europe have worked in training on site. As with other institutions from developing countries, international cooperation and collaboration is mandatory for successful development. Since 2002, TCK has collaborated with more than 20 universities and institutions, publishing companies, and others to help enrich its activities and knowledge. This successful international cooperation has been in the form of educational programs, videoconferences and seminars, lectures, consultation and other forms of mutual collaboration with universities in Europe, the United States, and other countries.

Live consultation between international academic sites in the United States and Europe and TCK are conducted using IP protocols or ISDN. Regional hospitals in Kosova are connected now with TCK and UCCK and provide a strong foundation for collaborative efforts.

As the only library for some 1,885 medical students, the Center has provided computer resources for all students and instruction in electronic resource. Formal and informal courses have been conducted with 100% participation of all medical students. More than 54,000 visits by doctors, students, nurses, and other healthcare providers have been registered in the TCK since January 2003. The electronic library has had 9,499 entries, since the start of HINARI program in November 2003. The entire electronic library has also been made available for each regional hospital of Kosova, where hospital personnel are undergoing training in electronic library use, computer use, and the English language. As part of Prishtina Summer University (2004) 36 medical, dental, pharmacy, engineering, and business students of University of Prishtina successfully finished a 3-week intensive telemedicine course, Telemedicine and Telehealth in Modern Medical Care. This course offered state-of-the-art telehealth education and hands-on knowledge of the equipment used in telemedicine. These graduated students represent a powerful cadre of individuals who can support and advance telemedicine in Kosova, ensuring sustainability of the telemedicine program.

The TCK has been utilized for 43 regional and international conferences in continuing medical education including live Web broadcasting of surgical procedures as of March 2005. The facility is well suited to connect to primary sites in Europe or the United States for classroom participation in Kosova. The sessions cover the spectrum of medicine and have largely served the staff of the UCCK. The leadership of UCCK continues to offer encouragement to the Center by serving as the heart of medical education for the university clinical center staff. The electronic library of the Center is also the main information resource of the hospital. The Center personnel have provided advice and leadership to connect different departments of the UCCK with telecommunications lines. This VPN, extended to the operating suites throughout the UCCK, is providing abilities for live broadcasting of general surgery procedures, endoscopic procedures as well as dental procedures and is offering telesurgical training and mentoring to a wider audience of local surgeons. Live and interactive teleconferences from the operating rooms are transmitted to a larger audience in one or more classrooms, instead of large groups of students crowding into operating rooms. This also adds significantly to the exposure of medical students to clinical education.

The establishment of telemedicine protocols, consultation policies, second opinions and development of other modes of collaboration between the UCCK and other regional medical centers in Kosova in the fields of dermatology, pathology, family practice, ear, nose and throat, ophthalmology, surgery, internal medicine, cardiology, and dentistry has been accomplished. A database of all clinical activities has been created and consultations within the region and to collaborators abroad have been accomplished.

This will include total access to telemedicine systems in Kosova from every hospital, health house centers and private medical practice in the country. These will be supported by IP, ISDN, or by wireless technology. These nine centers in Kosova will make arrangement for, and ensure the regional health house centers and medical practices will be included in the telemedicine network during the third phase of the project. Their local and regional programs will ensure that proper education is provided for those centers and individuals and make certain proper leadership is in place in preparation for the implementation of the third phase.

3. Back to the Future: Spring 2006

The June issue of Telemedicine and e-Health published a paper titled "The role of telemedicine and information technology in the redevelopment of Medical systems: the case of Kosova." [45] Just days before that we received the great news that the State Department, the Bureau of Education and Cultural Agency has granted the IVEH (than Kosova Foundation for Medical Development) $850,000 to finish the second phase of the project in Kosova and to introduce the telemedicine in other countries of the Balkans such as Montenegro, Albania and Macedonia. Things are coming together. I was the happiest man on earth. The dream was coming true.

We call the program: "Improving Health Care in the Balkans Using Telemedicine, Advanced Technologies and Cultural Exchange Program as a Platform" in attempt to improve health care delivery in the Balkans, and make this region of the world part of the global health and collaboration through structured educational curriculums and exchange programs. Forty-eight physicians, nurses, and technical professionals from Kosova, Montenegro, Macedonia and Albania are being trained in the US for three to four weeks intensive training. At the same time US experts are being sent to the region for work shops, seminars and other cultural and educational activities. When fully implemented, this program will create a powerful international medical education network in the Balkans for further collaboration and development. The medical and technical leadership created during these two years will provide a solid foundation for new changes in health care in the Balkans. This multi-institutional, multi-state, and multi country program represent a massive educational undertakings that will have significant impact in the health care of the Balkans. By creating new opportunities for partnerships of medical institutions from the region with many renowned institutions in the USA, this program will become a true ambassador of our medical advances, cultural diversity, and advances in technology. In addition, we hope it will help prevent brain drain of experts and intellectuals from these countries and ability for integration into interregional and international activities using technological advances and virtual communications.

By the time this book is published we will have finished the first year of this program. We have trained twenty-eight experts from the Balkan countries. And the training does not end the day they get the certificates. We call it the moment of great beginning.

The Balkans project of the International Virtual e-Hospital is coming together.

4. Instead of Post Scriptum

It appears that during this journey we almost had to go to Mars to establish something in the Balkans. And, yes we still have a way to go. But now we know how to do it, and most importantly we have learned from our mistakes and experiences what not to do.

Telemedicine and telehealth development have brought hopes to the developing countries and their most remote areas, yet has raised significant questions and anxiety among those forces hoping to maintain the status- quo of existing medical practice. Advanced technologies such as computers, diagnostic imaging, robotics, voice-activating machines, and remote controls have changed the hospitals and the operating theatres in the hospitals around the Western world. The patient has become an educated and informed consumer, that questions the decisions of the practitioner and demand explanations and evidence based medicine approach, validates his or her expertise through the web sites and other forms, and requires that the doctor offers care that is current world standard. He or she can consult any expert in the field, in any country of the world, at any time. The geography and the distance have become an abstract nouns and a meaningless entity. At the same time, the world equilibrium has not followed the punctuation of the industrial world directed by the broad bandwidth rush.

As we move toward next decades and toward a perfect future and electronic globalization, it is hoped that the gap between our imagination and achievements will narrow significantly, if not be eliminated entirely. While applying telemedicine and telehealth technology, we will be able to deliver and manage medical care in Mars, here down on earth, or wherever there is the need for radical changes of the configuration of medical care. Kosova and other developing countries are perfect example of situation, where education and health related issues have lagged significantly behind other development for at least 4–5 decades. These countries need modern health information system and advanced technology in order to become part of global community of medical practice and are in need for radical changes. The concept of the International Virtual e-Hospital, while it has to grow and be enriched with content, offers such necessary radical changes. Telemedicine and e-health overall, is changing the delivery of medical care by bringing together a coalition of new partners with innovative visions, especially for countries and in those that have been devastated by war, suffering or political neglect. This concept has been accepted, adopted and has raised more sincere hopes than questions in Kosova. For now, it is viewed as the penetrating eye of the future and of the unconventional, and as such has become the Balkan's Center of Excellence for Telemedicine, Telehealth and Telesurgery.

It is up to us to add more content and richness to the programs.

As Kosova becomes part of the independent nations in the Balkans and in the world, it will become a true partner in the global development—a true partner, if not one of the main leaders in this field. It should and it will.

5. Looking Back

Five years ago when telemedicine program in Kosova became a reality, Kosova was ravaged by war, and had no medical standards, policies and practice management guidelines or simply had really bad management. Although these elements are still present for the most part, telemedicine program is making a difference, albeit very small. There is one other very important element for the need of Telemedicine in Kosova and the other Balkan countries. Although the region is relatively small, non-the-less there is a tremendous traffic of patients from one country to the other, from one hospital to another, from one physician to another in the search for the best medical care. In this vertigo-like search from patients and their families to obtain the best medical care and sometimes to just obtain any kind of care, it is not unusual that the patients will travel thousands of kilometers from one side to another needlessly. So if and when we will have wide distribution of telemedicine and technologies networks between the hospitals and physicians in one country and at the same time these networks will communicate from one region to another and one country to another. The collaboration between physicians and hospitals will culminate in much better care for the patient and for the entire region. This way the Balkans will become part of the globalization and part of the medical care around the world. Also telemedicine does not deal exclusively with patient care and consultations but with massive education of physicians, nurses, and other health care providers. Application of telemedicine in this region in particular will create similar standards from one site to another and there will be no significant discrepancies in the care between the regions. I recently visited Kosova, Macedonia, Montenegro and Albania and it is unbelievable how many discrepancies exist in patient care even in those very small countries that are relatively a very short distance from each other. No wonder that patients travel frantically so frequently between the Balkans, Central Europe or even to Asia and other countries in search of better medical care. Due to the existence of telemedicine program in Kosova today any expert from anywhere in the world can lecture, educate, propagate information in the medical and other arenas to students, residents, doctors, other healthcare providers in Kosova. As of right now, this program of has become a prime example of successful programs in developing countries and more. Last year, the Council of Europe adopted a resolution where this program is recognized as the best program of Telemedicine in Southeastern Europe.

We have put together a proposal which has been adopted by the Council of Europe that calls for the creation of the Southeastern European Telemedicine and Virtual Education Network that will involve all the countries of South Eastern Europe and more.

Overall, however, we have so much to do in the developing countries such as the Balkans, we have so many things that are so beautiful and so many things that are so sad and awful. We need to change the sad things to beautiful things and we need to become part of the world. We can do it and we need to change the notion in the world that the only thing we are good at and for is to fight and shed blood. Creating a sustainable medical system is the only way we can provide good medical care for people. And telemedicine can help. Our program has demonstrated that.

On personal note, my involvement in telemedicine has been one great adventure. Intellectually and spiritually very fulfilling! Rich.

Hopefully some else will get inspired and chase the same rainbow I did. One thing has become very clear that when it comes to telemedicine there are no limits. The only limit is your will and your passion. If you do not have these two, you are in trouble.

References

[1] Latifi R, Muja Sh, Bekteshi F, Reinicke M. The impact of telemedicine project of Kosova in the Balkans reaches far beyond the telemedicine applications. ATA annual meeting, Ft. Lauderdale, Florida, May 2-5, 2004.

[2] Latifi, R. The Anatomy of War and Destruction of Kosova: An Alumni view on restructuring health care. Final Conference of G-8, Global Applications Health project, Berlin, May 3-5, 2000.

[3] Latifi R. The anatomy of war and destruction in Kosova: An alumni surgeon's view on restructuring health care. European Health Telematics Observatory web site (www.ehto.org), June, 2000.

[4] Latifi R, Doarn C, Merrell RC. International Virtual e-Hospital of Kosova. First International Symposium: Medical Emergencies during Military Conflicts. Prishtina, Kosova, September 28-30, 2000.

[5] Latifi R, Muja Sh, Merrell RC. An urgent need for creation of an organized trauma system in Kosova. First International Symposium: Medical Emergencies during Military Conflicts. Prishtina, Kosova, September 28-30, 2000.

[6] Latifi, R, Nerlich M, Richardson R, Doarn RC, Al Nuaim AA, Range P, Merrell RC. International Virtual e-Hospital of Kosova. International Society for Telemedicine, The 5th International Conference on the Medical Aspects of Telemedicine and the 2nd Annual Meeting of the International Society for Telemedicine, October 2-4, 2002, Montreal, Canada.

[7] Latifi R. Telemedicine networks: Telemedicine in under developed countries. International Society for Telemedicine, The 5th International Conference on the Medical Aspects of Telemedicine and the 2nd Annual Meeting of the International Society for Telemedicine, October 2-4, 2000, Montreal, Canada.

[8] Darenkov IA, Latifi R, Russell MK, Lavrentyev VA, Kapoor V, Doarn CR, Merrell RC. Multinational Distance Learning Project Utilizing Low Bandwidth Internet. International Virtual e- Hospital of Kosova. International Society for Telemedicine, The 5th International Conference on the Medical Aspects of Telemedicine and the 2nd Annual Meeting of the International Society for Telemedicine, October 2-4, 2000, Montreal, Canada.

[9] Latifi, R. Telemedicine in Kosova: Where do our priorities and responsibilities to our fellow European citizens' lie? First EHTEL conference, Lillie, France, November 16-17, 2000.

[10] Latifi R. Telemedicine in Kosova: Where do our responsibilities and priorities to our European citizens' lie? www.ehtel.org, December 21, 2000.

[11] Latifi R. Multinational Distance Learning Project Utilizing Low Bandwidth Internet as a Tool to International Collaboration: MITAC Experience. The 12th International Scientific Congress of the Egyptian Medical Syndicate and First International Telemedicine Conference of Arabic Telemedicine Society. Cairo, Egypt, January 8-11, 2001.

[12] Latifi, R. From Mars to Kosova Round Trip: Telesurgery and International Virtual e-Hospital of Kosova. The 12th International Scientific Congress of the Egyptian Medical Syndicate and First International Telemedicine Conference of Arabic Telemedicine Society. Cairo, Egypt, January 8-11, 2001.

[13] Latifi, R. International Virtual e-Hospital of Kosova. American Military Base Bondsteel, Ferizaj, Kosova February 2, 2001.

[14] Latifi R. From Mars to Kosova Round Trip: Telesurgery and Internet. The First International e-health Association Conference, Jeddah, Kingdom of Saudi Arabia, May 5-8, 2001.

[15] Latifi R. Virtual e- Hospitals. The First International e-health Association Conference, Jeddah, Kingdom of Saudi Arabia, May 5-8, 2001.

[16] Latifi R. Virtual e-Hospital. 2nd International Congress of Emergency Medicine of Malaysia. Kuala Lumpur, Malaysia, October 15-17, 2001.

[17] Latifi R. Management of intra-abdominal injuries in morbidly obese patients: New trends. 2nd International Congress of Emergency Medicine of Malaysia. Kuala Lumpur, Malaysia, October 15-17, 2001.

[18] Latifi R. Management of elderly trauma patients. 2nd International Congress of Emergency Medicine of Malaysia. Kuala Lumpur, Malaysia, October 15-17, 2001.

[19] Latifi R, Doarn CR, Merrell RC. Kosova's International Virtual e-Hospital: Putting it all together. The ATA 6th Annual Meeting Fort Lauderdale, Florida, June 3-6, 2001

[20] Latifi R, Doarn CR, Merrell RC. Kosova's International Virtual e-Hospital: Putting it all together. Telemed Jour and e-Health 2001; 7(2); 139.

[21] Latifi R. The International virtual e-hospital of Kosova and Telesurgery: Where do we stand? 42nd Congress of Austrian Surgical Society, Graz, Austria, June 14-16, 2001.

[22] Latifi R, Merrell RCM. From Mars to Kosova round trip: The international Virtual e- Hospital from inception to reality. 6th International Telemedicine Conference of International telemedicine society, Upsala, Sweden, June 18-21, 2001.

[23] Latifi R. The situation of Telemedicine in the Balkans. European Society for Telemedicine Scientific meeting. Paris, France, January 28, 2002.

[24] Latifi R. 10th European Endoscopic Congress, Lisbon, Portugal June 2002.

[25] Latifi R. International Virtual e-Hospital. 2nd International Congress of Emergency Medicine of Malaysia. Kuala Lumpur, Malaysia, October 15-17, 2001.

[26] Latifi R. Establishing Telemedicine in Third World Countries: Kosova as an Example presented at the 7th International Conference on the Medical Aspects of Telemedicine Integration of Health Telematics into Medical Practice, Regensburg, Germany, and September 22-25, 2002.

[27] Latifi R. Establishing Telemedicine in Third World Countries: Kosova as an Example Eur J Research 2002; 7 (Suppl); 43.

[28] Latifi R. International Virtual E-Hospital and Telesurgery. The Curriculum Reform in Medical Faculties of South East Europe Universities, 2nd Conference, Zagreb, Germany, November 16-18, 2002.

[29] Latifi, R. Use of telemedicine as an educational tool: Can it help with infection control. Annual Meeting of Egyptian Infectious Society, Cairo, Egypt, January 8-11, 2001.

[30] Latifi R. Telemedicine centre of Kosovo and international virtual e-hospital network at the end of the first phase of development: Ahead of the Game. Tromsø Telemedicine Conference, Tromsø, Norway, September 16, 2003.

[31] www.iveh.org.

[32] Latifi R. E-health education: Challenges and the future in the changing world. The European Space Agency Symposium on Satellite Application in Telemedicine, Frascati, Italy, July 4, 2004.

[33] Latifi R, From Berlin to Prishtina via Mars: Establishing Telemedicine in the Balkans, International Telehealth Conference, Anchorage, Alaska, March 2004.

[34] Latifi R, Can virtual reality help reduce brain drain in developing countries: Kosova as an example. ATA Meeting, May, 2006.

[35] Latifi R. Telepresence and Telemedicine in Trauma and Emergency Management: Lessons from Space and Changing the Paradigm (Keynote Speaker) at 9th Annual Spirit of Marshfield Conference, Trauma Care: A Team Approach. Marshfield, Wisconsin, August 13, 2004.

[36] Latifi R. International Telehealth—Challenges & Reality Checks. Four Corners Telemedicine & Telehealth Planning Conference, Tucson, Arizona, August 23-24, 2004.

[37] Latifi R. Key Note address: International Virtual e-Hospital: Building bridges and improving the quality of healthcare in developing countries. International Telemedicine Conference, Bangalore, India, March 17-19, 2005.

[38] Latifi R. Inaugural Address at the Astronautical Society of India and Indian Space Research Organization of the International Telemedicine Conference, Intelemedindia Bangalore, India, March 17, 2005.

[39] Latifi R. International Virtual e-Hospital Initiative, The International Trade Event and Conference for eHealth, Telemedicine and Health ICT, Luxembourg, April 6-8, 2005.

[40] Latifi R. The Role of Disruptive Technology in Redevelopment of Medical Systems: Telemedicine of Kosova as an Example. 10th Congress of the International Society for Telemedicine and eHealth and the 2nd Congress of the Brazilian Council of Telemedicine and Telehealth, Sao Paulo, Brazil, October 23-26, 2005. (Microsoft Scientific Award Recipient.)

[41] Latifi R. Virtual reduction of brain drain in developing countries using telemedicine as platform: what does it take? XVII PanAmerican Trauma Congress, VII Ecuadorian Trauma Congress, Guayaquil, Ecuador, November 16-18, 2005.
[42] Latifi R. Transforming Current Medical Care to Higher Standards using Disruptive Technologies and Telemedicine as a Platform. UN-OOSA/UN-ESCAP Workshop on Tele-Health Development in Asia and the Pacific Region. Co-sponsored by the China National Space Administration, China Ministry of Health and Asia Pacific Multilateral Cooperation in Space Technology and Applications, Guangzhou, China, December 5-9, 2005.
[43] Latifi R. Brain gain for developing countries using telemedicine, Poster, SFT-6: 6th International Conference on Successes and Failure in Telehealth, Brisbane, Australia, August 24-25, 2006.
[44] Latifi, R. International Virtual e-Hospital as Model in Rebuilding medical System in developing Countries. United nation/India/USA Pilot Project "Telemedicine in the reconstruction of Afghanistan", August 29-31, 2006, Kochi, India.
[45] Latifi R, Muja S, Bekteshi Fl, Merrell RC. The Role of Telemedicine and Information Technology in the Redevelopment of Medical Systems: The Case of Kosova. Telemedicine and eHealth. June 2006.
[46] Latifi, R. Case Report: Kosova. International Telecommunication Union Report on Application of Telecommunication in Health Care. Edited by National Institute of Information and Communications Technology, Japan. October, 2005. pp. 202-207.

II. Creating and Integrating Telemedicine and e-Health Systems

Current Principles and Practices of Telemedicine and e-Health
R. Latifi (Ed.)
IOS Press, 2008

Integrating Telemedicine and Telehealth: Putting It All Together

Ronald S. WEINSTEIN, MD [a,b], Ana Maria LOPEZ, MD, MPH [a,b,c],
Elizabeth A. KRUPINSKI, PhD [a,d], Sandra J. BEINAR [a,b], Michael HOLCOMB [a,d],
Richard A. McNEELY [a,e], Rifat LATIFI, MD, FACS [a,f]
and Gail BARKER, MBA, PhD [a,b,g]

[a] Arizona Telemedicine Program
[b] Department of Pathology
[c] Arizona Cancer Center
[d] Department of Radiology
[e] Department of Biomedical Communications
[f] Department of Surgery
[g] University of Arizona College of Medicine-Tucson Campus, Department of Financial
Affairs, University of Arizona College of Medicine-Phoenix Campus

Abstract. Telemedicine and telehealth programs are inherently complex compared with their traditional on-site health care delivery counterparts. Relatively few organizations have developed sustainable, multi-specialty telemedicine programs, although single service programs, such as teleradiology and telepsychiatry programs, are common. A number of factors are barriers to the development of sustainable telemedicine and telehealth programs. First, starting programs is often challenging since relatively few organizations have, in house, a critical mass of individuals with the skill sets required to organize and manage a telemedicine program. Therefore, it is necessary to "boot strap" many of the start-up activities using available personnel. Another challenge is to assemble a management team that has time to champion telemedicine and telehealth while dealing with the broad range of issues that often confront telemedicine programs. Telemedicine programs housed within a single health care delivery system have advantages over programs that serve as umbrella telehealth organizations for multiple health care systems. Planning a telemedicine program can involve developing a shared vision among the participants, including the parent organizations, management, customers and the public. Developing shared visions can be a time-consuming, iterative process. Part of planning includes having the partnering organizations and their management teams reach a consensus on the initial program goals, priorities, strategies, and implementation plans. Staffing requirements of telemedicine and telehealth programs may be met by sharing existent resources, hiring additional personnel, or outsourcing activities. Business models, such as the Application Service Provider (ASP) model used by the Arizona Telemedicine Program, are designed to provide staffing flexibility by offering a combination of in-house and out-sourced services, depending on the needs of the individual participating health care organizations. Telemedicine programs should perform ongoing assessments of activities, ranging from service usage to quality of service assessments, to ongoing analyses of financial performance. The financial assessments should include evaluations of costs and benefits, coding issues, reimbursement, account receivables, bad debt and network utilization. Long-range strategic planning for a telemedicine and telehealth program should be carried out on an on-going basis and should include the program's governing board. This planning process should include goal setting and the periodic updating of the program's vision and mission statements. There can be additional special issues for multi-organization telemedicine and telehealth programs. For example, authority management can require the use of innovative approaches tailored to the realities of the organizational structures of the participating members. Inter-institutional relations may introduce additional issues when competing health care organizations are utilizing shared resources. Branding issues are preferably addressed during the initial planning of a multi-organizational telemedicine and telehealth program. Ideally, public policy regarding telemedicine and telehealth within a service region will complement the objectives of telemedicine and telehealth programs within that service area.

Keywords. Integrating Telemedicine and Telehealth, Business models for telemedicine, evaluation of costs and benefits, coding issues, reimbursement, planning of a multi-organizational telemedicine and telehealth program, public policy

Introduction

In 1996, the Arizona State Legislature gave the state's only medical school, the University of Arizona College of Medicine headquartered in Tucson, Arizona, the opportunity to develop a statewide telemedicine program [1–6]. A legislative proponent of telemedicine, State Representative Robert "Bob" Burns (R-Glendale, now a State Senator) spearheaded the legislative initiative to create an eight-site pilot telemedicine program [2]. Over a decade later, he remains the Arizona Telemedicine Program's strongest proponent. By coincidence, an early adopter of telepathology, the first author on this chapter (RSW), was the Pathology Department Head at the University of Arizona at the time and was willing to serve as the Founding Director of the Arizona Telemedicine Program on a part time basis. Dr. Weinstein had trained in pathology at the Massachusetts General Hospital (MGH) in Boston, Massachusetts in the 1960s when the world's first multi-specialty telemedicine program was established at that institution. Although he was not personally involved in the MGH program he was well aware of it, since it was widely publicized in the press. He subsequently invented robotic telepathology in 1986, for which he was granted U.S. patents, and published many papers and books on telepathology [7–12]. He was on the international lecture circuit as a speaker on telemedicine and telepathology before the Arizona State Legislature developed its interest in supporting a pilot project [13]. For over a decade, he has had a dual role as Head of Pathology and Director of the Arizona Telemedicine Program [2]. Today, Senator Burns and Dr. Weinstein continue to work closely together on the development of statewide and regional telehealth programs (Fig. 1).

The initial collaboration of a key legislator and a medical school department head with a special interest in telemedicine led to the immediate development and implementation of statewide telemedicine and telehealth public policies [3]. Since then, these public policies have served as the framework for developing many additional telemedicine and telehealth initiatives in Arizona. Being able to start with a clean slate and address a multiplicity of program requirements, such as that of creating a new statewide broad band telecommunications infrastructure, allowed the Arizona Telemedicine Program to develop an unusually inclusive multi-organizational program from the bottom up, while documenting lessons learned as part of the process [1]. These lessons learned form the basis for this chapter. Although many of these lessons grew out of this specific program, they may be broadly applicable to other programs as well.

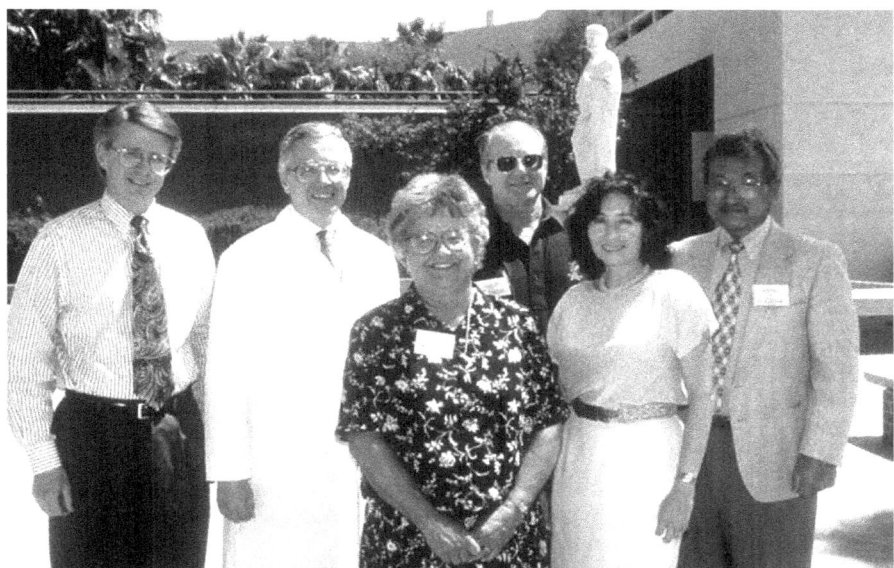

Figure 1. Founders of the Arizona Telemedicine Program at their initial organizational meeting, held at the University of Arizona College of Medicine, Tucson, Arizona, in June 1996. The photograph was taken in an open area outside of the Arizona Health Science Center Library. Left to right: Richard A. McNeely, Founding Co-Director of the Arizona Telemedicine Program and Director of Biomedical Communications at the Arizona Health Sciences Center; Ronald S. Weinstein, M.D., Founding Director of the Arizona Telemedicine and Professor and Head of the Department of Pathology, University of Arizona College of Medicine; State Representative Lou-Ann Preble, from Tucson, an early advocate of telemedicine; State Representative Robert "Bob" Burns, (now Senator Burns) who started the statewide telemedicine initiative in Arizona and has chaired its governing body, the Arizona Telemedicine Council, since the beginning; Rachael Anderson, an Associate Director of the Arizona Telemedicine Program and Director of the Arizona Health Science Center Library; and John J. Lee (deceased), Deputy Budget Director at the Joint Legislative Budget Committee of the Arizona State Legislature. Mr. Lee played a major role in creating the governance structure for the Arizona Telemedicine Program and in helping the Arizona State Legislature and the University of Arizona College of Medicine to develop a shared vision for this statewide telemedicine and telehealth enterprise. A statue of Hippocrates (background) adds a sense of history to the event.

1. Current Developments: Evidence-Based Practice

Good telehealth public policy is obvious when you see it. At the time of the organization of the Arizona Telemedicine Program, eight public policies were proposed by Dr. Weinstein as components of his "start up package." These were immediately endorsed by influential leaders in the Arizona State Legislature [3]. The policies were authored as a package of public policies and presented as a unit. The authoring of the policies was completed in four hours by Dr. Weinstein. Endorsement by the Co-Chairs of the Joint Legislative Budget Committee of the Arizona State Legislature took place within days. Since then, these telemedicine policies have provided the framework for the development of many of the telemedicine and telehealth activities in Arizona. It is doubtful that these policies would have been accepted on a piecemeal basis since they make the best sense when viewed in their entirety. These policies have been described elsewhere [3] and are summarized as follows.

- To have, as a goal, the creation of a single statewide multi-service telemedicine program.
- To establish a program governance framework with an overarching authority structure to support the unique missions of a statewide telemedicine organization.
- To operate the program as a virtual organization that would be inclusive and create incentives for all health care organizations to participate in a statewide single telemedicine program.
- To provide access to the program's telecommunications infrastructure for all legitimate health care organizations in the state.
- To encourage the development of interoperability of all telemedicine facilities
- To develop an open staff model for participation of telephysicians as service providers for multiple health care organizations.
- To promote best practice guidelines that are evidence-based and supported by clinical research.
- To have the state legislature encourage all state agencies, including the Arizona Department of Corrections and the Arizona Department of Health Services, to participate in the program [3].

The governance issue was addressed by the creation of the Arizona Telemedicine Council, a so-called non-statutory overarching authority. This Council has approximately 25 members from government, both the public and private sectors of the health care industry, and community members. It has been chaired by Mr. Burns since its creation 11 years ago. The Council meets quarterly for a two hour luncheon meeting at the State Capital Campus in Phoenix. Mr. Burns, the Council Chair, and Dr. Weinstein, the Director, have attended all 43 meetings to date.

At the first meeting of the Arizona Telemedicine Council in 1996, the Director proposed broadening the scope of the Arizona Telemedicine Program as it was outlined initially by the State Legislature in its enabling legislation. The Director wanted to develop a "comprehensive telemedicine program" (Fig. 2). He thought that this was essential in order to achieve sustainability of the program. Also, he regarded many of the then available applications of telemedicine as unproven health care delivery systems at the time. Implementation of the statewide program would take place along with on-going assessments of the candidate telemedicine technologies. His proposal was for a telemedicine program with five components: 1- telemedicine services; 2- a technology assessment division (i.e. clinical research division); 3- on-going telemedicine training programs; 4- distance education; and 5- the development of a telemedicine infrastructure, including a shared telecommunications network and standardized telemedicine clinical facilities throughout Arizona (Fig. 2). Establishment of interoperable telemedicine clinics in independent health care facilities across the state was regarded as key to success. Strong branding of the Arizona Telemedicine Program was also thought to be important. Initially, legislative leaders had concerns about encouraging clinical research within the program due to their apprehension that this might distract academic physicians from the telemedicine program's primary mission of patient care. This concern dissipated as the program's staff competed successfully for federal grants and proved to state leaders that it was fully committed to making telemedicine services effective throughout the state.

Today, the Arizona Telemedicine Program serves as an umbrella organization for 55 independent health care organizations located in communities throughout Arizona,

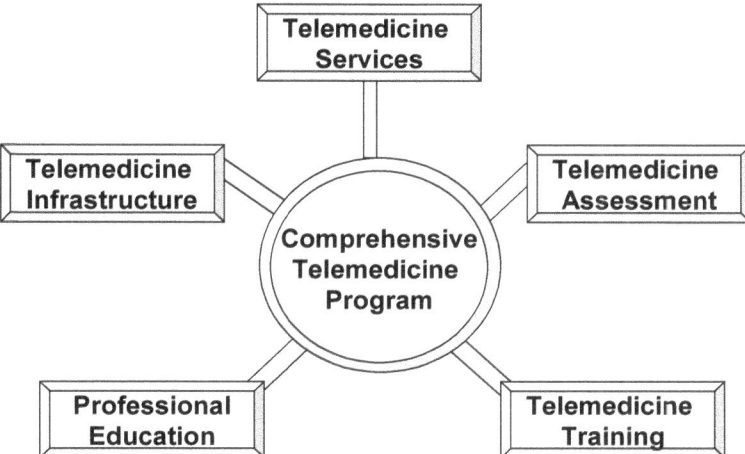

Figure 2. The components of the comprehensive telemedicine program developed by the Arizona Telemedicine Program. The program integrates telemedicine and telehealth services with clinical research and distance learning activities. In addition, the Arizona Program operates the broad band Arizona Telemedicine Network. Introduced at the second meeting of the Arizona Telemedicine Council in the Fall of 1995.

adjacent states, and in other countries. Health care facilities in both urban and rural communities, on Native American reservations (i.e., the Navajo, Hopi, and Apache Nations, among others), in all of Arizona's 10 state prisons, and in community health centers and schools are members of the Arizona Telemedicine Program. The Arizona Telemedicine Program owns (Arizona Board of Regents is the actual owner) and operates a private health care broad band telecommunications network, the Arizona Telemedicine Network, that links 171 sites in 71 communities ranging in size from 280 people to 1.9 million people (Fig. 3). It operates an Application Service Provider (ASP) business which offers a wide range of services and facilities to the Arizona Telemedicine Program ASP members [5]. This ASP business is critical to the sustainability of the program.

Telehealth services are offered over the Arizona Telemedicine Network in over 60 subspecialties of medicine and nursing. For example, twenty-eight hospitals in the region receive teleradiology services 24/7 provided by university-based physicians in Tucson. Over 2500 patients have received teledermatology diagnoses by store-and-forward teledermatology. Telepathology services are delivered to rural communities either by robotic telepathology, in some communities, or virtual slice telepathology, (i.e. whole slide digitization), the most advanced technology in the field, in other communities. It is estimated that 80 per cent of the specialty consultations for the 36,000 prisoners housed by the Arizona Department of Corrections are delivered directly into the prisons by telemedicine, thus avoiding tens of thousands of miles of travel by guarded prisoners every year. Prisoner and service provider satisfaction with the correctional telemedicine services in Arizona is high. There are also several affiliated telepsychiatry networks in Arizona. In total, there have been over 40,000 telepsychiatry patient sessions to date. Tallying all specialties combined, 500,000 Arizona patients have received telemedicine services since the inception of the program. Many

ARIZONA TELEMEDICINE NETWORK

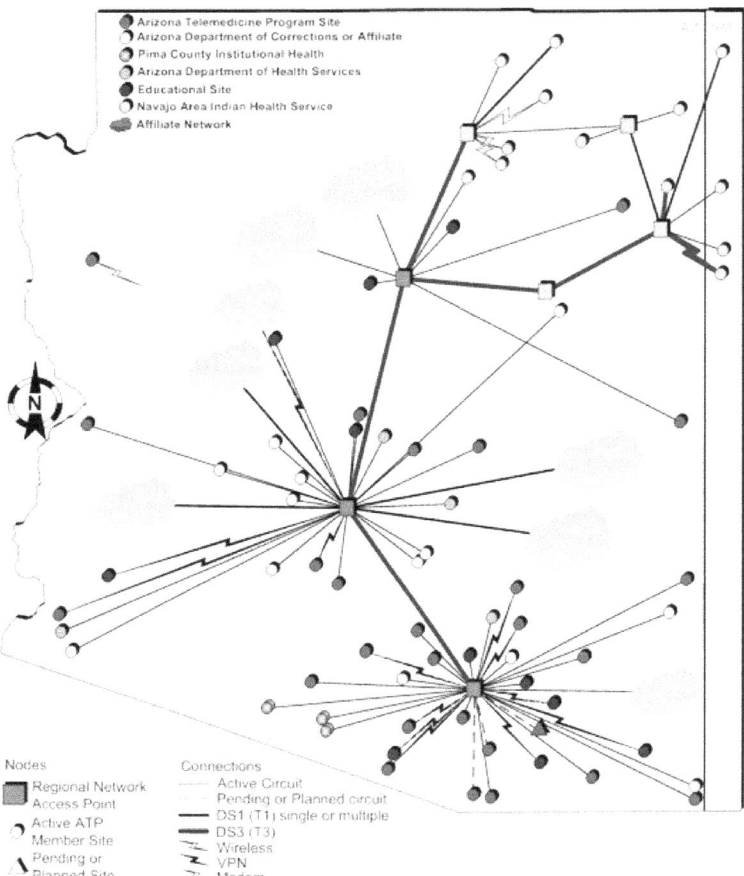

Figure 3. Arizona Telemedicine Network is staffed by the Arizona Telemedicine Program engineers. The network equipment is owned by the Arizona Telemedicine Program.

of these patients are in rural areas of the state. However, the numbers of urban telemedicine and telehealth cases are on the rise in Arizona [2].

With regard to technology transfer activities, funding for clinical research and the development of innovative telehealth services has exceeded expectations. The Arizona Telemedicine Program and its affiliates have been awarded 61 extramural grants totaling over $23,000,000. There are two telemedicine spin off companies from the University of Arizona and the Arizona Telemedicine Program, DMetrix, Inc., and UltraClinics, Inc. [13–18]. The return-on-investment for the state has been very good at over 2.3 times the original investment. To date, the Arizona Telemedicine Program and its staff have won nine national and international awards, including awards as a top telemedicine program, for distance education over a telemedicine network, and for clinical research, including technology assessment [2].

Table 1. Components of a Telemedicine and Telehealth Program

Category	Comment
Strategic Planning	Critical component of early stage planning
Facilities Design and Implementation	Facility interoperability is a major goal
Authority Management	Challenge especially in multi-organization programs
Practice Management	Impacted by organizational structures
Health Care Services	Establish potentially high volume services first
Network Operations	Services including maintenance must be of high quality
Risk Management	Largely a local matter except on network issues
Legal and Regulatory	Must be abreast of latest developments
Financial and Business	Policy can drive reimbursement
Inter-institutional Relations	Branding requires creativity and strong leadership
Marketing and Public Affairs	Substantive achievements make good news articles
Governmental Affairs	Government can be a natural partner for regional telemedicine and telehealth programs

2. Barriers and Issues at Hand

For many health care organizations with an interest in developing a telemedicine program, a critical question is "where to start?" How does an organization start a telemedicine and telehealth program in the absence of any local telehealth activities? Is the current health care environment likely to be receptive to innovative health care delivery models? [19–26] Arizona was faced with this challenge a decade ago.

To help independent health care organizations address this challenge, the Arizona Telemedicine Program sponsors regularly scheduled introductory courses on telemedicine, held at its headquarters at the Arizona Health Sciences Center campus in Tucson. Those courses have been popular and well attended for years. There are one and two day versions of the courses. These provide an overview of telemedicine and telehealth, discuss strategies and road maps for starting programs, and provide a limited amount of hands-on experience. The courses emphasize that telemedicine services require many of the same components that would be needed to start other multi-specialty health care services. The process of developing these components begins with strategic planning (Table 1).

Typically, only larger health care organizations have all of the core competencies needed to establish a successful telemedicine and telehealth program, yet the greatest need for access to telehealth services are often at smaller health care organizations. The Arizona Telemedicine Program's ASP business model was designed to provide a mechanism for its member organizations to obtain otherwise difficult to obtain services through in-sourcing directly from the Arizona Telemedicine Program [5]. The ease with which this can be arranged and the cost of the low annual membership fee has enabled dozens of independent health care organizations to get involved in telemedicine and telehealth with relatively little effort and without significantly increasing the numbers of IT or financial personnel at their organizations. The Arizona Telemedicine Program also serves an important advocacy role for telemedicine and telehealth at Arizona state agencies, such as the state Medicaid program. It is an effective neutral broker for members interested in participating in a wide range of extramurally funded projects [19].

Another challenge for new programs is recruiting a permanent director. Since telemedicine and telehealth are relatively new, the pool of qualified candidates available to direct new telemedicine programs is limited [24].

3. Suggested Solutions to Overcome Barriers

For many rural hospitals interested in joining regional telemedicine and telehealth programs, personnel with experience in a number of critical areas could be lacking. The Arizona Telemedicine Program's ASP business model accommodates many of those needs by providing a menu of these services from which member organizations can select the specific services they need [5,19]. Telemedicine and telehealth offerings range from turn-key solutions to simple program connections to other fully developed sites on the Arizona Telemedicine Network for access to Arizona Telemedicine Program's sites.

Starting a telemedicine and telehealth program in a health care organization with little prior experience with the concepts and technologies of telemedicine is challenging [23,24]. Nevertheless the future level of success of a new telemedicine and telehealth program can be influenced by the clarity and accuracy of the early vision for the program. The challenge is to align the program's vision (i.e., determined locally) with the vision of the program director, especially when that individual is an outside recruit. Simultaneously developing a vision statement and recruiting a program director requires skillful management of the start-up processes by the program initiators. It can be beneficial to insert highly respected community leaders into this process early on, in order to provide a strong guiding hand for the process.

We recommend that the process of starting a telemedicine and telehealth program, or adding an additional community to an established regional program, start with the naming of a local Planning Group and the selection of an official facilitator. Often, a highly respected member of the community, such as a former mayor, a respected business leader, or a member of the hospital's board can fill this role. The facilitator will then chair the ad-hoc group that will take on the task of drafting an initial list of outcome expectations for the new program. A telemedicine and telehealth consultant, preferably an individual with personal prior experience managing a telemedicine and telehealth program, can be invaluable in assisting the facilitator in establishing goals and outcome expectations. This consultant, or a separate search firm, can be given the assignment of recruiting a permanent program director. The consultant then works with the planning group on developing the initial business plan for the new enterprise (Fig. 4).

The selection of a qualified program director can be critical to the eventual success and sustainability of a telemedicine and telehealth program. In order to be successful, telemedicine and telehealth program directors need a broad range of skill sets. In addition, they frequently assume an additional role as spokesperson due to the inherently public nature of multi-organization telemedicine and telehealth programs. Multi-specialty telemedicine and telehealth programs have a public face and their communities will have an appetite for updates. The telemedicine program director may also become a local spokesperson for health care innovation in general, as well as the local expert on health care access disparities.

Planning Telemedicine Programs

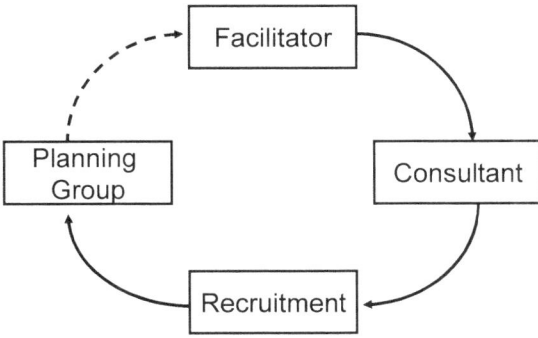

Figure 4. A strategy the Arizona Telemedicine Program developed to help member sites recruit a director or medical director for their telemedicine and telehealth program.

A challenge may be to gain adequate community support for establishing a community-based telemedicine and telehealth program. Establishing enthusiastic support can help the program director recruitment process. The lack of prior familiarity with telemedicine and telehealth in communities without access to such services can become its major barrier to acceptance. It is helpful to develop public support for welcoming telemedicine and telehealth services into a community. At a later stage of implementation, community support can be used to influence reimbursement policies of insurers, to give patients complete confidence in the services, and to provide opportunities to highlight the advantages of in-sourcing subspecialty health care services into geographically isolated communities as opposed to having people travel great distances for subspecialty medical services.

There are a number of other reasons for having communities enthusiastically support local telemedicine and telehealth programs. Distance learning, at many levels of education, can be carried out over the telemedicine program's network. Programs designed to interest local students in health care careers can be implemented. The sponsoring institution can also be proactive in educating community leaders about telemedicine. A community intern program can bring health care industry leaders from many organizations, business leaders, and government leaders to the program for a two-day immersion experience in medical center activities, including telemedicine. Also, a telemedicine program should consider sponsoring one and two day introductory courses on telemedicine. The Arizona Telemedicine Program has done this for years and has had over 600 graduates from over 50 independent health care organizations and agencies in its region. Attendees represent a broad-range of constituents ranging from patient case managers, to chief financial officers, to community leaders.

The Arizona Telemedicine Program has developed a process for initiating a telemedicine program. Many, but not all, elements have been used in Arizona.

In Phase 1, a preliminary list of telehealth services is generated. By the end of the Facilitator Phase, a tentative vision for the program will have emerged. This helps guide the Planning Group to an outside consultant appropriate to the type and scope of the telehealth program envisioned locally. It also builds in a mechanism for early reality testing by the program's early advocates and invites the making of a crucial "go-no-

Table 2. Phases in a Telehealth Program Start-up

Phase	Activity	Goal
1	Facilitation	Drafts the initial vision and outcome expectations documents for the telemedicine and telehealth program, aimed at providing the outside consultant with local information and perspective (Fig. 3).
2	Consultation	Helps design the telemedicine and telehealth program; lists and prioritizes key tasks including the recruitment of a permanent director.
3	Recruitment	Recruitment of the permanent director for the program. The director typically becomes a "champion" for the program, although this role should be shared with key government officials and high profile community leaders. There are many other possible candidates for the "champion" role.
4	Planning & Implementation	Move from concept through start-up and ramp-up of the new telemedicine and telehealth organization.

go" decision by the leadership group. It is important to understand that a "one-size-fits-all" approach does not work for all sites. Only those telemedicine or telehealth services identified as necessary should be initially implemented. An expansion of services can be added as needs arise.

In Phase 2, the consultant works with the Planning Group and the Facilitator on designing some of the specifications of the program and generating a sample list of tasks for the "soon to be" recruited director.

Phase 3 involves the recruitment of the permanent director of the program and bringing that individual on board.

In Phase 4, the director may choose to incorporate members of the initial Planning Group into task forces that will work on further exploration of telemedicine and telehealth applications, urgent branding issues, a business plan and a host of other start-up activities.

Planning a telemedicine and telehealth program is a complex process and involves developing shared visions at a number of levels. The levels will include the leadership of the organization that will house the program, (i.e., board of directors, deans for universities if applicable, etc.) the management team, the customers of the health care system, and, ideally, the general public. Ultimately, the success of innovative health care solutions may rest on achieving some level of support at each of these levels within the community.

Tracking progress in creating a community-wide shared vision for a new telemedicine and telehealth program can be challenging but a reward for doing so can be the attracting of strong political support. Political leaders tend to admire cohesive visions of technology-based programs.

The Arizona Telemedicine Program has developed a methodology to guide a member organization through a process aimed at developing shared visions for telemedicine and telehealth within their own enterprise. There are many categories of so called "shared visions." These include such things as: shared visions of how to start a new program; shared visions on the goals of a program; shared visions on resource and risk sharing; and shared visions on the workplace environment. There are many more. The following example concerns the development of a shared vision on the creation of a new telemedicine and telehealth program.

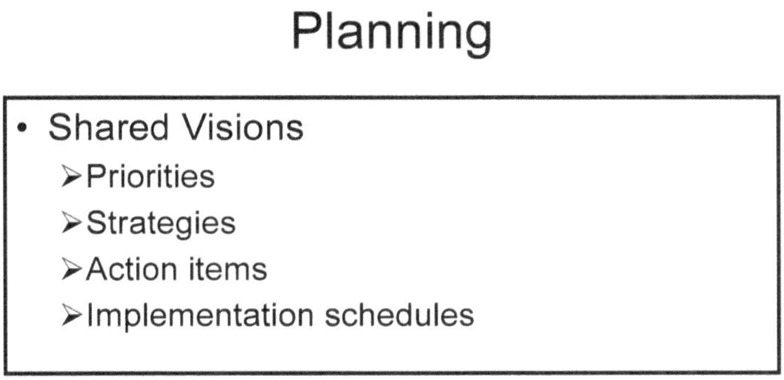

Planning

- Shared Visions
  - ➢Priorities
  - ➢Strategies
  - ➢Action items
  - ➢Implementation schedules

Figure 5. This figure lists components of the target shared visions for the start-up activities for a comprehensive telemedicine program. For a large, multi-organization program, this shared vision should periodically be updated and reconciled with the constantly evolving visions of the member health care organizations.

Planning

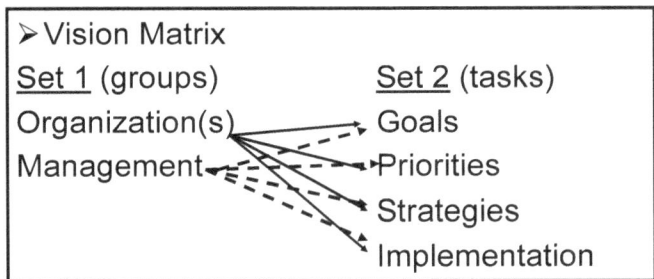

Figure 6. A vision matrix that can be used as a tool for designing and implementing telemedicine and telehealth programs. This methodology also identifies concerns and barriers as perceived separately by the organization leaders and their management team.

In Arizona, as part of our planning process, we go through an exercise, which we call a "Vision Matrix" exercise, in which leaders of each participating health care organization and, at separate sessions, managers, discuss a series of tasks: goal setting; establishment of priorities; articulation of a strategy to achieve each goal; and the development of formal implementation plans and schedules. Ideally, separate documents generated by organizations' leaders and their managements teams are then reconciled and a joint vision statement (leaders plus management) is generated and circulated (Fig. 6).

The process involves having two separate groups: the organization leadership (including Board members, senior corporate officers, and possibly other senior stake holders from the community, such as the CEO of a major company; and the organizations' management teams, including the Vice Presidents and division directors, meet to discuss the proposed multi-organization telemedicine and telehealth initiative in broad terms. Ideally, both service provider institutions and service user institutions are represented. Under certain circumstances, the Vision Matrix exercise would take place twice, initially with the designated Facilitator and the Consultant co-chairing the meetings and a second time, after the Program Director has been recruited and can personally attend the meetings. The primary goal of these meetings is to begin to develop shared visions with regards to what telemedicine and telehealth might achieve in the service area and to nurture the concept that there is plenty of room for collaboration among other-wise competing institutions in the health care industry. We find that telemedicine and tele-health are natural conduits for communication among organizations which can be an unexpected benefit of a program.

In it's full implementation, during the Vision Matrix exercise, the two groups, or-ganizational leadership and management, go through an agenda involving discussion of four topics: goals; priorities; strategies; and implementation. These four topics are dis-cussed in sequence. Generally, each topic is discussed for about 20 minutes with the Facilitator listing the participants' points on a flip chart. The resulting list is then dis-cussed by the group for about 10 minutes before the group moves on to the next topic. The Facilitator should understand that each of these topics is broad and could be dis-cussed for half a day or more, but be willing to resist temptation and stay with the time line for the exercise. After these four topics have been discussed in the allotted time, the groups break for an hour. They then reconvene for wrap-up comments and a discus-sion of next steps.

Our experience in Arizona is that many participants of planning sessions and train-ing events, although from the same geographic area, will be meeting one another for the first time. They come away from such in-person sessions with an unexpectedly high level of respect for the talent within the health care industry in their service area. Many long term acquaintances have been established at Arizona Telemedicine Program train-ing programs and program planning events over the years. This has benefited both in-dividuals, in terms of career development, and the health care industry, in terms of cre-ating a shared sense of mission for the health care industry in Arizona [2,3,19].

Why use the Vision Matrix exercise format? Telemedicine and telehealth are very broad topics. In our experience, it is valuable to give health care executives and manag-ers a highly structured environment in which to hear about telemedicine and telehealth, to begin conceptualizing its processes and to begin to understand the potential benefits to their organizations, and to provide peer-to-peer settings in which to develop the shared sense of mission that can make a regional telemedicine and telehealth collabora-tive successful and sustainable.

With respect to the administrators of telemedicine and telehealth programs, the program directors of such enterprises have complex jobs. They must have a clear vision of what they want their program to become from the outset, since all of the early stake-holders will look to them for guidance and will remember early promises, as they should. This does not preclude future growth beyond the original vision. Since tele-medicine is an extension of each of the participating member organizations, each entity needs to have confidence in the director from the outset. The director should be highly credible, with a reputation preferably based upon a solid track record of distinguished accomplishments. Controversial individuals or individuals without suitable credentials are disadvantaged when it comes to managing such public undertakings. Missionary zeal and entrepreneurial spirits are desirable attributes. Individuals in leadership posi-tions in the telehealth world should demonstrate an unusually high level of passion for what they are doing and function under the halo of idealism whenever possible. Creat-ing the future can appear intoxicating for the leaders of the charge for a new health care technology. This is fine. On the other hand, hyper-enthusiasm should be balanced with a willingness to be constantly challenged by technology skeptics. Political acumen is especially important for the telemedicine and telehealth program director in this regard. Within the shifting sands of today's health care industry, there are streams of disparate messages that come to telemedicine program directors. Given the tense atmosphere within the health care industry in the United States today, a program director needs finely tuned antennae to pick up on subtle messages from numerous sources on an on-going basis and deal with them proactively and with fortitude.

The Planning Group should also weigh in on the selection of the location of a new telemedicine and telehealth program within its organization. This may be especially important for a university-based program since many diverse functional units may choose to compete for the program. A common error in establishing a telemedicine and telehealth program is to place it administratively in an inappropriate administrative unit. It must be emphasized that telemedicine and telehealth program are, first and foremost, clinical services. At universities, a new telemedicine and telehealth program should be assigned administratively to a clinical department. In our opinion, it would be suboptimal to have a telemedicine and telehealth program administered within a non-service entity such as a School of Public Health, although there can be extenuating circumstances. A telemedicine and telehealth program's business activities must be handled by a competent medical business office, with personnel experienced in dealing with billing and coding issues. At many universities, such business offices are housed in clinical departments.

The reader is warned that, in most cases, the program director should not be a physician whose only special credential is an interest in computers. The successful candidate should have experience that would qualify him or her to be a medical service chief. The area of medical specialization is remarkably unimportant. However, prior experience in implementing and operating clinical services and overseeing medical business offices is important. As part of the business and operations activities, contracts and grants, reimbursement, procurement, licensure, and a wide spectrum of regulatory issues require attention. Generally, the program director should be an M.D. with an active medical license.

Today, given the current stage of technology diffusion of telemedicine and telehealth, it is helpful for the program director to serve the dual role of the program director and program "champion." This is somewhat analogous to the desirability of having health care system CEOs serve as both the public face and champions for their organizations. Championing a regional telemedicine and telehealth program can be demanding. Many stakeholders will lack a frame of reference in which to judge what is going on and to understand the many hurdles being overcome simultaneously. Readers of these comments a decade from now might find this observation outdated and even confusing but it all makes sense in terms of the fragmentary nature of telemedicine and telehealth programs during start-up and ramp-up stages of implementation today.

Staff training programs should be instituted early on in the development of telemedicine and telehealth programs. Although some of the training program components may be applicable to other types of health care services, it is important that many topics specific to the practice of telemedicine be incorporated in the training programs. The telemedicine training programs should cover special topics including: core competencies of telehealth providers; team building; outreach strategies; and the culture of "virtual communities." The virtual community concept will be new, and even somewhat mystifying to many employees being assigned to a telemedicine and telehealth program for the first time.

Training should include information on parameters that will be used as measures of success for the telemedicine and telehealth program under construction. These should include: meeting needs; achieving specific clinical outcomes; provider and service user satisfaction; and cost effectiveness. Financial performance can be considered in terms of: revenue; coding issues; accounts receivables; patient mix; bad debt; and network utilization. It should be understood, from the outset, that long-range strategic planning for telemedicine and telehealth programs is important and includes market assessment, goal setting, and the need for periodic updating of the program's vision and mission statements. Case studies can be effectively used in telemedicine and telehealth training programs in order to provide context for the didactic material.

4. Future

In the future, it is likely to say that telemedicine and telehealth services will become commonplace and ubiquitous. In medical imaging fields, such as teleradiology and telepathology, this may become the preferred way of delivering services. As these teleimaging services move into the mainstream of medical practice, the "tele-" prefixes might disappear. "E-health" has already become a term of choice by some practitioners but that could become antiquated as well. Telemedicine may become synonymous with medicine.

Telemedicine and telehealth may emerge as global industries. Since the United States has a fragmented health care system, it will not necessarily be the top international player in the telemedicine and telehealth industries, either in terms of technologies or service volumes. However, health care's superstar physicians, based in the United States, may have advantages and be aggressively marketed as "big name" brands within health care niches. Advertising dollars may pour into promoting the reputations of prestigious physicians who will carry a brand's flag.

We also anticipate that patients will increasingly utilize direct access health care services [19]. Service integrators may play an increasingly important role in aggregating health care services for patients [25]. High quality telemedicine and telehealth services will be readily available over standard broad-band telecommunications networks. High prestige institutions, such as John Hopkins, the "Harvard Hospitals" and the Cleveland and Mayo Clinics are currently leveraging their well-established brand names into international telemedicine and telehealth industries. They are advantaged by their international reputations. Also, these high quality programs train many fellows from other countries. They may return home to practice and become a source of referrals.

5. Conclusion

Telemedicine and telehealth organizations are not "business as usual." The media of telemedicine, including video conferencing and still imaging, magnify personalities and performances, frame scenes, and effectively focus communication. The technologies of telemedicine may also foster unexpected levels of cooperation and partnering with the health care industry.

In Arizona, the Arizona Telemedicine Program brand is advertised as standing for resource sharing and seamless technical interoperability among the state's large numbers of independent health care organizations. These notions resonate well in the Arizona State Legislature and in other governmental agencies. The success of the Arizona Telemedicine Program's ASP business models shows that economies of scale can be achieved in the health care industry by bringing independent health care organizations under a shared umbrella [5,19]. Although access to our telecommunications infrastructure may provide the largest single economic benefit of membership for Arizona Telemedicine Program members, the availability of telemedicine and telehealth services are the drivers of the membership model.

References

[1] www.telemedicine.arizona.edu (last opened May 2007).
[2] K. Blanchet, "Innovative Programs in Telemedicine. The Arizona Telemedicine Program". Telemedicine & e-Health 11, 633-640 (2005).
[3] R.S. Weinstein, G. Barker, S Beinar, M. Holcomb, E.A. Krupinski, A.M. Lopez, A. Hughes, and R.A. McNeely. "Policy and the Origins of the Arizona Statewide Telemedicine Program". In: Understanding Health Communications Technologies, P. Whitten, D. Cook, eds. Jossey-Bass, San Francisco, pp. 299-309 (2004).
[4] K.M. McNeill, R.S. Weinstein, and T.W. Ovitt. "Project Nightingale: A Geographically Distributed, Multi-Organizational Integrated Telemedicine Network Infrastructure". In: Computer Assisted Radiology and Surgery. H.U. Lemke, M.W. Vannier, K. Inmara, A.G. Farman, eds, Elsevier, Amsterdam, pp. 550-553 (1999).
[5] G.P. Barker, E.A. Krupinski, R.A. McNeely, M.J. Holcomb, A.M. Lopez, and R.S. Weinstein. "The Arizona Telemedicine Program Business Model". J Telemed Telecare 11, 397-402 (2005).
[6] K.M. McNeill, M.K. Carroll, M.J. Holcomb, M.M. Frost, P. Yonsetto, P. Schwarts, and K. Haber. "Teleradiology as a Driver for Regional-Scale, Multi-Organizational, High-Volume Telehealth Services". In: Proceedings of SPIE: Medical Imaging 2003: PACS and Integrated Medical Information Systems: Design and Evaluation. H.K. Huang and O.M. Ratib, editors, SPIE Press, Billingham, WA. Volume 5033, 155-159 (2003).
[7] R.S. Weinstein, Prospects for Telepathology. (Editorial) Human Pathol 17, 433-434 (1986).
[8] R.S. Weinstein, K.J. Bloom, and L.S. Rozek, "Telepathology and the Networking of Pathology Diagnostic Services". Arch Path Lab Med 111, 646-652 (1987).
[9] R.S. Weinstein, A.K. Bhattacharyya, A.R. Graham, and J.R. Davis. "Telepathology: A Ten-Year Progress Report". Human Pathol 28, 1-7 (1997).
[10] E. Krupinski, R.S. Weinstein, K.L. Bloom, and L.S. Rozek. "Progress in Telepathology: System Implementation and Testing." Advances in Path Lab Med 6, 63-87 (1993).
[11] R.S. Weinstein, M.R. Descour, C. Liang, A.K. Bhattacharyya, A.R. Graham, J.R. Davis, K.M. Scott, L. Richter, E.A. Krupinski, J. Szymus, K. Kayser, and B.E. Dunn. Telepathology overview. From concept to implementation. Human Pathol 32, 1283-1299 (2001).
[12] K. Kayser, J. Szymas, and R.S. Weinstein. "Telepathology and Telemedicine: Communication. Electronic Education and Publication in e-Health". VSV Interdisciplinary Medical Publishing, Berlin, pp. 1-257 (2005).
[13] R.S. Weinstein, A. Bhattacharyya, B.E. Halliday, Y.-P. Yu, J.R. Davis, J.M. Byers. A.R. Graham, and R. Martinez. "Pathology Consultation Service via the Arizona-International Telemedicine Network". Arch Anat Cytol Pathol, 43, 219-226 (1995).
[14] www.demtrix.com.
[15] www.ultraclinics.com.
[16] R.S. Weinstein, M.R. Descour, C. Liang, G. Barker, K.M. Scott, L. Richter, E.A. Krupinski, A.K. Bhattacharyya, J.R. Davis, A.R. Graham, M. Rennels, W.C. Russum, J.F. Goodall, P Zhou, A.G. Olszak, B.H. Williams, J.C. Wyant, and P.H. Bartels. "An Array Microscope for Ultrarapid Virtual Slide Processing and Telepathology. Design, Fabrication, and Validation Study". Hum Pathol. 35, 1303-1314 (2004).
[17] R.S. Weinstein, M.R. Descour, C. Liang, L. Richter, W.C. Russum, J.F. Goodall, P. Zhou, A.G. Olszak, and P.H. Bartels, "Reinvention of Light Microscopy. Array Microscopy and Ultrarapidly Scanned Virtual Slides for Diagnostic Pathology and Medical Education". In: Virtual microscopy and Virtual Slides in Teaching, Diagnosis and Research, J. Gu and R.W. Oglivie, editors CRC Press, pp. 9-35 (2005).

[18] A.M. Lopez, C. Venker, A. Howerter, G.P. Barker, A. Bhattacharyya, K.M. Scott, M.R. Descour, L.C. Richter, E.A. Krupinski, and R.S. Weinstein. "Demonstration of an expedited breast care (EBC) clinic" (abstract). J. Clinical Oncology 24, 661s (2006).

[19] R.S. Weinstein, A.M. Lopez, G.P. Barker, E.A. Krupinski, M.R. Descour, K.M. Scott, L.C. Richter, S.J. Beinar, M.R. Holcomb, P.H. Bartels, R.A. McNeely, and A.K. Bhattacharyya. "The innovative bundling of teleradiology, telepathology, and teleoncology services". IBM Systems Journal 46, 69-84 (2007).

[20] R.E. Herzlinger, "Consumer-Driven Health Care. Implications for Providers, Payers, and Policymakers". Jossey-Bass, pp. 1-197 (2004).

[21] B.J. Marcotte, "How Employers Can Make Consumer-Driven Health Care a Reality". In: R.E. Herzlinger, Ed. "Consumer-Driven Health Care. Implications for Providers, Payers, and Policymakers". Jossey-Bass, (2004), pp. 213-223.

[22] B.T. Ferrari, "Where Will Consumer-Driven Health Care Take Hold?" In: R.E. Herzlinger, Ed. "Consumer-Driven Health Care. Implications for Providers, Payers, and Policymakers". Jossey-Bass, (2004), pp. 403-409.

[23] M.M. Maheu, P. Whitten, and A. Allen, "E-Health, Telehealth and Telemedicine. A Guide to Start-Up and Success". Jossey-Bass, San Francisco, pp. 1-380 (2001).

[24] A.W. Darkins and M.A. Cary, "Telemedicine and Telehealth. Principles, Policies, Performance and Pitfalls", Springer, Publishing Company, New York, pp. 1-316 (2000).

[25] R.E. Herzlinger, "Why Innovation in Health Care is So Hard". Harvard Business Review, May (2006), 58-66.

[26] R.S. Weinstein, B.E. Dunn, and A.R. Graham, "Telepathology Networks as Models of Telemedicine Services by Cybercorps". New Medicine 1, 235-241 (1997).

The Do's and Don't's when You Establish Telemedicine and e-Health (Not Only) in Developing Countries

Rifat LATIFI
Professor of Clinical Surgery
Trauma, Surgical Critical Care and Emergency General Surgery
Department of Surgery, The University of Arizona, Tucson, Arizona, USA
Associate Director of Arizona Telemedicine Program, Telesurgery and International Affairs
President, International Virtual e-Hospital Foundation
Director, Telemedicine Program of Kosova

Abstract. One may face obstacles in implementing technological advances in our environment or exporting technology and knowledge by disseminating telemedicine and e-health in the rural areas or to the developing countries, or just by simply trying to advance already established medical systems. Dr. Weinstein et al have eloquently put all you need to know it order "to put it all together," however I wanted to alert you to few other issues may become important as you proceed. So let's talk first about obstacles as they vary. They may be as simple as ignorance, or as complex as political or national lack of vision, and leadership. Frankly, there are no obstacles that cannot be overcome, and there are no valid reasons that will justify failure to start and failure to succeed. We need to adopt the slogan "Failure is not an option." Determination to succeed is often associated with serious difficulties and growing pain, but that is not a good reason why you should stop.

Introduction

Obviously Telemedicine is not new, however, as in the case with many innovations it taking decades for telemedicine to enter the mainstream as a healthcare delivery system. Nonetheless telemedicine and telehealth development have brought real hope to developing countries and many of the remote areas and yet has raised significant questions and anxiety among those forces hoping to retain the status quo of current medical practice.

While most developments in telemedicine and other technologies in the medical field are being implemented among the developed world and prominent universities and institutions, the developing countries are the perfect examples where the telemedicine, e-health and relevant technologies are in great need. These countries need modern health information systems and advanced technology in order to become a part of the global community of medical practice. There is a need for significant medical and radical changes. So today, telemedicine is basically applied and is used from one continent to the other and one can find some elements of telemedicine in almost every part of the world. The penetration of the internet into the global scene has made this very possible. Transmission of medical information through the internet, as an attachment, enables consultation of doctors from one corner of the world is possible through these technologies. Today, the patient and the physician should not be alone anywhere in the world as long as there is some form of technology present and acceptable.

For the last seven years that I have been involved in telemedicine, I have learned many new things. The most important things that come to mind are that one needs to identify the issues that need to be recognized and resolved, even before one takes on creating and establishing telemedicine and e-health programs in any community or country, especially in a developing country. However dealing with telemedicine administration where multiple players with different backgrounds, cultures, education, goals and mentalities are involved could be very challenging and interesting to say the least. Personally, I have learned a great deal of how to deal with people, what to do, but mostly what not to do. Managing and administering telemedicine program has been a humbling experience. As trauma surgeon I have everything I need to take care of the patient at the time I need. All I need to do is be there and know how to take care of the patient with complex stab wounds, gun shot wounds or any other surgical emergencies. That is really easy. We walk into the trauma room or operating room and everything is there, the patient, the nurse, and the equipment. So all I need to know is how to operate and save someone's life. Managing complex telemedicine programs could represent a real challenge if one is not ready to face all the issues.

These issues maybe seem simple, but if not addressed properly and completely to the last detail, they will make the development and implementation of any program painful, if not impossible. These issues, at the beginning of the project, are not known to most of us. Nonetheless they are of outmost importance. They reveal their relevance as we painfully make mistakes of not addressing and resolving them upfront. Many of us assume, albeit wrongly, that the business philosophy of "build-operate-transfer" of technology boom in few developing countries may be applied in e-health and telemedicine field as well. So, why does the "build-operate-transfer" philosophy not apply entirely? Well, this is far more complex than setting up "a call center" in India or in Bangladesh, thus that business philosophy does not apply entirely, although the goal is the same: "build-operate-transfer."

1. Project Leadership

One of the most common question that comes to mind is who should lead the project and for how long? Let's say that you have an idea, you obtained the funds, and you are running the project and working hard with every one involved. When do you say: OK, now the time is right – you take it from here!

The answer to this question cannot be simple either. But, in my opinion, while every bit of the entire process is directed by "you," the program should be build by "locals" if it is to succeed and be recognized. The locals are the Kosovars, the Mizorams, the Cambodians, the villagers in southern Arizona, or Eskimos in Alaska. They are wherever the project is located. Without strong involvement of local citizens, the program will not become successful. Their involvement will ensure the key elements responsible for success of any e-health and telemedicine program because it is based on the sense of pride, operability, interoperability. All these ingredients are "must have" elements in order to ensure sustainability.

2. Telemedicine Program Is Not a Factory

We should not see creating telemedicine and telehealth systems in any region, but especially in developing countries, as creating few profitable call centers, or building a factory in the middle of nowhere. The motives have to be different, deeper, and certainly, more transparent and may be more complex, as the profitability is not the order of business and may not be visible for many years or decades. Remember, however, that you will eventually leave that institution, perhaps leave the entire region or the country, move on, but the operation that you have established will need to stay on, function, operate, and the "locals" will and should continue to benefit from it.

2.1. Unpredicted Problems

I am almost certain that as you go through different phases of the project, you will encounter different issues that none of the authors of this book have thought of, or perhaps did not think it is important enough to be mentioned in this volume. There are no "guidelines" to walk you through the pain and joy, since these "guidelines" lack many uncovered or recognized elements.

2.2. Can We Predict Success?

We continue to struggle finding the best approach and best solution to ensure success, and not fail, and so on. Predicting success is difficult, if not impossible. This is not the same as the Injury Severity Score (ISS) that predicts the mortality and morbidity of trauma patients. For this, I have generated few must "do's" and "don't's" that have helped me over the past seven years. These do's and don'ts are not evidence based and are not the best recognized practices by our peers. These are simply opinions. These are common senses, but you and I know that common sense may not prevail in the best business world.

3. The Must Do's

1. Know your stuff – be an expert and be honest.
2. Make sure you have the support and commitment of your institution and your family, as this will take you from your professional and family time. This is particularly important if telemedicine is not your main occupation.
3. Work very closely with local governments, especially if working in another country. You must be invited (best from the government itself) or from an institution such as a University. Check the credibility and the motives for involvement in the project of any one who invites you.
4. Identify local champions and work with them in close partnership. Do not rush identifying this person, or group of people. Take your time to make this decision. It will be the most important decision that you have made for the life of the project.
5. Identify the goals and objectives of your program and stick to them, although you may have to be flexible. As technology advances, and changes, things may change as well.

6. Perform the feasibility study and analysis of your geography of operation. In other words, decide where your project will be implemented, what space it will cover, how many people will be involved, what territory will be covered.
7. Secure the space from where you will operate and identify the political and physical geography of the operation.
8. Secure the budget for the project at least for the first three to five years – and be as detailed as possible.
9. Create the business model to ensure sustainability. Involve as many experts as possible when you create this. If you make big mistakes at this stage, you will have significant problems and may put the entire project in jeopardy.
10. Identify technical infrastructure and have a solid plan, but be ready to change if needed and as technology changes.
11. Acquire state of the art equipment: do not compromise on quality – consult the technical experts what technology you should adopt.
12. Ensure interoperability between your telemedicine and telehealth project with long term goals for transforming health care information technology of the hospital, region or the country you working.
13. Total transparency is crucial. Plan and spell out every detail of the project – no secrets in your plan. Send a copy of your plan to every one involved.
14. Make your plan public. Publish it in the local paper. Ensure good public relations for the project. Use media when ever possible to educate the public about your project.
15. Ensure continuous education of all members of the team. This is the most valuable time and expense that you will spend on the project.
16. Maintain continuous international presence. Invite your expert friends to give talks and have them speak out in public about the program. This adds a great deal of credibility to the program.
17. Report on the project collectively – when you write a paper on the project, make sure everyone's name is on the paper. Have them review the data and make them part of the process.
18. Keep a close eye on the project and maintain line of accountability – leadership of the projects should not be relaxed. Make sure you change the local leadership if need be. You have to be firm and open.
19. Make sure that every one on the project knows their job description and their obligation. Go over their duties often and ask for their input as often as possible.
20. Adapt, respect the local tradition, culture and environment, and be very sensitive to their tradition and culture.

4. The Don't's

1. Do not promise things that you will not be able to deliver.
2. Do not take sides in local politics – stay indifferent in local politics.
3. Do not sweat the small stuff – keep the big picture on your mind. This will help you overcome the difficulties with project.
4. Do not get discouraged; few things are destined to fail or go wrong.
5. Do no take part in anything that will compromise you and the project, especially bribes and gifts that may be offered to you.

6.   Do not allow repeated mistakes – intervene early. Early interventions will prevent failure of the projects, especially if you picked the wrong team the first time! You should be able to change the team or members of the team. Do not be afraid to do that.
7.   Do not abandon your private life and your family. If you do you will lose everything else. Try to make them part of your project, but do not pay for any of them.
8.   Do not lose your autonomy; stay in charge.
9.   Do not take all the credit for the work done in the project; the true leader shares the glory.

5. Conclusion

I expect the next three to five years we will have the telemedicine projects in the developing countries such those in the Balkans the way I have envisioned it some years ago. The physicians and nurses from different countries and hospitals will be on the same screen talking about the same patient and will offer different approaches. The biggest winner on this will be the patient and humanity. This fall, we will have the Second Intensive Balkans Telemedicine Seminar, this time in Tirana. The next one will be in Macedonia and then Montenegro and, so on. We will continue to build bridges, we will continue to put technology in every health "house" and, every where patients are in that region. The lessons that we are learning in this process are invaluable for other parts of the world. We will need to keep writing this up so the world can share our lessons our success as well as our failures. By then, the list of do's and don'ts will probably grow. And I hope it will get easier.

Reference

Latifi, R. Editor. Establishing Telemedicine in Developing Countries: From Inception to Implementation. IOS Press, 2004, Amsterdam.

Current Principles and Practices of Telemedicine and e-Health
R. Latifi (Ed.)
IOS Press, 2008

The Last Challenges and Barriers to the Development of Telemedicine Programs

Charles R. DOARN, MBA
Deputy Director
Advanced Center for Telemedicine and Surgical Innovation
Executive Director Center for Surgical Innovation
Administrative Director Minimally Invasive Medical Technologies Center
Associate Professor Department of Surgery and Biomedical Engineering
University of Cincinnati

Abstract. Over the past several decades the concept of telemedicine has evolved to be more commonplace with many unique applications. These applications have been made possible by overcoming challenges and barriers that have been present for most of telemedicine's development. The application of telemedicine continues to undergo growth and scrutiny. However, the rapid infusion of technology continues to serve as a catalyst for adoption and validation. Looking into the future requires a review of the past. Overcoming barriers and challenges has not been easy. Many have been minimized, in part because of technologies rapid flow and diffusion. Yet there are still significant challenges that must be overcome. In many parts of the world, healthcare and education are limited because of access. This has been driven by many influences, which continue to have an impact, albeit in many cases, minimal. Future generations of telemedicine users will look back at this period as one of transition. The first 30 years or so of telemedicine implementation were fraught with barriers and challenges. The next 30 years will see and entirely different paradigm of practicing medicine, including consumerism and smart systems.

Keywords. Telemedicine, Barriers, Challenges, Opportunities, Consumerism

Introduction

Several years ago, I wrote a chapter for the first publication of this book 'Establishing Telemedicine in Developing Countries: From Inception to Implementation'. The chapter was entitled 'The Challenges and Barriers to Development of Telemedicine Programs'. It outlined numerous challenges and barriers to not only the development of telemedicine but to the adoption and utilization of it as well. These for the most part remain the same. Some of them have been exacerbated and some have been ameliorated, yet they remain formidable to wide adoption and integration of telemedicine. Change and in many cases the lack of change has been affected by many influences, including the actions of different sectors of industry and government. Over these past several years, technology development, validation, and implementation has continued unabated. What was once insurmountable is no longer such. Telemedicine continues to grow the world over.

Table 1. Barriers and Challenges Facing Telemedicine Implementation

Barriers/Challenges
Limited or untimely access to definitive care
Distance and geography
Telecommunications
Limits in diagnosis, treatment
Language, Culture, Religion
Automony
Extreme environmental conditions
Financial – economic
Legislative – policy
Technology accessibility
Attitudes
Standards (interoperability)
Business plans – models
Consumerism

Many challenges that we have observed in the practice of medicine have come about by demand, either consumer driven or through ease-of-use. In the military and in space exploration, the challenges of providing healthcare are daunting, yet these are overcome [1]. These same barriers impact healthcare for the general population, but they are not as easily overcome. Telemedicine, three decades ago, faced an uphill battle, predicated on government funding for survival. Today, consumer electronics at the local audio technology outlet are being sold with capabilities for supporting medical monitoring – consumers are looking for it! Home healthcare and remote health services are rapidly moving forward and it seems there is no end in site to the plethora of applications in telemedicine [2]. Bandwidth capabilities are far greater each passing year, and the cost has become more economical, opening new markets and opportunities.

As technology has marched forward, what was once a barrier is now perhaps better defined as a boundary to wider adoption and application in mainstream healthcare. What was once a challenge is now an opportunity. Yet many of the old barriers and challenges that limit telemedicine's reach stubbornly remain across the great expanse of the globe [3,4].

To address these new challenges and barriers, we must first understand earlier challenges and how they have been diminished. These barriers share common characteristics across many cultures and varying stages of economic development. Often there is resistance to change. The way technology diffuses is significant and its acceptance is often challenged [5,6]. We will find that many of these early characteristics remain the same (Table 1). Barriers and challenges to the adoption of telemedicine delineated in Table 1 are not in any particular priority.

1. Foundation for Change – Removing the Gauntlet

Each of the 14 elements, highlighted in Table 1, provides us with a foundation for what is in the way or a barrier to the development, adoption and integration of telemedicine in healthcare delivery. As we have moved forward in the development and adoption of telemedicine, there has been significant growth in telemedicine programs at national and international levels. Government and commercial vendors have moved forward with programs and products to meet customer demand and to look at niche markets, which continue to grow. Much like the Berlin Wall that separated a people, the barriers to telemedicine – those that keep it from wide spread proliferation are slowly ebbing away.

1.1. Current Practice – Evidence-Based Practice

For the past 13 years, the scientific literature has produced an abundance of knowledge, illustrating that telemedicine works. Before this time, there were limited sources on telemedicine activities. Those that existed prior to the 1990s were funded in large part through governments and were not sustainable. These programs did not produce a plethora of knowledge that was publishable. Since the early 1990s however, there has been significant contributions to the scientific literature. The *Telemedicine and e-Health Journal* and the *Journal of Telemedicine and Telehealth*, the world's leading journals in telemedicine have published in excess of 1,000 peer-reviewed articles on various programs and efforts in telemedicine [7]. Other journals have published manuscripts related to this field as well. A large portion of these manuscripts illustrate the empirical evidence scientifically and statistically that telemedicine works and is a significant tool.

The largest trade organization for telemedicine, the American Telemedicine Association (ATA), has established special interest groups (SIG) to address many of the issues facing telemedicine today. Other organizations also look at various elements of emerging healthcare technologies, including the International Society for Telemedicine and e-Health (ISfTeH) and an ever growing list of national-based telemedicine associations. These activities help shape policy at all levels of healthcare across the globe. The gauntlet is coming down.

The definitions for telemedicine, although upgraded to reflect new technologies remain essentially the same. There are many definitions for telemedicine. Sood et al. recently reported that there are 105 different definitions cited in the literature [8]. It often depends upon who you are talking to, what country you are in or what you want to do with telemedicine. For the purposes of this paper, telemedicine is simply defined as "the integration of telecommunications and information systems in the delivery of healthcare."

2. Challenges and Barriers – It's in the Details

The challenges and barriers to telemedicine must be addressed against the backdrop of a more global issue and that is the need to address global health. Telemedicine, through health information technology, must play a role in disaster response [9]. The application of telemedicine has already been shown to be useful in natural disasters during the response to the massive earthquake in Soviet Armenia in 1989 [10–12]. There are predictions of impending pandemic and there is always the threat of deadly disease crossing species or being introduced into the ecosystems intentionally (bioterrorism) or naturally. Nations must work together to overcome differences to promulgate corrective and humanitarian response effectively, efficiently, and rapidly to minimize risk to the human population.

This is where the earlier challenges and barriers become new challenges and barriers. Many of the earlier characteristics remain. Their influences have diminished in part because of technology and wider distribution. Yet they remain, often shackling program growth or even program or project inception.

2.1. Attitudes

Previously referenced as arrogance, this barrier still remains. Whether it is a patient's mistrust, misunderstanding or unwillingness to change or it is a physician, other care giver or it's a government, attitudes and perceptions can be a significant barrier to acceptance. If a government is unwilling to permit access say to web-based health sites via the Internet, then there is a barrier or a wall erected that can have a negative impact on the general public health. In times of a pandemic, nation states could find themselves in situations similar to that of the Dark Ages. Open lines of communication and accurate information will lead to attitudinal changes. History has clearly shown that the lack of information on issues affecting public health can be devastating.

There remains today, in many parts of the world, those who do not believe that telemedicine works. They think it is not cost effective. Physicians believe the way they were trained and the way they practice works; and they are reticent to change. Although many patients are excited about technology and telemedicine, many still feel the need to be in the same room as their healthcare provider.

Such attitudinal change will also be brought about through consumerism and education. This has been the general observation over the past several years. As a frequent international traveler, it amazes me how cell phone distribution is across the globe. This inexpensive device is proving to be a valuable tool for sharing information, some of which we would prefer not being shared on YouTube. Nevertheless, attitudes still poses a significant barrier. They are changing, but there is still much work ahead [9–11].

2.2. Consumerism

Emerging challenges and perceived barriers include the demand for consumer products. There are a number of consumer electronics that are available at retail outlets around the world that are being used to support healthcare. Consider the digital camera, the cell phone, wireless sensors, wireless networks, or even the very popular Apple IPOD. Today's economy has created more choices and more disposable income. In the United States, the aging baby boom population, those born in the years after World War II (1946–1962), is increasingly looking for technologies to enhance the lives of their families and themselves. Health is no exception.

An increasing number of Americans look to the Internet for health information. This new kind of technology will drive the next generation of self-care by allowing patients to manage their own health conveniently and proficiently [12]. The issue for the consumer is how valid is the information [13]. Consumers are more affluent today and have more disposable income with which to shop around for healthcare services. There is more technology available in healthcare services. Hip joints can be replaced, organs can be transplanted safely with a high survivability, and robotic systems are now used to conduct a wide variety of surgical procedures.

The wide spread of technology is not limited to the developed world. In a global economy where news travels instantaneously, the populations that were once isolated now demand more goods and services. New economies are being built because of immediate access to information. Consider the outsourcing of radiology film readings being done in Bangalore, India. Patient films are obtained at a hospital in one country and transmitted through a secure network to a highly skilled team of radiologists in Bangalore. The films are read, a diagnosis is rendered and sent back to the referring physician [14]. Thus providing a sustainable and stable business model.

Consumerism is more of an opportunity than a barrier to wide spread adoption of telemedicine. However, some challenges to consumerism remain. These are interlinked with other barriers discussed herein, including attitudes, financial, access, etc. All play a significant role in consumerism.

2.3. Distance and Geography

Geographically speaking the world is a huge place. Yet, with 21st century telecommunications technologies you can pretty much connect with everyone, wherever they are. So the barriers of distance and geography are not as significant perhaps as they once were. However, challenges remain. On the battlefield, wounded American combat soldiers from Iraq or Afghanistan are treated highly effectively in theater but it takes more than 10 hours for them to be airlifted to Germany, and then another 10 hours to the continental United States (CONUS). In the space program, both American and Russian, medical care is provided in orbit, but there is no immediate return or access to definitive care [1]. The same can be said about individuals who are located in places that are far removed from definitive care. This implies that distance is a challenge. There are large populations around the world that are isolated by distance, which is not necessarily due to geography. It may in fact be merely the distance from one building to another in large cities like New York or Bangalore. This of course is more an attribute of access than geography.

Communications and health information technology are permitting more virtual presence, where patient and healthcare provider can be linked. This has had a tremendous impact on access, thus diminishing – not eliminating the barrier of distance and geography.

2.4. Access

Access to resources can be a significant barrier to telemedicine. There are many things that influence access, including the other barriers presented here. Global access can be defined as the ability for anyone to gain access to health information and medical expertise that pertains to their needs regardless of where they are located in relation to the information. Today, the Internet is the most realistic platform to support this. In the past, libraries and journals were the portals for information. However, access to them is limited because they are physical assets and often located somewhere else. The 'bricks and mortar' concept prevents access just because it is not located where the user is. The Internet is universally virtual. It is everywhere.

Imagine visiting the Louvre Museum in Paris or Red Square in Moscow without actually being there. Imagine reviewing ancient manuscripts on your own computer, wherever you are. This is the importance of access. Patients and healthcare providers can literally be connected to one another without the need for being in the same room.

Fundamentally, access is then integrated with consumerism. If a consumer can use simple communications tools like their cell phone or even dial-up Internet, they can gain access to a plethora of information and expertise. Their interest or needs can be gratified much faster as access to what the want is at their finger tips. Access comes about much faster than ever before.

2.5. Telecommunications

Telecommunication is of course the key to any successful telemedicine activity. Tele-communication tools have been limited in both time and rate or could be absent for periods of time. Telecommunications are of vital importance to the future of healthcare. Those individuals who find themselves in a remote location may experience delays in telecommunications or not have it at all. For many years, telemedicine was supported by dedicated telecommunication assets – plain old telephone systems (POTS), satellite-based, etc. Today, there is a wide diversity in telecommunication tools available, in-cluding the Internet, Voice over Internet Protocol (VOIP), etc. The fastest growing segment is cellular phone technology. Manufactures and retailers provide services that seemed unrealistic just a few years ago, including transmission of data, transmission and receipt of video, and global positioning using the cell phone.

Telecommunications services support synchronous (real-time) and asynchronous (store-and-forward) interactions. These two modalities provide a wide variety of capa-bilities, including video teleconferencing, VOIP, and transmission of still photography and radiology images.

Telecommunications in healthcare is impacted by bandwidth. The more bandwidth available for applications the better the outcome is. For instance, a synchronous interac-tion – a videoconference – at a low bandwidth would be very difficult to participate in. Although, this may be of value, a higher bandwidth would make the interaction much better, and more importantly impress upon participants the importance of continuing. Telecommunications and bandwidth have not been the only challenge that has helped telemedicine flourish. It has, however, been a dominant reason. The choice of tele-communications solutions must be driven by requirements, costs, availability, quality of service, and consumer expectations.

Telecommunications, although a barrier, is not the barrier it once was. New tech-nologies and inexpensive telecommunications options continue to grow.

2.6. Limitations in Diagnosis and Treatment

An environment that has appropriate telecommunications connectivity, a population base that can support telemedicine, and needs may be limited in what it can do simply because the diagnosis and treatment modalities may be limited. For example, the tele-medicine consult may occur with little or no problem, be deemed a success, but the recommended treatment and follow-up could not happen because the capabilities at the patient site are limited. The telemedicine system designed and deployed must take this into consideration. This is more of a challenge than a barrier, and, therefore, will al-ways remain as such.

2.7. Language, Culture, Religion

Language and culture are of significant issue for many reasons. The ability to commu-nicate in a common language is important. English seems to be the common language for telemedicine. Depending on the country one finds themselves in, obtaining medical attention can be highly challenging because either the patient or the healthcare delivery system does not speak the same language, or there are nuances of language that can alter the treatment of the ability to treat. In some instances language can drive culture. Certainly, there are numerous cultural differences in the practice of medicine. This has been well known in the space program as well as in ground-based telemedicine projects such as the Space Bridge projects [1,16–19].

Many telemedicine programs and much of the healthcare information available today can be obtained from the Internet. If this venue is the infrastructure by which information can be obtained, then there are real challenges for those populations located in nations that limit access to the Internet. There are many countries that limit access, principally due to religion or politics. Countries like China use Internet filters to eliminate searches on key words through a search engine like Google. Access in China to many education sites for instance is not permitted [20]. The same is true in Saudi Arabia [21]. Access to healthcare information in a time of crisis may be stymied in a predominately Muslim country if individuals lack access to the Internet and its vast amounts of data. This issue remains a significant challenge to wider adoption in many parts of the world.

2.8. Extreme Environmental Conditions

Remote medical capabilities, regardless of location, often times have limited diagnostic tools, limited treatment capabilities, and limited pharmaceuticals. This can be a significant challenge in addressing medical care because these limitations may in fact further exacerbate the situation. Limited resources can be of significant impact in implementing telemedicine. Emerging telemedicine applications, however, have shown the healthcare and surgical intervention can be addressed in remote and extreme environments. Space, the battlefield, ships at sea, individuals located in the alpine areas and the jungle (both natural and concrete) are but a few environments that have seen successful applications of telemedicine. Although, these kinds of environments remain, the challenges are diminished because of technological innovation in telecommunications, information systems, sensor technologies, and robotics.

Significant work has been accomplished in the application of telemedicine in the extremes of disasters. Telemedicine has played a significant role in natural disasters such as earthquakes and the battlefield [16,23–26].

2.9. Financial – Economic

The biggest challenge to telemedicine implementation is the cost of capital investment and operations. If these costs cannot be recovered, then the barrier of implementation is very high. Many international programs, linked between the United States or Europe and developing nations face this issue. On one side, there is a tremendous amount of resources set aside for healthcare per capita, where as in a developing country like Kosova, where per capita expense is low. This is where telemedicine can add the most value [27,28].

Reimbursement and other funding profiles must be considered as grants and philanthropy cannot sustain telemedicine. Otherwise this barrier remains significant.

2.10. Standards (Interoperability) Technical/Clinical

In order for telemedicine to work, there must be standards for technical and clinical areas. There are many efforts underway to develop standards. This has been more prolific for the technical than the clinical. These remain a challenge more than a barrier.

2.11. Legislative – Policy

Legislation is important to telemedicine regardless of location. Each country's health department or ministry works to develop policies that address telemedicine. These policies can have an impact on the success of telemedicine implementation and ultimately access. Access can also be impacted by the capability and availability of technology. In some countries technology oozes out of the corner store. In other countries, it may take months to acquire what is needed to do the simplest of tasks.

2.12. Business Plans – Models

As sure as technology is made available one day it becomes obsolete the next. As the 21st Century begins, new technologies in computers, imaging systems, and telecommunications lead paradigm shifts in healthcare. Such systems include informatics components that permit continued growth in data collection and useful databases. This is very important as medical informatics is the foundation or fabric of the future of medicine and healthcare delivery. The future looks bright for all people regardless of their location on Earth or where ever they may be.

This future must be tempered with robust business models that meet the patient and caregiver's requirements. Through a thorough needs assessment and system design telemedicine can be integrated and have added value. This takes a champion and strong evidence the purports success and cost savings. A word of caution, however, cost savings can be intangible or difficult to measure monetarily.

3. Future

The future of telemedicine is extremely bright. The sky is the limit as to the applications that are being developed and deployed. The barriers are ebbing away at different rates. This will permit wider adoption and more applications. Remote health services, where patient's health is monitored from their homes will see a huge increase in growth world wide. The application of telemedicine in surgery, telesurgery, will become more widely distributed. Access to healthcare and health information worldwide will become more widely available. Telemedicine will become a vital tool, national and international, for responding to disaster response and education. Telemedicine kiosks, similar to free standing blood pressure monitoring stations at the pharmacy will spring up at the workplace, on cruise ships and other points of service. This kiosks will be linked with health departments for easy monitoring of the health of the population.

4. Conclusion

Where does that leave us? Well telemedicine is no longer a novelty. It is no longer a demonstration. The "Mission is Complete." Telemedicine has become a useful tool in the delivery of healthcare. The technologies used, transcend culture, time and geography. It has the potential of touching every human life. The integration of medicine with information and telecommunications technologies has provided a strong foundation for change in health care. Simple technologies can be used to bring help to remote regions where there was nothing but despair and frustration.

The concepts of telemedicine are here to stay. As time goes by, it becomes a proven technology and paradigm for medicine that will have gone through more vigorous review and evaluation than any other technology before it and perhaps after it. Indeed the future is bright.

References

[1]   Doarn CR, Nicogossian AE, Merrell RC. Application of telemedicine in the United States Space Program. *Telemed J* 1998; 4(1):19-30.

[2]   Haselkorn A, Coyle M, Doarn CR. The future of remote health services: Summary of an expert panel discussion. *Telemed and E Health.* At Press.

[3]   Doarn CR. Challenges and Barriers to Development of Telemedicine Programs. *Establishing Telemedicine. Developing Countries: From Inception to Implementation.* R Latifi (Ed) IOS Press. Amsterdam. 2004; 104:41-48.

[4]   Federal Strategy is Needed to Guide Investment. US Government Accounting Office. GAO/NSIAD/ HEHS97-67 Telemedicine. Feb 1997.

[5]   Whan P, Brown NA, Wootton R. A bibliographic snapshot of the telemedicine citation literature. *J Telemed Telecare* 2006; 12(Suppl 3):95-102.

[6]   Stanberry B. Telemedicine Barriers and Opportunities in the 21st Century. *J Intern Med* 2000; 247(6):615-28.

[7]   Paul DL, Pearlson KE, McDaniel RR. Assessing technological barriers to telemedicine: Technology-management implications. *IEEE Transactions on Engineering Management* 1999; 46(3):279-88.

[8]   Sood S, Jugoo S, Dookhy R, Mbarika V, Prakash N, Merrell, RC, Doarn, CR. What is telemedicine?: 104 peer-reviewed perspectives and theoretical underpinngs. Telemed and e-Health, At press.

[9]   Higgins CA, Conrath DW, Dunn EV. Provider acceptance of telemedicine systems in remote areas of Ontario. *J Fam Pract* 1984; 18(2):285-9.

[10] Miller EA. Telemedicine and doctor-patient communication: an analytical survey of the literature. *J Telemed and Telecare* 2001; 7(11):1-17.

[11] Hu PJ, Chau PY. Physician acceptance of telemedicine technology: an empirical investigation. *Top Health Inf Manager* 1999; 19(4):20-35.

[12] Forkner-Dunn J. Internet-based patient self care: The next generation of healthcare delivery. *J Med Internet Res* 2003; 5(2):e8.

[13] Hesse BW, Nelson DE, Kreps GL, Croyle RT, Arora NK, Rimer BK, Viswanath K. Trust and Sources of Health Information. The Impact of the Internet and Its Implications for Health Care Providers: Findings From the First Health Information National Trends Survey. *Arch Intern Med.* 2005; 165(22): 2618-24.

[14] Kalyanpur A, Neklesa VP, Pham DT, Forman HP, Stein ST, Brink JA. Implementation of an International Teleradiology Staffing Model. *Radiology* 2004; 232(2):415-19.

[15] Chan TC, Kileen J, Griswold W, Lenert L. Information Technology and Emergency Medical Care during Disasters. *Acad Emerg Med* 2004; 11(11):1229-36.

[16] Houtchens BA, Clemmer TP, Holloway HC, et al. Telemedicine and international disaster response: medical consultation to Armenia and Russia via a telemedicine spacebridge. *Prehosp. Disaster Med* 1993; 8(1):57-66.

[17] Doarn CR, Lavrentyev V, Orlov OI, Grigoriev A, Nicogossian AE, Ferguson EW, Merrell RC. Evolution of telemedicine in Russia: Influences from the space program. A ten-year summary. *Telemed J E-Health* 2003; 9(1).

[18] Williams DR, Bashshur RL, Pool SL, Doarn CR, Merrell RC, Logan JS. A strategic vision for telemedicine and medical informatics in space flight. *Telemed J E-Health,* 2000; 6(4):441-448.

[19] Holloway HC, Nicogossian AE, Stewart DF (Editors); Dervay JP, Doarn CR, Teeter R (Co-editors). First International Telemedicine/ Disaster Medicine Conference, Proceedings. NASA Publication NP-107. Washington, DC: NASA Headquarters, 1993.

[20] Empirical Analysis of Internet Filtering in China at http://cyber.law.harvard.edu/filtering/china/ (last accessed April 3, 2007).
[21] Empirical Analysis of Internet Filtering in Saudi Arabia at http://cyber.law.harvard.edu/filtering/saudiarabia/ (last accessed April 3, 2007).
[22] Teich JM, Wagner MM, Mackenzie CF, Schafer KO. The informatics response in disaster, terroism, and war. *J Am Med Inform Assoc* 9(2):97-104.
[23] Mandil SH. Telematics in Health Care in Developing Countries. *J Med Sys* 1995; 19(2):195-203.
[24] Poropatich RK, DeTreville R, Lappan C, Barrigan CR. The The U.S. Army telemedicine program: general overview and current status in Southwest Asia. *Telemed J E. Health* 2006; 12(4):396-408.
[25] Meliev T, Cram B, Hunsaker D, Deniston W, Caola L. A retrospective evaluation of the development of a telemedicine network in a military setting. *Mil Med* 2002; 167(6):510-515.
[26] Abbott KC, Mann S, Dewitt D, Sales LY, Kennedy S, Poropatich RK. Physician to physician consultation via electronic mail: the Walter Reed Army Medical Center Ask a Doc System. *Mil Med* 2002; 167(3):200-204.
[27] Latifi R, Muja S, Bekteshi F, Merrell RC. The role of telemedicine and information technology in the redevelopment of medical systems: The case of Kosova. *Telemed J E Health* 2006; 12(3):332-40.
[28] Merrell RC, Lee A, Kwankam SY, Mwape B, Chinyama C, Latifi R, Piso MI, Serban F. Satellite applications for telehealth in the developing world. *J Telemed Telecare* 2006; 12(6):321-4.

Current Principles and Practices of Telemedicine and e-Health
R. Latifi (Ed.)
IOS Press, 2008

55

Creating Telehealth Networks from Existing Infrastructures

Brett HARNETT, MS-IS
Research Assistant Professor, University of Cincinnati
Department of Surgery, Cincinnati, Ohio

Abstract. Implementing a telehealth program from the technical standpoint can be an engineering and financial challenge due to associated costs such as hardware, software, networking, administration and human expertise. To maximize potential and minimize costs, it makes sense to leverage existing telecommunications infrastructures and tailor the program based on what is available. This is especially critical in developing nations where funding is often limited.

Keywords. Telehealth, telecommunications, networks, bandwidth, topologies

Introduction

The ability to reach remote areas with modernized medicine has been traditionally handled by short-term visits by medical professionals in specially outfitted vehicles for primary care or even surgery [1]. However, much of the medical care that is needed can be accomplished – at least to a reasonable level of quality – through the use of telemedicine. By designing systems that utilize the existing and nascent telecommunications capabilities within a given region, a sustainable telehealth network can be achieved.

One of the most profound advances in telecommunications in the past 10 years has been wireless. Voice over IP (VOIP) has also made a significant impact by lowering communication costs even from fixed, legacy systems. The former is considered an infrastructure technology while the latter is considered to be a platform technology. By combining an evolving infrastructure technology with a revolutionary platform technology new and immense opportunities are created [2].

These will have positive effects on heath care throughout the world. The digital divide is despairingly wide for millions of people. International groups, relief agencies and other non-governmental organizations (NGOs) play a role in addressing the needs of the people on the fringes of the digital divide. Attempts to apply global governance have fallen woefully short of the actual needs [3]. Using telecommunications, the barrier of geography can indeed be overcome.

Although still enormous, the digital division between developed and developing world, it is changing. The gap for fixed lines has decreased from 14:1 in 1992 to about 5:1 in 2002. Changes in cellular comparisons are more dramatic, from 30:1 to 5:1 [4].

While the telecommunications gap is rapidly shrinking, it is still considered too wide. Of the one billion fixed telephone lines installed throughout the world, over 50 percent are found in the 29 richest countries, even though these countries only account for 15 percent of the world's population. Furthermore, it is estimated that only ten percent of the world's population uses the Internet and 72% of those live in developed countries. This statistic points out an interesting irony. If we look back at the wired world it seems evident that the integration of telehealth services would follow the lead of developed countries. An interesting phenomenon is occurring however where telehealth programs are increasingly being deployed in the developing nations. When implemented well, telemedicine may allow developing countries to leapfrog over their developed neighbors in successful telehealth delivery [5].

The wide availability of information technology and telecommunications has raised expectations and concerns throughout the world for increased levels of quality healthcare [6]. Costs for these technologies continue to decline. However, the decision to implement telehealth services for a given region requires considerable attention to available telecommunications technologies. Therefore, to engineer an economical means of achieving national health policy objectives requires comprehensive assessments of available resources and planning for scalability.

1. Current Developments

International telecommunications is an extremely dynamic topic. Since the early days of electronic communications in the mid 19th century, global communications have evolved in leaps and bounds. During those years, developed nations in particular, benefited from the ever-growing installation base of copper, fiber, terrestrial wireless and satellite communications. Underdeveloped nations lagged behind in telecommunications and in many cases, were simply nonexistent. In some cases where services were available, only the military and government officials had access. The most basic of telecommunications services, a simple telephone was not available to the masses.

Because of the high costs of pulling copper, laying fiber or even installation of towers for fixed wireless systems such as microwave, these developing nations found themselves increasingly behind the curve in not only telecommunications infrastructures but also industry and commerce which rely heavily on communications. The gap simply grew.

As technology continues to gain momentum and becomes more affordable, telemedicine practices are beginning to show that engaging in multidisciplinary collaboration by healthcare professionals can be beneficial [7–11]. This implies that areas such as developing nations can find ways to benefit as well. According to the International Telecommunication Union (ITU), developing nations are experiencing the fastest growth in wireless communications [12]. This is a positive step. National Ministries of Health and communications providers need to work together to leverage investments multilaterally. Involving medical universities usually located in major metropolitan areas can be an added value [13]. Even the use of standard email mechanisms can prove effective [14]. In areas where funding is nominal, installation and improvements to communications is often cost prohibitive or not possible. What may be available is all that may be used.

There are some basic issues that need to be addressed when determining the networking architecture for telemedicine. Here are some of the more commonly used technical terms when describing telemedicine network design:

Telecommunication is defined as any transmission, emission or reception of signs, signals, writing, images and sounds or intelligence of any nature by wire, radio, optical or other electromagnetic systems.

Bandwidth is the capacity of a network segment to carry data. The term bandwidth stems from the early days of radio where it literally meant "width of the band" with regard to the particular frequency. In network jargon, it refers to the amount of data that can pass a given point over time, measured as "bits per second."

Availability is the likelihood that the network will be available for usage and performing at its design specification, often the term Quality of Service (QoS) is used to gauge availability.

Latency is the time required for an individual packet to traverse the network from one point to another. Latency stems from two primary factors, physical distance and routing mechanisms, i.e. hardware devices such as routers and switches.

Security addresses a wide range of issues, but in terms of packet switched networks, it refers to the confidentiality, integrity and authentication of the information sent between point A and point B.

Ubiquity is the measurement of accessibility to network resources. This means both availability for the masses to the network and access to specific resources on that network.

An "infrastructure" can be loosely compared to a topology. A topology is defined as "the arrangement in which the nodes of a network are connected to each other." Due to the nature of telehealth design, a topology is the infrastructure of a system. This is the critical element. Topology dictates the type of physical infrastructure(s) that are used to bridge two points. The earliest applications of telemedicine simply used standard or legacy telephones [15].

Legacy phone systems are based on "circuit switched" technology. This is what your regular telephone uses. When a call is initiated, the phone company opens a line between you and your destination. This "circuit" is dedicated to the two parties until the conclusion of the call the circuit is released and then available to others. (Most modern switching is now digital.) In contrast, the Internet uses a "packet switched" technology more commonly called TCP/IP (Transmission Control Protocol/Internet Protocol). Here, lines are shared and the information (this could be asynchronous content such as the text of an email message or synchronous content such as video and voice) is broken into packets, addressed and forwarded along the shared topologies and natively unsecure. (See Security Considerations later in this chapter). TCP/IP can be compared to the traditional old fashioned letter and post office. The TCP [packet] is like the letter; it has on the outside the destination, the sender and sometimes informational data such as "FRAGILE". IP is akin to the postal system. Here, there is a system in place to receive the letter, read its destination, labels and deliver it. If it is non-deliverable, the sender's address is also there so the letter can be returned. The protocol of the system says if you do not get the letter returned to you, you can assume it reached its destination. TCP/IP works the very same way, packets (that make up the entire message) are sent, if there is a problem, you will be notified [typically]. An example is how an email with a bogus email address will be returned to the sender.

There are many technical differences between circuit and packet switched networks. But from a strategic standpoint, the primary differences are capability, cost, ubiquity and availability. Furthermore, the Internet is not a centrally controlled entity; it is a loose consortium of inter-networked partners. Because of this, there is no definable Quality of Service (QoS), rather, it is considered a "best effort" network. There is no central authority overseeing the network unlike a network administrator at a single organization. TCP/IP is now being used at both the Local Area Network (LAN) and Wide Area Network (WAN) scenarios. This common protocol helps to ensure interoperability with global partners. This is possible because TCP/IP is a highly routable protocol meaning it can easily span the globe. This was of course the original idea of TCP/IP.

In the early days, a WAN was typically configured as a virtual circuit where semi-dedicated lines connected remotes sites. The Internet now provides the topology for the more contemporary WAN using existing IP routing to dynamically connect remote sites at a much lower cost. Creating a secure connection is often accomplished using a Virtual Private Network (VPN) through either hardware, software or both. Whether it is a corporate headquarters and a regional office or a hospital and a remote clinic, the technology is the same. In a WAN, multiple topologies may be used from one point to another. For example, a remote clinic may only have a plain old telephone system (POTS) and a dial up Internet service provider such as America Online (AOL). The connection to AOL will first utilize POTS until it reaches the local telephone exchange; this segment is referred to as the "local loop" and is usually copper wire. Once at the local telephone exchange, the circuit may continue along terrestrial links, which may be copper or perhaps fiber. This can continue great distances towards the eventual destination or perhaps be routed to a geostationary communications satellite. This space segment would be considered another topology. Once the circuit is downlinked to an earth station, it may be sent to a microwave link, yet another topology, and again back to fiber or copper until it reaches the exchange of the remote participant and eventually the final destination.

These commercial transport topologies are usually invested in and installed by telecommunications companies that interconnect with other telecommunications companies through peering arrangements. These arrangements dictate how voice traffic and data flow to and from each carrier's systems as well as tariff agreements for financial charges that are assessed to the users. These long haul telecommunications circuits – which may span multiple topologies and multiple carriers – are known as backbones.

Between the end user and the backbone is another important consideration to network resource management – the amount of bandwidth the local Internet Service Provider (ISP) has access to. See Fig. 1. To connect to the Internet, an end user must first connect to a "Point of Presence" (POP) – a gateway that routes traffic to the Internet – this gateway/POP is usually the ISP. It is the ISP that assigns the user an address and routes traffic to the Internet. An ISP pays fees to backbone provider(s) for a specified amount of bandwidth. This could be availability of a few hundred kilobits to many megabits. Depending on the amount of bandwidth and the number of users or customers, that "pipe" can become saturated especially at peak periods. The local ISP's capacity vs. commitment must be assessed because it will affect the capabilities at the remote sites.

2. Barriers and Issues at Hand

As mentioned in previous chapters, telehealth services are generally categorized as either real-time or store-and-forward. Some, such as videoconferencing require significant bandwidth while email requires very little. In most cases, the level of service will

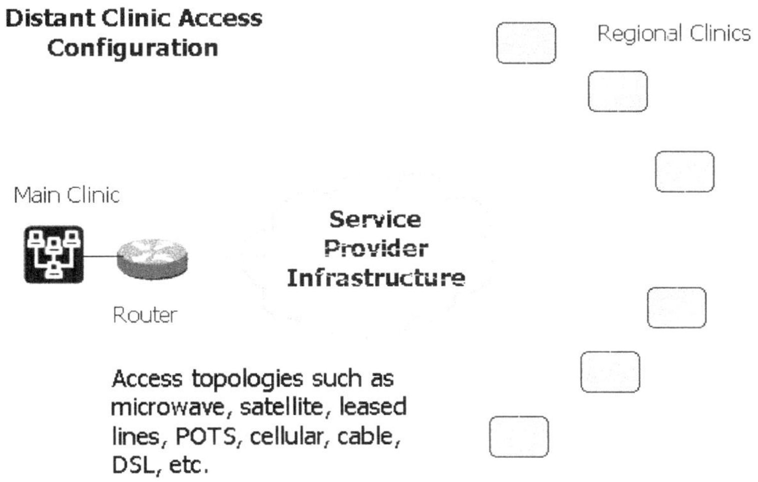

**Distant Clinic Access
Configuration**

Regional Clinics

Main Clinic

**Service
Provider
Infrastructure**

Router

**Access topologies such as
microwave, satellite, leased
lines, POTS, cellular, cable,
DSL, etc.**

Figure 1. Example of how remote clinics might connect to the main clinic.

be dictated by the availability of bandwidth. But this statement requires dissection; while there may be bandwidth available to certain locations such as large cities, telemedicine, again by definition, requires two or more distant points; if there is copious bandwidth at an urban hospital and very little at the rural clinic, the exchange of information will be transported at the rate of the "lowest common denominator" – the level of bandwidth at the rural clinic. This final leg or extension to the exterior site is known as the "last mile." It is this last mile and the aggregate bandwidth of the local ISPs that often create the largest challenges for implementers of telehealth programs.

When designing the wide area network for a telehealth system, careful review of available resources and planning for future growth is imperative. Issues that should be considered are:

Transport protocol: The primary protocol will be TCP/IP for store-and-forward data while User Datagram Protocol/Internet Provider is typically used for real-time conferences.

Topology assessment: Determining the availability of types of telecommunications infrastructures and access to them.

Circuit/bandwidth requirements: This is an assessment based on what is available and how it can be utilized.

Forecast for future capacity demands: Based on a broad assessment of a particular region and available clinical resources.

Web services/medical informatics: A key to maximizing the capabilities of the system, storage of and access to stored data.

Education/Training: A telehealth network's value can be enhanced by using for not only clinical application but also as a platform for distance education.

Security considerations: Patient information is becoming increasingly more important so stored information and data in transit must be addressed using tools such as firewalls, secure servers and Virtual Private Networks (VPNs).

When people talk about telemedicine, they often use videoconferencing as a synonymous term. This is understandable but technically inaccurate. In the early days of telemedicine – before proliferation of packet switched networks – videoconferencing was the primary component. Remote patients consulted with a distant specialist in live, face-to-face interactions that usually led to a higher-level quality of care [16–18]. This is still true today, but videoconferencing is only a component, not the core. Most of these early telemedicine programs funded by government or private institutions relied on dedicated lines and videoconferencing equipment [19–21]. After the funding ran out, the consults stopped; this model is not sustainable and not practical for developing nations [22,23]. Monies may be better invested towards local infrastructure and network services. While outside funding is advantageous to get started, it cannot be relied upon for ongoing programs.

Early videoconferencing sessions relied on the Integrated Services Digital Network (ISDN). This all digital topology – developed in the 1970's – is available in limited areas around the world. ISDN often uses dedicated hardware and topologies to provide a QoS needed for synchronous transfer such as videoconferencing which is reliable but not widely available and relatively expensive [24].

One major advantage of the ISDN architecture is its dynamic bandwidth allocation feature also known as bandwidth-on-demand. Through inverse multiplexing and channel aggregation, dynamic bandwidth allocation is the process of combining the individual (or B) channels into a single larger circuit. Videoconferencing using ISDN adheres to a standard called H.320. This allows disparate manufacturers' equipment to interoperate. It is unlikely developing nations have ISDN, many have limited regular telephone service. This is why a telehealth system needs to first embrace Internet technology which is much more ubiquitous and affordable. An existing standard, H.323 describes how videoconferencing over IP networks interoperate. Another protocol that can route IP video is called Session Initialization Protocol (SIP). Unlike text or static image transfer that uses TCP, H.323 uses User Datagram Protocol (UDP), which reduces overhead by eliminating unnecessary tasks such as error correction and flow control. There is no need to resend lost packets from a video session due to the synchronous nature of a conversation. H.323 can operate using inexpensive desktop cameras and free software or more expensive hardware and embedded applications. It is important to note that H.323 can be implemented inexpensively over Internet links while H.320 requires an ISDN infrastructure.

In some locations, a mixture of topologies may be available for medical use. An increasingly popular option for IP connectivity is a technology called Digital Subscriber Lines (DSL). There are different flavors of DSL, but they all rely on increasing the bandwidth capabilities of existing copper phone lines. While portions of the link must include a digital connection, other aspects such as distance from the central office will dictate the capacity of the circuit. DSL can be an affordable technology to embrace, but again, is based on the infrastructure of the local carrier. See Table 1 for a comparison of topologies.

No matter what topology is selected, the system must be designed to match the available bandwidth. Through comprehensive assessments of both the expected demand and future network availability, an equitable balance of capability and cost can be realized.

Table 1. Chart estimating typical network topologies available to end-users

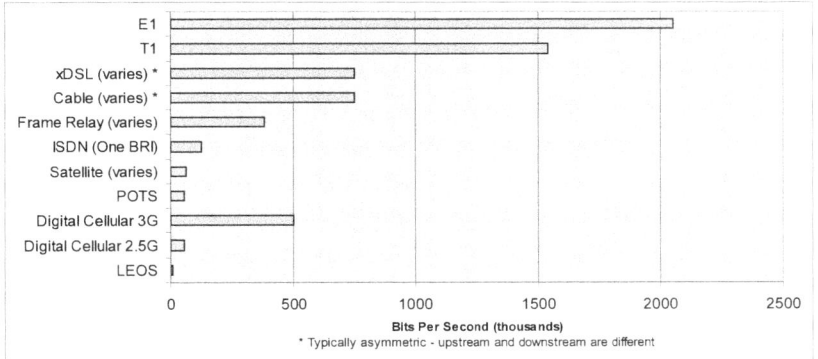

3. Suggested Solutions to Overcome Barriers

To fund a program with finite resources requires vision and must be designed with sustainability and scalability in mind [25]. This is why it is so important to design systems using the lowest common denominator and existing infrastructures. In certain cases it may be necessary to install a single access point such as a microwave tower on a hill to connect an isolated region over the ridge of a mountain range. An investment like this is a matter of strategic implementation and economic return. By attempting to install a network of towers, tail circuits and switching equipment will likely be cost prohibitive and possibly illegal. Any infrastructure installation or augmentation must be coordinated with the local ministry of communications and any existing telephone carriers.

Unfortunately, existing infrastructure may only provide low data rates as mentioned earlier. This is why is becomes important to embrace technologies and techniques that properly utilize low bandwidth to ensure availability and scalability. Certain capabilities such as videoconferencing may not be a viable option but transfer of electronic medical records are. This exchange of information – in the form of text (such as ASCII or eXtensible Markup Language (XML)) – becomes powerful a tool for regions that had no tools in the past [26–28]. By using the concept of existing infrastructure, the cost of building and maintaining a telehealth network are minimized. Use of standard personal computers at the client level permits leveraging of the installed base rather than requiring purchases of new, high-end workstations. Traditional network design requires a type of network redundancy, but in some cases this will not be an option or the cost may be prohibitive. Services must be designed as non-mission critical in the event the link goes down.

The new paradigm for last mile telecommunications infrastructures in underserved areas is clearly wireless. The demonstrated success of cellular networks and relatively low cost of installation is allowing developing nations the ability to provide telecommunications where there were once none. Completing skipping over the stringing of wire, these nations (and rural areas of developed countries) have been able to provide much needed services [29–31]. While these emerging cellular networks provide voice communications with reasonable coverage, much of the capability is still based on analog transmission. Digital services represent only a percentage of installations in developing nations but this is changing [32]. As digital footprints are expanded and added, use of cellular topologies in these areas for data transfer become apparent.

Wireless systems are categorized as generations (G). Early analog systems referred to as Advanced Mobile Phone Services (AMPS) were considered first generation or 1G. 2G services included early digital capabilities such as Cellular Digital Packet Data (CDPD). We are currently in a transition between 2.5G and 3G that includes technologies such as TDMA, CDMA, GSM and iDEN. Fourth Generation services (4G) are just a matter of time.

Although the digital services that will be offered will be increasingly available, the data rates are still very low. 2G–2.5G services provide from 9,600 bps to 56,000 bps, this limited bandwidth is considered too low for synchronous telemedicine consults [33–35]. As 3G services are deployed in developing nations, this will change dramatically with data rates approaching 128–768 Kbps or more. This level of service is being deployed across the globe. Because developing countries are making huge advances in basic services and planning to incorporate data services over cellular, there is optimism for implementing telehealth – albeit slow. Once again, this addresses the problem with the last mile.

Any program that involves use of, modification of or augmentation of existing technology will require permission from the controlling body. In most cases this is a governmental agency that oversees telecommunications such as the Ministry of Communications. Most every country in the world has ties to the international community through the ITU. The ITU provides a multilateral forum where governments and the private sector work together to forge the standards and policies that lead to cooperative installation and upgrading of telecommunications. The ITU can provide information about member countries as well as contacts with respective governments. The annual ITU Trends in Telecommunication Reform publication is recognized as an invaluable reference document for policy makers, regulators and industry players [36]. While the ITU does not control these areas, they can assist with issues such as tariff agreements, radio frequency usage and governance.

The ITU also plays a vital role in facilitating communications within and between countries. One of the challenging business rules is that of peering. Carriers must interconnect to other carriers' infrastructures to facilitate end-to-end connections. In an effort to reduce costs and encourage more seamless international communications the ITU has published a cost sharing recommendation. This addresses the rapid growth of the Internet and Internet protocol-based services.

Realizing that international connections are subject to commercial agreements between carriers, the ITU is encouraging continued negotiations between those carriers to agree to bilateral communications arrangements enabling IP traffic to traverse the carriers Points of Presence (POP). This type of arrangement must take into account the possible need for unequal financial compensation based on traffic volume, flow, discreet routes, geographical coverage and operational costs [37].

The World Bank Group's Global Information & Communication Technologies (GICT) Department plays an important role in developing and promoting access to information and communications technologies in developing countries. The GICT brings together investment practice and the public sector of the World Bank to provide governments, private companies and community organizations with the capital and expertise needed to develop, implement and foster development in regions that need it most.

4. Future

Telemedicine continues to advance as a healthcare delivery mechanism. While the United States struggles with cross-state licensure, compensation and liability issues, developing nations continue to press ahead with operational programs. However, positive steps have been taken to create a more seamless, interconnected telehealth network such as the National Emergency Telemedical Communications Act of 2002 [38].

The ITU is instrumental in helping to integrate the world's 49 most marginalized countries into the global telecommunication network through its special program for Least Developed Countries (LDCs). Most of these countries have very poor telecommunication networks resulting in teledensities below one per 100 inhabitants. Such pilot programs are exemplified in Asia/Commonwealth of Independent States, Africa and the Americas. Since 1998, ITU has implemented a large number of telemedicine projects in partnership with different stakeholders.

In the next few years we can expect to see increased growth in telehealth programs. Part of the drive will be fueled by simple necessity. These programs will be easier to deploy as telecommunications infrastructure become more available and ubiquitous. There is a fear that as the network layers become more robust, the applications will demand more bandwidth. This is the case with computer power and application development. As the computers get faster with more capacity the applications crave more power and memory space. Fortunately the telemedicine community has learned valuable lessons about applications and network throughput that is well documented. While some areas continue to demand more disk space, others have lost weight though new compression algorithms and lightweight markup languages that quickly move information across even limited bandwidth WANs. The information is becoming more portable and interoperable.

Clearly, the costs to install fixed wired telecommunications infrastructures are daunting. For developing nations it is likely not possible. Perhaps in the urban areas where there are existing copper infrastructures, technologies like DSL will enhance network communications. Wireless technology however has advanced to a point where deployment is within reach and this is extremely evident in the rural and remote areas that never had *any* type of telecommunications. The costs to install cellular towers are significantly less and becoming the defacto installed base in many countries [39]. Cellular towers along with digital services provide enough bandwidth and coverage to solve many of the last mile issues thereby providing end-to-end communications for sustainable telehealth services.

5. Conclusion

Unlike many developed areas on earth, most of the world's population is underserved in terms of telecommunications. Implementing telehealth in these areas at an affordable cost is a challenging task. By leveraging existing infrastructures and installed bases of computing hardware, a telemedicine program can be built and functional. Although broadband communications will likely be non-existent or prohibitively expensive, low band topologies can be utilized to provide basic but powerful services, even to very remote locations and more importantly, those that need it the most.

References

[1]   Rosser JC, Bell RL, Harnett BM, Rodas E, Murayama M, Merrell RC. Use of mobile low-bandwidth telemedical techniques for extreme telemedicine application. Am Coll Surg J 1999;189(4):397–793 404.

[2]   Telemedicine Systems and Telecommunications. Telemedicine Systems and Telecommunications. ISBN: 1-85315-677-9 Wootton, R. (Ed) Publisher: Royal Society of Medicine Press, London, England. Chapter 2, Pgs 15-34.

[3]   Godden DJ. Rural health care in the U.K.: a rapidly changing scene. J Agric Saf Health 2005 May; 11(2):205-10.

[4]   http://www.itu.int/ASIA2004/media/development.html [Accessed October 15, 2006].

[5]   Mitka M. Developing countries find telemedicine forges links to more care and research. JAMA 1998; 280: 1295-1296.

[6]   Wright D. Telemedicine and developing countries. A report of study group 2 of the ITU Development Sector. J Telemedicine Telecare 1998;4 (suppl 2):1-85.

[7]   Bashshur RL, Reardon TG, Shannon GW. Telemedicine: a new health care delivery system. Annu Rev Public Health 2000;21:613-37.

[8]   Wootton R. The possible use of telemedicine in developing countries. J Telemed Telecare 1997;3(1): 23-6.

[9]   Zhao Y, Nakajima I, Juzoji H. On-site investigation of the early phase of Bhutan Health Telematics Project. J Med Syst 2002 Feb;26(1):67-77.

[10] Norris TE, Hart GL, Larson EH, Tarczy-Hornoch P, Masuda DL, Fuller SS, House PJ, Dyck SM. Low-bandwidth, low-cost telemedicine consultations in rural family practice. J Am Board Fam Pract 2002 Mar-Apr;15(2):123-7.

[11] Lacroix A, Lareng, L, Padeken D, Nerlich M, Bracale M, Ogushi Y, Okada Y, Orlov O, McGee J, Wootton R, Sanders JH, Doarn CR, Prerost S, and McDonald I. International Concerted Action on Collaboration in Telemedicine. Recommendations of the G-8 Global Healthcare Applications Subproject 4. Telemed J and e-Health 2002;8(2):149-57.

[12] High WA, Houston MS, Calobrisi SD, Drage LA, McEvoy MT. Assessment of the accuracy of low-cost store-and-forward teledermatology consultation. J Am Acad Dermatol 2000 May;42(5 Pt 1): 776-83.

[13] Latifi R, Muja S, Bekteshi F, Merrell RC. The role of telemedicine and information technology in the redevelopment of medical systems: The case of Kosova. Telemed J E Health. 2006 Jun;12(3):332-40.

[14] Cooke FJ, Holmes A. E-mail consultations in international health. Lancet 2000; 356: 138.

[15] Benschoter, R.A. Educational Broadcasting; CCTV-Pioneering Nebraska Medical Center, Oct. 1971; 1-3.

[16] Darkins A, Fisk N, Garner P, Wootton R. Point-to-point telemedicine using the ISDN. J Telemed Telecare 1996;2 Suppl 1:82-3.

[17] Baruffaldi F, Mattioli P, Toni A, Klutke PJ, Englmeier KH. Low-cost ISDN videoconferencing equipment for orthopaedic second opinions. J Telemed Telecare 1999;5 Suppl 1:S37-8.

[18] Chan FY, Whitehall J, Hayes L, Taylor A, Soong B, Lessing K, Cincotta R, Cooper D, Stone M, Lee-Tannock A, Baker S, Smith M, Green E, Whiting R. Minimum requirements for remote realtime fetal tele-ultrasound consultation. J Telemed Telecare 1999;5(3):171-6.

[19] Stensland J, Speedie SM, Ideker M, House J, Thompson T. The relative cost of outpatient telemedicine services. Telemed J 1999 Fall;5(3):245-56.

[20] Lobley D. The economics of telemedicine. J Telemed Telecare 1997;3(3):117-25.

[21] Picot J. Towards a methodology for developing and implementing best practices in telehealth and telemedicine. Stud Health Technol Inform 1999;64:23-8.

[22] Wright D, Androuchko L. Telemedicine and developing countries. J Telemed Telecare 1996;2(2):63-70.

[23] Wright D. The sustainability of telemedicine projects. J Telemed Telecare 1999;5 Suppl 1:S107-11.

[24] Wu TK, Liu JL, Tschai HJ, Lee YH, Leu HT. An ISDN-based telemedicine system. Digit Imaging 1998 Aug;11(3 Suppl 1):93-5.

[25] Wright D. Telemedicine and developing countries. A report of study group 2 of the ITU Development Sector. J Telemed Telecare 1998;4 Suppl 2:1-85.

[26] Della Mea V. Internet electronic mail: a tool for low-cost telemedicine. Telemed Telecare 1999; 5(2):84-9.

[27] Worth ER, Patrick TB, Klimczak JC, Reid JC. Cost-effective clinical uses of wide-area networks: electronic mail as telemedicine. Proc Annu Symp Comput Appl Med Care 1995;814-8.

[28] Patterson V, Hoque F, Vassallo D, Farquharson Roberts M, Swinfen P, Swinfen R. Store-and-forward teleneurology in developing countries. J Telemed Telecare 2001;7 Suppl 1:52-3.

[29] Istepanian RH, Woodward B, Balos PA, Chen S, Luk B. The comparative performance of mobile tele-medical systems based on the IS-54 and GSM cellular telephone standards. J Telemed Telecare 1999; 5(2):97-104.
[30] Reponen J, Ilkko E, Jyrkinen L, Karhula V, Tervonen O, Laitinen J, Leisti EL, Koivula A, Suramo I. Digital wireless radiology consultations with a portable computer. J Telemed Telecare 1998;4(4):201-5.
[31] Yamamoto LG. Wireless teleradiology and fax using cellular phones and notebook PCs for instant access to consultants. Am J Emerg Med 1995 Mar;13(2):184-7.
[32] Orlov OI, Drozdov DV, Doarn CR, and Merrell RC. Wireless ECG Monitoring by Telephone. Telemed J and e-Health 2000;7(1):33-38.
[33] Frost & Sullivan. World Digital Cellular Infrastructure Market Overview: Market Report August 1999.
[34] Rosser JC, Bell RL, Harnett BM, Rodas E, Murayama M, Merrell RC. Use of Mobile Low-Bandwidth Telemedical Techniques for Extreme Telemedicine Application. American College of Surgeons J, 1999;189(4):397-404.
[35] Broderick TJ, Harnett BM, Merriam NR, Kapoor V, Doarn CR, and Merrell RC. Impact of Varying Transmission Bandwidth on Image Quality in Laparoscopic Telemedicine. Telemed J and e-Health 2001;7(1):47-53.
[36] http://www.itu.int/ITU-D/treg/index.phtml [Accessed 24 October 2006].
[37] http://www.ct-magazine.com/archives/ct/1100/148_backbone.htm [Accessed 24 October 2006].
[38] http://thomas.loc.gov/cgi-bin/query/z?c107:S.2748.IS [Accessed 24 October 2006].
[39] http://www.itu.int/ITU-D/ict/statistics/at_glance/Africa_EE2006_e.pdf [Accessed 24 October 2006].

Current Principles and Practices of Telemedicine and e-Health
R. Latifi (Ed.)
IOS Press, 2008

Network Design for Telemedicine – e-Health Using Satellite Technology

Georgi GRASCHEW, Theo A. ROELOFS, Stefan RAKOWSKY
and Peter M. SCHLAG
Surgical Research Unit OP 2000, Robert-Roessle-Klinik and Max-Delbrueck-Centrum,
Charité – University Medicine Berlin, Lindenberger Weg 80,
D-13125 Berlin, Germany

Abstract. Over the last decade various international Information and Communications Technology networks have been created for a global access to high-level medical care. OP 2000 has designed and validated the high-end interactive video communication system WinVicos especially for telemedical applications, training of the physician in a distributed environment, teleconsultation and second opinion. WinVicos is operated on a workstation (WoTeSa) using standard hardware components and offers a superior image quality at a moderate transmission bandwidth of up to 2 Mbps. WoTeSa / WinVicos have been applied for IP-based communication in different satellite-based telemedical networks. In the DELTASS-project a disaster scenario was analysed and an appropriate telecommunication system for effective rescue measures for the victims was set up and evaluated. In the MEDASHIP project an integrated system for telemedical services (teleconsultation, teleelectro-cardiography, telesonography) on board of cruise ships and ferries has been set up. EMISPHER offers an equal access for most of the countries of the Euro-Mediterranean area to on-line services for health care in the required quality of service. E-learning applications, real-time telemedicine and shared management of medical assistance have been realized. The innovative developments in ICT with the aim of realizing a ubiquitous access to medical resources for everyone at any time and anywhere (u-Health) bear the risk of creating and amplifying a digital divide in the world. Therefore we have analyzed how the objective needs of the heterogeneous partners can be joined with the result that there is a need for real integration of the various platforms and services. A virtual combination of applications serves as the basic idea for the Virtual Hospital. The development of virtual hospitals and digital medicine helps to bridge the digital divide between different regions of the world and enables equal access to high-level medical care. Pre-operative planning, intra-operative navigation and minimally-invasive surgery require a digital and virtual environment supporting the perception of the physician. As data and computing resources in a virtual hospital are distributed over many sites the concept of the Grid should be integrated with other communication networks and platforms.

Keywords. Real-time telemedicine, interactive video communication, satellite-based networks, emergency services, maritime telemedicine, e-learning, virtual hospital

Introduction

Networks for Telemedicine enable the integration of distributed medical competence and contribute to the improvement of the quality of medical care, to the cost-effective use of medical resources and to quick and reliable decisions. For optimal performance of telemedical applications, the networks and communication tools used must be opti-mised for medical applications, both with respect to the Quality-of-Service (QoS, a set of parameters characterising the performance of the communication channel per se, such as transmission bandwidth, delay, jitter, data loss, etc.) as well as to the Class-of-Service (CoS; a set of terms specifying the medical services offered in the network, like Telesurgery, Telepathology, Telesonography, Tele-Teaching, -Training & -Education, etc.).

Telemedicine aims at equal access to medical expertise irrespective of the geo-graphical location of the person in need. New developments in Information and Com-munication Technologies (ICT) have enabled the transmission of medical images in sufficiently high quality that allows for a reliable diagnosis to be determined by the expert at the receiving site [1,2].

Through Telemedicine patients can get access to medical expertise that may not be available at the patients' site. The use of specifically designed networks for telemedi-cine (distributed medical intelligence) contributes to the continuous improvement of patient care. Experience over the last decade has shown that the goals of Telemedicine are not automatically reached by the introduction and use of singular new technologies per se, but rather require the implementation of *integral services*.

At the same time, however, these innovative developments in ICT over the last decade bear the risk of creating and amplifying a digital divide in the world, creating a disparity in the quality of life, e.g. between the northern and the southern Euro-Mediterranean area [3–5].

In recent years different projects have demonstrated how the digital divide is only one part of a more complex problem: the need for integration [6–9].

1. Current Developments: Evidence Based Practice

During the last years OP 2000 (Operating Room of the future; [10]) has designed, de-veloped and validated various modules for interactive telemedicine services [11,12]. One of the key elements is the interactive telecommunication module WoTeSa/ WinVicos: WoTeSa, a dedicated Workstation for Telemedical applications via Satellite that uses the communication software WinVicos (Wavelet-based interactive Video communication system). WoTeSa is a PC with sufficient processing capacity (≥ 3 GHz Pentium IV, ≥ 512 MBytes RAM, etc.), one or more Osprey video capture boards (Os-prey 100 or Osprey 500), a camera with F-BAS and S-Video output as live source (e.g. Canon VC-C4); a second camera as document camera for transmission of non-digital images; standard headset or microphone with small loudspeakers. The different video inputs of the Osprey video capture card can be used for direct connection to various medical equipment. WoTeSa serves quasi as a medical video hub. WinVicos is an all-software high-quality interactive video communication system, supplying real-time video, still-image and audio-transmission. WinVicos is especially designed for tele-medicine applications (e.g. telesurgery, teleradiology, telepathology), using a hybrid speed-optimised wavelet-codec that is based on the concepts of *Partition, Aggregation and Conditional Coding* (PACC; Patent DE 197 34 542 A1 from "Deutsche Telekom," Darmstadt, Germany). Other Codecs are under development. WinVicos communicates IP-based and allows for online scaling of the transmission parameters (bit rate, frame size, frame rate). Besides high quality live video transmission using moderate band-widths (0,5–1 Mbit/s) it also allows for still-image transmission. In both the video win-

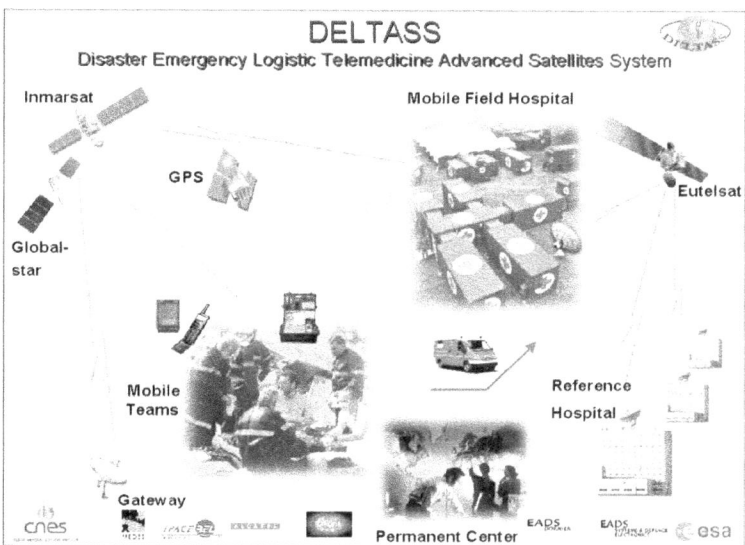

Figure 1. DELTASS System Architecture: Mobile Teams, Permanent Center (PC), Mobile Field Hospital (MFH) and Reference Hospital (RH) are interconnected via several satellite systems with different bandwidths. Additionally terrestrial communication channels support the data exchange between the PC and the RH.

dows and the still-image windows WinVicos supports the use of common cursors shared by the conference partners. WoTeSa and WinVicos have been described in more detail elsewhere [13,14].

Other telemedicine systems are used e.g. for tele-ultrasound in rural areas where telementoring by live videoconferencing allowed to guide the ultrasound technician to record additional images of the patient [15], for clinical assessment of pediatric burns which showed a good agreement between the face-to-face consultation and seeing the patient via videoconference [16] and for home telecare services likely to improve quality of health services [17]. Other systems are described in [18–20].

1.1. Disaster Emergency Logistic Telemedicine Advanced Satellites Systems – DELTASS

In the DELTASS-project [21] a disaster scenario was analysed and an appropriate telecommunication system for effective rescue measures for the victims was set up and evaluated (see http://telecom.esa.int/telecom/www/object/index.cfm?fobjectid=6324). Satellite-based systems are well suited for these circumstances, where generally ground infrastructures are partly or even totally destroyed. In such situations, even on a large geographic area or isolated area, space-based services can be easily and quickly deployed. DELTASS demonstrates operational performance of various services, covering the different aspects/phases of disaster emergency medicine. According to these phases, the DELTASS system is made up of the various corresponding subsystems (Fig. 1).

1.2. Mobile Teams

Mobile teams are deployed on the disaster site for search, identification, triage and evacuation of victims. They communicate with the coordination- and medical- teams located in Permanent Centre or Mobile Field Hospital via low-rate (Globalstar, 9.6 kbps) and medium-rate (Inmarsat, 64 kbps) satellite telecommunication systems. Their positions are tracked via the established Global Positioning System (GPS satellite system).

1.3. Permanent Centre

The Permanent Centre is located outside the disaster area. The Permanent Center constitutes a new element in the architecture of support systems for disaster emergencies and is unique to the DELTASS system. In conventional set-ups the mobile teams at the disaster site are coordinated and supported by the staff of a Mobile Field Hospital deployed at or close to the disaster site. However, complete deployment of such a Mobile Field Hospital takes at least ~6 hours, usually ~12 hours, and consequently the activities of mobile teams in these first, highly critical hours, are ill-coordinated and far from optimal. To improve this bottleneck, DELTASS has a designated Permanent Center that is in control of coordination and medical support to the mobile teams from time zero on. The Permanent Center is equipped with terrestrial gateways to the Globalstar and Inmarsat satellite systems through which it receives all data from the mobile teams. It coordinates all actions of the mobile teams and manages all medical and logistic data, *thus assuring efficient operation during the first critical phase*. All data received at the Permanent Center are processed, appropriate Reference Hospitals (RH; see below) are identified and the logistic and medical data are transferred to these RH via terrestrial telecommunication links.

1.4. Mobile Field Hospital (MFH)

A Mobile Field Hospital (MFH), which will be deployed at or close to the disaster site, provides all activities related to the co-ordination of the mobile teams on the disaster site, the victims medical triage, reception, first aid treatment, conditioning for transportation, further medical expertise for some patients by teleconsultations between MFH and Reference Hospital(s).

1.5. Reference Hospital (RH)

The Reference Hospital(s) (RH), located outside of the disaster area, acts as an expert center by providing telemedical services to the MFH using the high-bandwidth satellite link (VSAT, 2 Mbps). These services consist of off-line and on-line telediagnosis, access to external medical databases, as well as real-time interactive telemedical services such as live teleconsultations, live telesonography, intraoperative virtual reality simulation and interactive telemicrobiology (Figs 2–3). Statistics show that in cases of disaster emergency medicine, approx. 40% more amputations are performed, as compared to normal situation. One of the aims of providing live second opinion by remote experts is to reduce this number of unneeded amputations, manipulations and subsequent complications substantially, by expert support during triage, diagnosis and medical treatment.

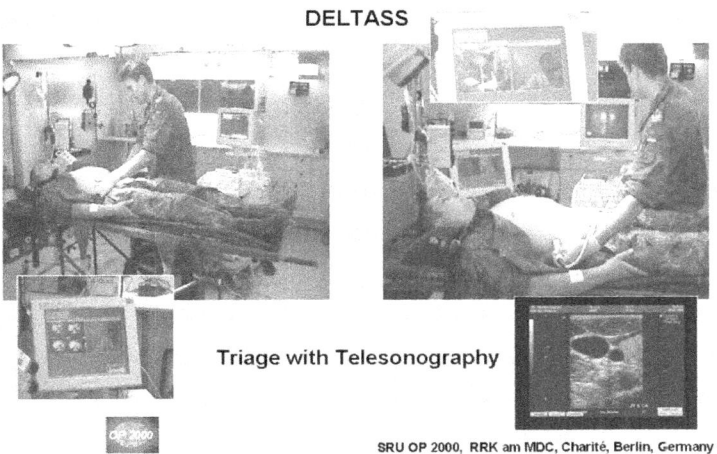

DELTASS

Triage with Telesonography

SRU OP 2000, RRK am MDC, Charité, Berlin, Germany

Figure 2. Live Telesonography: The ultrasound video data stream (insert right bottom) is transmitted live via WoTeSa / WinVicos to the experts of the RH (insert right top). Additionally the signal of a room camera (e.g. for telementoring; insert right top) as well as further medical data (e.g. X-ray, CT, etc.; insert left bottom) can be transmitted live to the RH.

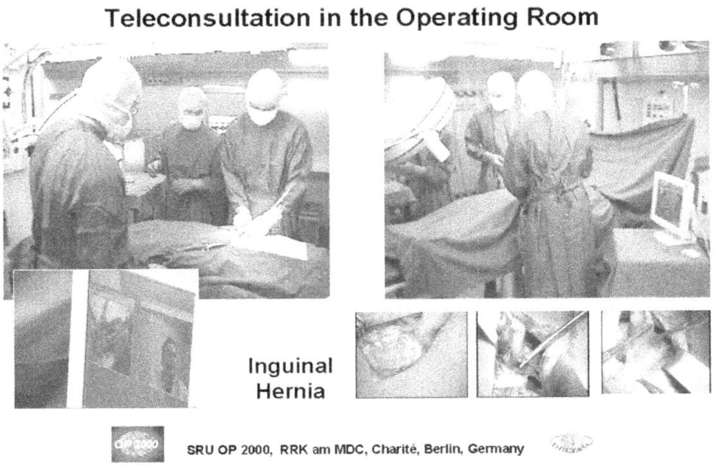

Teleconsultation in the Operating Room

Inguinal Hernia

SRU OP 2000, RRK am MDC, Charité, Berlin, Germany

Figure 3. Live Telesurgery of Inguinal Hernia: During the surgery the video data stream of a camera integrated in the centre of the surgical light can be transmitted live to the experts in the RH using WoTeSa/WinVicos (insert left bottom). In this way these experts receive a live video of the situs of surgery (insert right bottom) and can advise the colleague in the MFH.

These interactive telemedical services between the MFH and the RH are realised using a dedicated WoTeSa (Workstation for Telemedical Applications via Satellite) with the communication software WinVicos (Wavelet-based interactive Video communication system). WoTeSa/WinVicos combines the user-friendliness and flexibility of IP-based communication protocols with the security and sufficiently-high quality of the

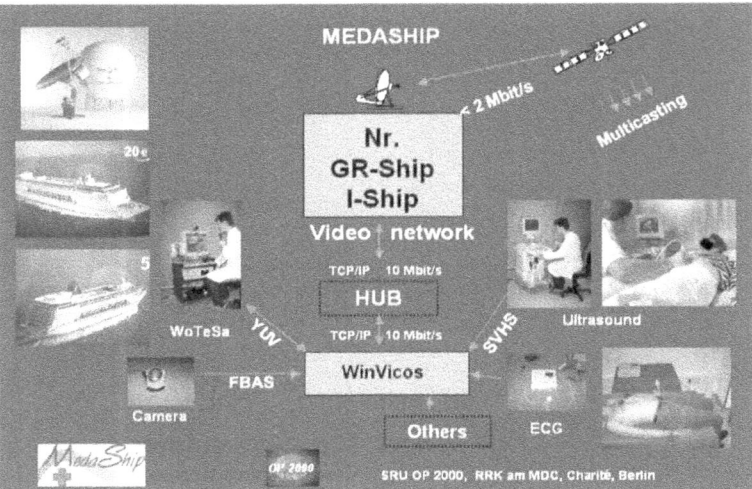

Figure 4. Video network on-board of the ships. Video camera, ultrasound- and electrocardiography-equipment are connected with the satellite modem via WoTeSa/WinVicos.

live video transmission at a satellite bandwidth of only up to 2 Mbps. Medical experts at the RH support the medical treatments in the MFH and enable a quick and reliable decision concerning treatment and/or evacuation of the patient/victim. In this way, the quality of the provided medical service during and after disaster emergencies is strongly improved. The performance of the DELTASS system has been shown during various full-size live demonstrations.

1.6. *Medical Assistance for Ships* – MEDASHIP

The main objective of the service developed by the MEDASHIP project is to supply integrated solutions for medical consultations on-board of ships [22]. The satellite-based telemedicine services address both passenger ships and merchant vessels and are intended to provide passengers and crew members with an effective medical assistance in cases of emergency and in all those cases where the on board medical staff requires second opinion. During the validation phase the service was tested on board of three ships with the possibility to have it connected to three land medical centers (Fig. 4).

In addition to the standard medical equipment aboard the ships, two video cameras, an electrocardiograph (ECG) and an ultrasound (US) equipment are used. With this equipment the following telemedical services have been realized using satellite transmission at a bandwidth of 512 kbps up to 1 Mbps offering the required high quality of images and video transmission:

1.7. Teleconsultation

The live camera on-board of the ship can be used to transmit the image of the doctor who is leading the examination on-board of the ship or the image of the patient when being questioned by the land-based expert. It can also be used to show the land-based expert an injured part of the patient's body which he needs to see for his consultation. Thus a very realistic and effective live communication is possible.

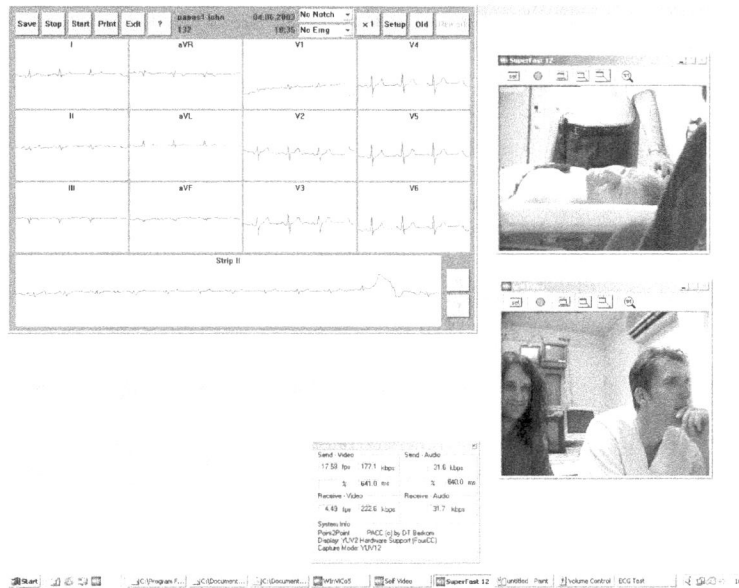

Figure 5. Tele-electrocardiography: the live signals of the 12 channels of the ECG-device on-board of the ship are transmitted to the reference hospital. All functions of the ECG-device can be remotely controlled.

1.8. Electrocardiography

The ECG system is connected to WoTeSa on board the ship and can be controlled by the physician from this workstation. Via an application sharing software also the expert can control the ECG system from the land-based workstation. The main menu with all functions of the ECG as well as the patient's ECG are transmitted to the expert. Thus the expert and the physician on board can jointly acquire and analyse the ECG report (Fig. 5).

1.9. Telesonography

The S-video output of the US equipment is directly connected to the Osprey video capture board. Satellite transmission tests have shown that not only still images can be transferred but also live ultrasound investigations can be transmitted at 500–700 kbps.

With a Document camera analogous patient data can be captured and digitized by WinVicos as a document. For example X-ray or CT-images can be captured from an illumination board and displayed locally and transmitted using this document camera function.

1.10. Data Security

Respect for patient confidentiality is a clear requirement in the MEDASHIP system and the level of privacy protection has been addressed throughout the MEDASHIP project. In MEDASHIP, from the telemedicine platform viewpoint, the following requirements should be taken into account to prevent abuse and to safeguard the privacy and confidentiality of managed clinical and personal information of the patients.

- *Authentication*: Monitoring and verifying all the accesses to the information. A control over the users should be carried out at each access to the system, by utilising the users' credentials (username and password) in order to verify that the user is who he/she claims to be.
- *Encryption*: Scrambling a sender's transmission according to an algorithm that the recipient then uses to unscramble and decipher the transmission. All the process is not visible to the user, the client software knows all it needs.
- *Access control*: Authorizing access to specific and clearly identified resources to certain users based on their company responsibilities and the security classification of the resources.
- *Integrity*: Developing or utilising applications and data management software that is secure from unauthorized modification of their code.
- *Confidentiality*: Developing or utilising applications and data management software that is secure from disclosure to unauthorized persons or programs.
- *Auditing and accounting system*: Monitoring the system and maintaining records of system and user activity.
- *Security policy*: Establishing clear security policies with customers and end-users.

Unlike open network satellite equipment technologies Linkway uses a proprietary acquisition and synchronisation technique making signal interception and decoding virtually impossible. Data Security will also be assured by the coding algorithm of the WinVicos software. The transmitted data can only be decoded by this software. As one member owns the software licence this provides an initial level of data security through the licence distribution.

1.11. Reduction of Cost

The costs for emergency interventions for removing a passenger from the ship and hospitalization abroad are not to be undervalued. The removal of a passenger in the Carribean can cost up to $11.000,- and the cost for hospitalization can range from 500,--1000,- € per day. Consequently market trends force passenger shipping lines to offer services that help to improve the response to on-board clinical emergencies, improve the customer satisfaction and the companies' image.

1.12. Euro-Mediterranean Internet-Satellite Platform for Health, medical Education and Research – EMISPHER

EMISPHER is dedicated to establish an equal access for most of the countries of the Euro-Mediterranean area to real-time and on-line services for healthcare in the required quality of service (see www.emispher.org). In the project an integrated Internet-Satellite platform has been set up on which three main areas of work have been realized: Virtual Medical University, Real-Time Telemedicine, and Medical Assistance [23]. The platform includes a bi-directional satellite network (up to 2 Mbps) between 10 Centres of Excellence in the Euro-Mediterranean region (Morocco, Algeria, Tunisia, Egypt, Cyprus, Turkey, Greece, Italy, France and Germany) (Fig. 6). For dissemination of the achieved results and for maximizing its impact, EMISPHER has organized international conferences at each of the Mediterranean partner sites.

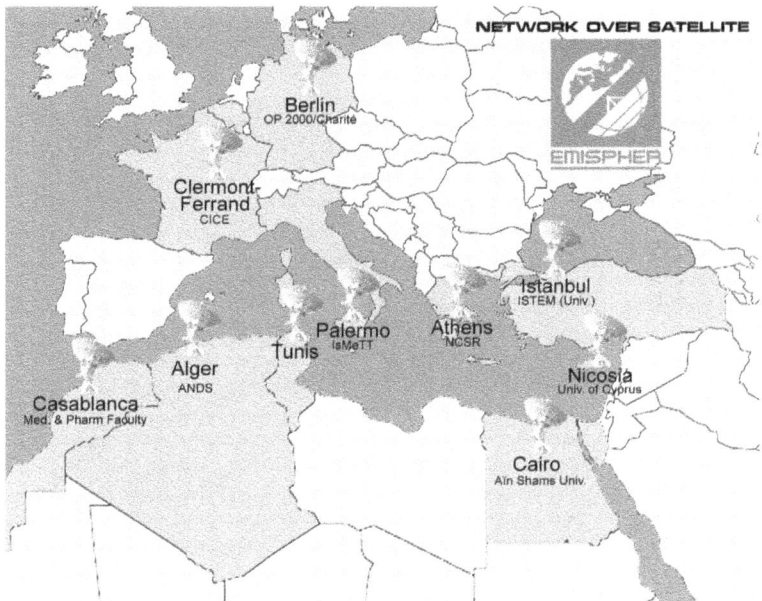

Figure 6. Medical Centers in the EMISPHER Network.

1.13. The EMISPHER Virtual Medical University

The formation and operation of the EMISPHER Virtual Medical University (EVMU) for e-learning (teleteaching) is one of the main efforts in the project. The EVMU uses real-time broadcast of lectures, live surgical operations and pre-recorded video sequences etc., as well as web-based e-learning applications. The target population of the EVMU is comprised of medical students (both undergraduate and postgraduate) hospital staff, general practitioners and specialists, health officers and citizens.

Each of the leading medical centers provides didactical material and modules for synchronous and asynchronous e-learning in their medical specialties. The central gateway to EVMU is the project's website: www.emispher.org.

Some of the multimedia teaching material needs to be presented in real-time. Live transmission of surgical operations from operating theatres, lectures, etc. from one site to one or several sites simultaneously (point-to-point or multipoint) are possible in the network between the 10 partners (Fig. 7).

1.14. Real-Time Telemedicine

EMISPHER has set up a satellite-based network using the combined WoTeSa and WinVicos modules for real-time telemedicine. In the field of real-time telemedicine the following categories of applications are offered: second opinion, teleteaching & teletraining (demonstration and spread of new techniques), telementoring (enhancement of staff qualification), and undergraduate teaching courses and optimisation of the learning curve. The leading medical centers in the project provide expertise in the following medical fields: open and minimally-invasive surgery, multi-organ transplantation, endoscopy, pathology, radiology, interventional imaging, neurology, infectious diseases,

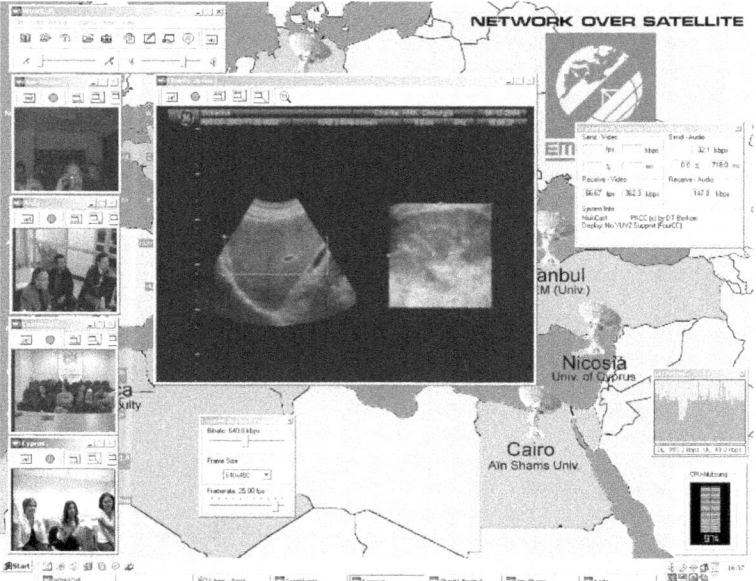

Figure 7. Interactive multipoint e-learning session with transmission of live ultrasound video data from Charité (Berlin) to Ain Shams University (Cairo), Agence Nationale de Sante (Algiers), Faculte de Medecine et de Pharmacie (Casablanca) and University of Cyprus (Nicosia).

oncology, gynaecology and obstetrics, reproductive medicine, etc. These real-time telemedical applications contribute to improved quality of patient care and to accelerated qualification of medical doctors in their respective specialty. The main target audience are specialist doctors (Fig. 8).

1.15. Medical Assistance

The third field of service operated in EMISPHER is medical assistance. As tourism constitutes a substantial economical factor in the Mediterranean region and because of the increasing mobility of the population, continuity of care through improved medical assistance is of major importance for improved healthcare in the Euro-Mediterranean region. Introduction of standardised procedures, integration of the platform with the various local communication systems and training of the medical and non-medical staff involved in the medical assistance chain allow for shared management of files related to medical assistance (medical images, diagnosis, workflow, financial management, etc.) and thus for improved care for travellers and expatriates.

1.16. User Evaluation

Two types of evaluation were performed for the EMISPHER satellite-internet platform and the services delivered from the platform. Firstly, the evaluation of all technical aspects of the platform and connecting services (WinVicos and MEDSKY) and secondly the evaluation of the operational elements of the system meeting the medical user requirements.

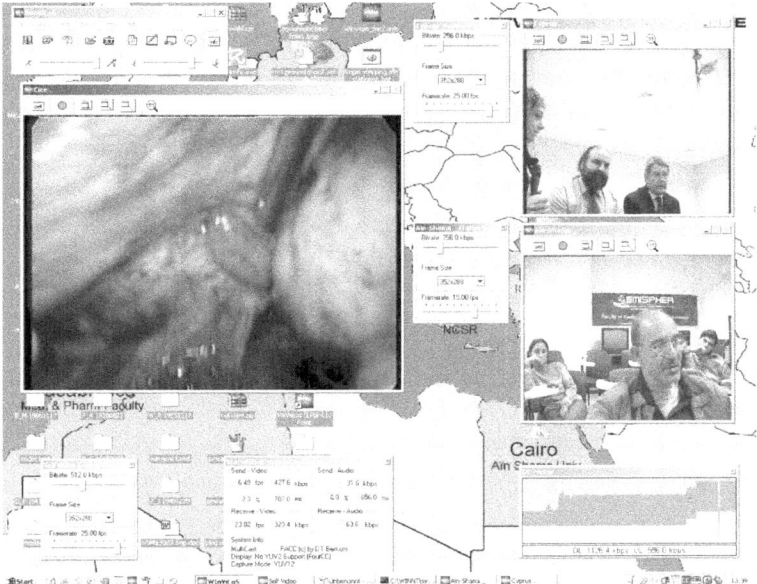

Figure 8. Interactive multipoint teleconsultation during laparoscopy between Charité (Berlin), Ain Shams University (Cairo) und University of Cyprus (Nicosia). A live video sequence of a laparoscopic investigation is transmitted and diagnosed by connected experts. The transmission bandwidth has been chosen asymmetrically to guarantee a high Quality of Service.

Overall point-to-point connections were successful with normal delays (~650 ms). Realised maximum bandwidths for symmetric point-to-point connections are 512–640 kbps in each direction. Up to these bandwidths the video and audio streaming is smooth. When going beyond these settings frozen images and audio problems start occurring. For asymmetric video bandwidth allocation (for example for e-learning applications) the maximum bandwidth settings for good operation are 768 kbps in one direction and 192 kbps in the other direction. For multipoint connections between three sites the maximum bandwidth settings for good operation are 384, 384 and 512 kbps. If the results presented above are compared with the nominal bandwidths required for the various services, it is clear that the EMISPHER platform provides sufficient bandwidth for most of the telemedicine applications with smooth video and audio streams in sufficient resolution.

During the first months of full operation of the network continuous evaluations have been performed and user-feedback was collected. This resulted in the upgrade of the WinVicos telemedical communication software as well as various upgrades of the MEDSKY software platform. The valuable user feedbacks were taken into account and have lead to even improved functionalities of the system and thus improved quality of medical work.

This demonstrates that the satellite platform with WoTeSa/WinVicos telemedical stations is very suited for the envisioned variety of medical services and is easy to learn for a wide range of medical professionals from the various countries.

2. Barriers and Issues at Hand

Although the market is promising and the technology ready (or nearly) to be used, the take-up and commercialisation of the telemedicine services is still uncertain due to a number of barriers:

External

- Decision-making in health is fragmented with respect to procurement policies, which hinders progression towards real integration.
- Establishing and building confidence with physicians takes time.
- It still seems that it will be a further 1–2 years before full deployment and therefore a critical mass can be built.
- How the services are packaged and attitudinal changes from within the health sector are also necessary.
- There are numerous organisational issues.

Economic

- It is difficult to predict the breakeven level of services and therefore to determine the minimum level of investment required for breakeven of the services.
- There is a lack of investment in health and therefore significant investment is still required.
- Considerable investment in improved management, training and education of personnel, re-designing of care and logistic processes is necessary.

Legal

- Ethical issues.
- Regulatory framework issues.
- Reimbursement issues.
- Lack of standardization.

Technical

- Software development is still evolving.
- IP levels of connectivity are also required as a minimum.
- All the services need to be fully integrated into one platform.

In various pilot projects, the technology has been put in place, the necessary applications have been developed and it had been proved that it can be used successfully and meet the needs of its end users. Yet numerous trials and demonstrations carried out during the projects have also highlighted a certain number of issues that could potentially hinder the commercialisation process of e-services in the medical sector.

In fact, a market analysis report, "The Emerging European Health Telematics Industry" (February 2000; prepared by Deloitte & Touche for the European Commission Directorate General for the Information Society), also insists on the fact that the telemedicine market growth will be dependent upon a number of vital conditions and enabling factors already noted above. The report also proposes that four key action lines should be initiated in parallel: consolidation on the supply side, technical integration, investment on the demand side and "accompanying measures" that could be the enabling factors required to allow the health telematics market to achieve substantial and exponential growth.

3. Suggested Solutions to Overcome Barriers

The solutions to such 'barriers' to commercialisation do not lie within the scope of the technology and appear to be generic to those 'up and running' tele-health activities worldwide. It is only in North America that new legislation has been introduced to respond to the particular needs of this practice and this legislation are not yet being applied on a federal level but rather on a state by state basis. However the organisational and cultural aspects that must accompany any new form of practice need the input of other actors both on the governmental, legal and political scale. Tele-health is not a simple extension of current health systems and cannot be perceived as such.

Solutions to the "barriers" can be consolidated under the following three main categories:

– Awareness of telemedicine and tele-health as integral part of medical practice;
– The need for common standards and policies;
– The need for specific legislation.

4. Future

The application of advanced telecommunications networks and services to health care practices is still evolving and maturing and hence telemedicine has yet to become an established part of day-to-day healthcare practice in many regions and countries. The main barriers to the development of the tele-health market relate to the organisation of healthcare services and, consequently, support to the connection to and usage of advanced telecommunications networks and services by healthcare establishments, which is primarily a matter for the public health authorities to consider.

However, the promise of telemedicine to provide equal access to medical expertise irrespective of the geographical location can only be met when not merely the patient's data are transferred but rather a telepresence is created bringing patient and remote expert together using ICT. Besides general interactivity between the two sites features like telehaptic, telesensation and remote control of medical devices (e.g. telerobotics) are prerequisite for a real telepresence.

The innovative developments in ICT over the last decade with the aim of realizing a ubiquitous or u-Health bear the risk of creating and amplifying a digital divide in the world. Therefore there is a need for real integration of the various platforms and services. A virtual combination of applications serves as the basic idea for the Virtual Hospital (VH) concept.

Based on the experience in the exploitation of previous European telemedicine projects and, in particular to activities carried out in the framework of the EUMEDIS programme, an open Euro-Mediterranean consortium has proposed the Virtual Euro-Mediterranean Hospital (VEMH) initiative [24].

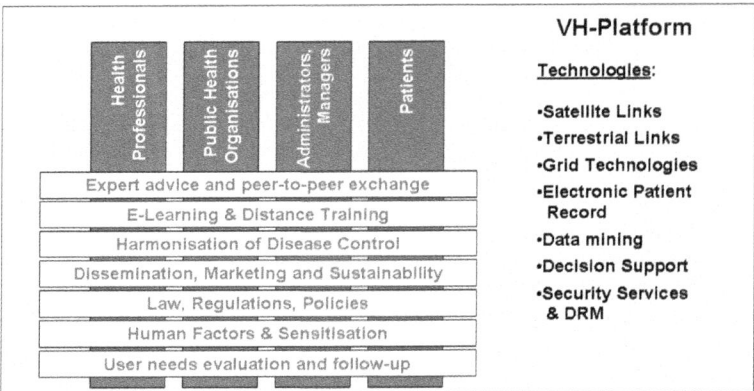

Figure 9. The technologies of the VH like satellite-terrestrial links, Grid technologies, etc. will be implemented as a transparent layer, so that the various user groups can use the services such as expert advice, e-learning, etc. on top of it, not bothering with the technological details and constraints.

VEMH will provide a heterogeneous integrated platform consisting of satellite links and terrestrial links for the application of various telemedical services: e-learning, real-time telemedicine and medical assistance, as well as Evidence-Based Medicine (EBM) (Fig. 9).

When it comes to the creation of telemedicine networks the following requirements need to be considered:

– traffic-intensive applications such as teleconsultation for diagnosis, and training, that require real-time interactivity of the audio and video stream;
– need for high quality of images and video transmission: min. 386 kbps up to 1 Mbps;
– need for guaranteed bandwidth: transmission of medical data does not allow for transfer delay and quality loss;
– guaranteed confidentiality of patient data.

Furthermore, grid infrastructures and services become inevitable for successful deployment of services like acquisition and processing of medical images (3D patient models), data storage, archiving and retrieval, data mining (especially for evidence-based medicine) [25,26]. In order to achieve this, conventional Grid technology has to be expanded to cover not only local computing resources but to a dimension of organisation-spanning integrated networks (Fig. 10).

5. Conclusion

The creation of a telemedicine and e-health network should be based on the current technological advances as well as on the need to get support from external experts, the improvement of the medical treatment by means of interactive telecommunication systems, as well as online documentation and hence improved analysis of the available data of a patient, contributing to an improvement in treatment and care of patients.

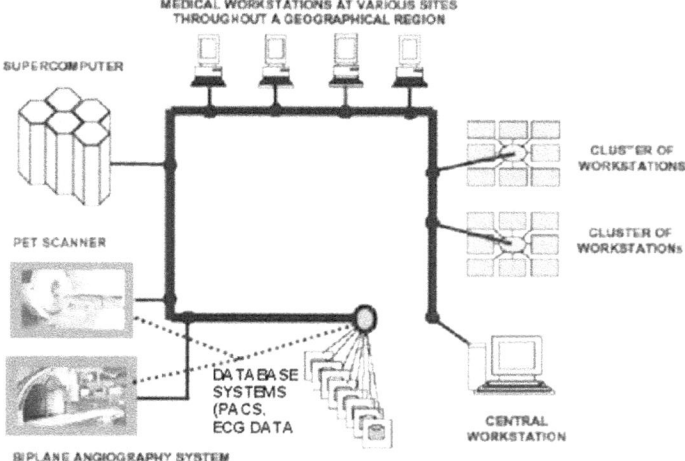

Figure 10. Grid Configuration for medical and clinical applications [25].

References

[1] R.U. Pande, Y. Patel, C.J. Powers, G. D'Ancona, H.L. Karamanoukian, *The telecommunication revolution in the medical field: present applications and future perspective*, Curr. Surg., Vol. 60, (2003), p. 636-640.
[2] Lacroix, L. Lareng, D. Padeken et al., *International concerted action on collaboration in telemedicine: recommendations of the G-8 Global Healthcare Applications Subproject-4*, Telemed. J. E-Health, Vol. 8, (2002), p. 149-157.
[3] G. Graschew, S. Rakowsky, T.A. Roelofs, P.M. Schlag, *Telemedicine as a Bridge to Avoid the Digital Divide World*, 8. Fortbildungsveranstaltung und Arbeitstagung Telemed 2003, Berlin, 7.-8. November 2003, Tagungsband (2003), p. 122-127.
[4] C. Dario, A. Dunbar, F. Feliciani et al., *Opportunities and Challenges of eHealth and Telemedicine via Satellite*, Eur J. Med. Res., Vol. 10, Suppl I, Proceedings of ESRIN-Symposium, July 5, 2004, Frascati, Italy, (2005), p. 1-52.
[5] G. Graschew, T.A. Roelofs, S. Rakowsky, P.M. Schlag, *Interactive Telemedicine as a Tool to Avoid a Digital Divide of the World*, In: L. Bos, (ed.) Medical Care and Compunetics 1, IOS Press, Amsterdam, (2004), p. 150-156.
[6] R. Wootton, L.S. Jebamani, S.A. Dow, *E-health and the Universitas 21 organization: 2. Telemedicine and underserved populations*, J. Telemed. Telecare., Vol. 11, (2005), p. 221-224.
[7] K.S. Rheuban, E. Sullivan, *The University of Virginia Telemedicine Program: traversing barriers beyond geography*, J. Long-Term Eff. Med. Implants, Vol. 15, (2005), p. 49-56.
[8] G. Graschew, T.A. Roelofs, S. Rakowsky, P.M. Schlag, *Telepresence over Satellite*, Proceedings of the 17th International Congress Computer Assisted Radiology and Surgery, London, 25.-28.6.2003, International Congress Series, Vol. 1256, ed. H.U. Lemke et al., (2003), p. 273-278.
[9] G. Graschew, T.A. Roelofs, S. Rakowsky, P.M. Schlag, *Broadband Networks for Interactive Telemedical Applications*, APOC 2002, Applications of Broadband Optical and Wireless Networks, Shanghai 16.-17.10.2002, Proceedings of SPIE, Vol. 4912, (2002), p. 1-6.
[10] G. Graschew, G. Bellaire, S. Rakowsky, F. Engel-Murke, D. Steines, P.M. Schlag, *OP 2000 – Interaktive Telekommunikation mit hochqualitativem Video, Fernsteuerung und intuitiven Benutzerschnittstellen für Telechirurgie und Simulationen chirurgischer Eingriffe*, In: A. Jäckel (Hrsg.), Telemedizinführer Deutschland, Ausgabe 2000, Bad Nauheim, (2000) p. 291-296.
[11] P.M. Schlag, T.K. Moesta, S. Rakowsky, G. Graschew, *Telemedicine – The New Must for Surgery*, Archives of Surgery Vol. 134, (1999), p. 1216-1221.
[12] G. Graschew, S. Rakowsky, P. Balanou, P.M. Schlag, *Interactive telemedicine in the operating theatre of the future*, J Telemedicine and Telecare 6, Suppl. 2, (2000), p. 20-24.

[13] G. Graschew, S. Rakowsky, T.A. Roelofs, P.M. Schlag, *OP2000 – Verteilte Medizinische Intelligenz in dem EU-Projekt GALENOS*, In: A. Jäckel (Hrsg.), Telemedizinführer Deutschland, Ausgabe 2001, Bad Nauheim, (2001), p. 269-273.
[14] G. Graschew, T.A. Roelofs, S. Rakowsky, P.M. Schlag, *GALENOS as interactive telemedical network via satellite*, In: *Optical Network Design and Management*, Xiaomin Ren, Tomonori Aoyama eds. Proc. of SPIE Vol. 4584, (2001), p. 202-205.
[15] S.K. O'Neill, D. Allen, P.D. Brockway, *The design and implementation of an off-the-shelf, standards-based tele-ultrasound system*, J. Telemed. Telecare, Vol. 6, suppl 2, (2000), p.52-53.
[16] A.C. Smith, R. Kimble, J. Mill, D. Bailey, P. O'Rourke, R. Wootton, *Diagnostic accuracy of and patient satisfaction with telemedicine for the follow-up of paediatric burns patients*, J. Telemed. Telecare, Vol. 10, (2004), p. 193-198.
[17] S. Guillen, M.T. Arredando, V. Traver et al., *User satisfaction with home telecare based on broadband communication*, J. Telemed. Telecare, Vol. 8, (2002), p. 81-90.
[18] C. Sable, *Digital echocardiography and telemedicine applications in pediatric cardiology*, Pediatr-Cardiol., Vol. 23, (2002), p. 358-369.
[19] R. Latifi, K. Peck, J.M. Porter, R. Poropatich, T. 3rd Geare, R.B. Nassi, *Telepresence and telemedicine in trauma and emergency care management*, Stud. Health Technol. Inform., Vol. 104, (2004), p. 193-199.
[20] L.H. Eadie, A.M. Seifalian, B.R. Davidson, *Telemedicine in surgery*, Br. J. Surg., Vol. 90, (2003), p. 647-58.
[21] G. Graschew, T.A. Roelofs, S. Rakowsky, P.M. Schlag and A. Lieber, U. Müller, R. Czymek, W. Düsel, *DELTASS – Disaster Emergency Logistic Telemedicine Advanced Satellites System – Telemedical Services for Disaster Emergencies*, International Journal of Risk Assessment and Management (in print).
[22] G. Graschew, S. Rakowsky, E. Balanos, T.A. Roelofs, P.M. Schlag, *MEDASHIP – Medizinische Assistenz an Bord von Schiffen,* In: A. Jäckel, ed. Telemedizinführer Deutschland, ed. 2004, Deutsches Medizin Forum, Ober-Mörlen, Germany (2004), p. 45-50.
[23] G. Graschew, T.A. Roelofs, S. Rakowsky, P.M. Schlag, *Überbrückung der digitalen Teilung in der Euro-Mediterranen Gesundheitsversorgung – das EMISPHER-Projekt*, In: A. Jäckel, ed. Telemedizinführer Deutschland, ed. 2005, Ober-Mörlen, Germany (2005), p. 231-236.
[24] G. Graschew, T.A. Roelofs, S. Rakowsky, P.M. Schlag, *VEMH – Virtual Euro-Mediterranean Hospital für Evidenz-basierte Medizin in der Euro-Mediterranen Region,* In A. Jäckel (Ed.), Telemedizinführer Deutschland, Ausgabe 2006, Medizin Forum AG, Bad Nauheim, (2006), p. 233-236.
[25] G. Graschew, T.A. Roelofs, S. Rakowsky, P.M. Schlag and P. Heinzlreiter, D. Kranzlmüller, J. Volkert, *Virtual Hospital and Digital Medicine – Why is the GRID needed?*, In: V. Hernandez et al. (Eds.) Challenges and Opportunities of HealthGrids, Proceedings of HealthGrid 2006, Valencia, 7-9 June 2006, IOS Press, Amsterdam, (2006), ISSN 0926-9630, p. 295-304.
[26] G. Graschew, T.A. Roelofs, S. Rakowsky, P.M. Schlag and P. Heinzlreiter, D. Kranzlmüller, J. Volkert, *New Trends in the Virtualization of Hospitals – Tools for Global e-Health*, In: L. Bos et al. (Eds.) Medical and Care Compunetics 3, Proceedings of ICMCC 2006, The Hague, 7-9 June 2006, IOS Press, Amsterdam, (2006), ISSN 0926-9630, p. 168-175.

Current Principles and Practices of Telemedicine and e-Health
R. Latifi (Ed.)
IOS Press, 2008
83

Changing from Paper to Paperless Hospitals in Busy Academic Centers

Keith SHELMAN, MD
The University Medical Center, Tucson, Arizona

Abstract. To decide to change from paper to a paperless hospital, one decides to go on a journey. This chapter will outline the destination, the reasons to make the journey and describe the best route to the destination. Becoming paperless is the route taken to the destination.

Keywords. Electronic workflows, User buy in, Leadership, Clinical champions

Introduction: Vision and Goals

The decision to change from paper based to electronic workflows must be founded on a clear sense of the problem or problems one seeks to solve with the migration to the paperless hospital. It is a common misconception that being paperless is a goal. Being paperless is a method of achieving a goal. A paperless solution is only worthy of pursuit if it is designed to solve a problem.

The problems typically addressed are those of clinical quality or basic business process. Some of these goals overlap. Example of clinical quality goals would be the reduction in hospital based adverse drug reactions, improved turn around time on pharmacy orders and improved compliance with the five *rights* of drug orders (right patient, right drug, right amount, right route and right time). To place these issues in context, 3.7% of hospitalizations are associated with error, and 13.6% of these led to death [1]. This is a problem worthy of solving and can motivate clinicians to modify their practices to make a difference. Medication errors are a leading cause of deaths per year [2] (see Fig. 1).

An example of improvement in basic business processes would be reduced cost or increased revenue.

These goals are not mutually exclusive. Adverse drug events increase hospital average length of stay by eight to twelve days and cost about $25,000 per incident [3].

It is important to understand the goals to be accomplished when adopting a paper free workflow (or any complex change). One physician CEO told me—"I know this is the right thing to do but I cannot justify the cost, at this time, on it being the right thing to do [4]." When juxtaposing the observation that greater than 50% of the $17–$29 billion national cost associated with medical errors is preventable when can begin to address operations costs in our goals sets [5].

A clear understanding of the goals of the effort is a prerequisite to the success of the effort to become paperless. If you do not know where you are going, you may end up somewhere else [6].

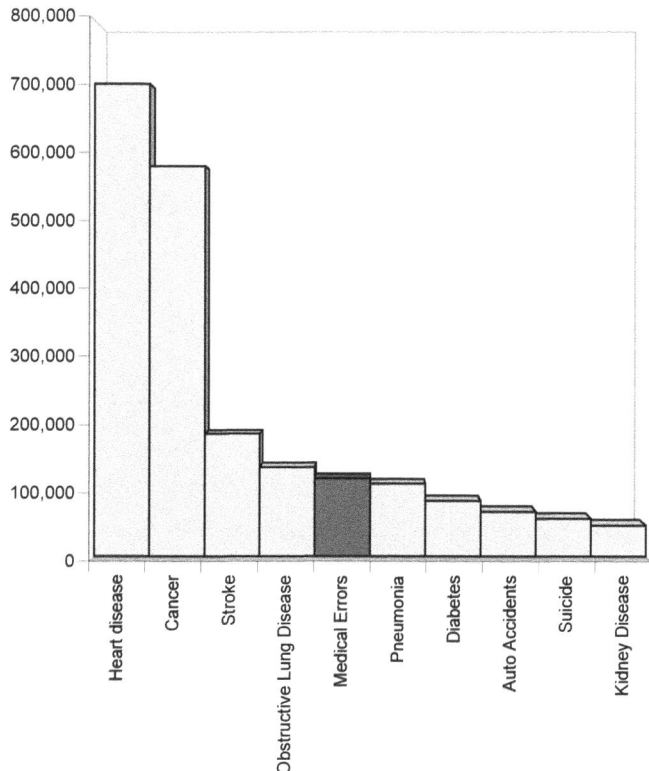

Figure 1. USA deaths by cause.

When we discuss paper free hospital process, we typically refer to Computerized Physician Order entry (CPOE). Please note the term is misleading because CPOE is not just for physicians. It is critical to understand the workflow implications. CPOE is not simply a niche computer system used by physicians in place of handwritten orders. Rather, it is the capstone of an entire process – that of order management. As such, it directly impacts not only physician ordering but also physician decision making (through the decision support features), care planning, pharmacist decision making and workflow, nursing workflow and documentation, and communication with ancillary services (laboratory, radiology, etc.). Implementing CPOE profoundly alters the way all of these stakeholders do their jobs. For the clinical stakeholders to achieve organizational change requires **consistent support from leadership**, plus **dedicated resources** and **commitment from all affected constituencies** [7].

Here CPOE connects previously disconnected silos of endeavor. Besides reducing handoffs and the errors and efficiency loss associate with those handoffs, new possibilities occur as a result of the new connections.

For example, connecting lab and pharmacy creates new possibilities in clinical management by connecting previously disconnected silos [8].

In addition, computerizing workflows exposes defects in those underlying processes. Be prepared to spend time and effort addressing these exposed problems. This is a significant opportunity to address previously *un*measurable process now that metrics are available as a direct result of computerization. Although unplanned effort will be required, unexpected benefits will be accrued.

The vision is the 'why' to answer the question, "why are we doing this?" The vision creates the demand for the transition to a paperless workflow and the vision will enable the stakeholder in the organization to connect the perceived losses associated with change with a worthy goal – enabling the change acceptance process.

1. Evidence Based Practice: Implementation

Successful implementation of an automated workflow (paperless process) requires the three key ingredients working together:

- end users and stakeholders
- the application (solution) vendor or developer
- the information technology department

1.1. End Users and Stakeholders

User buy in is critical. Implementations where an electronic solution is forced or imposed on the system users are not only fraught with difficulty are also more expensive. They require greater time and resource, and are more likely to fail.

To create user buy in, share the vision and communicate the problem to be solved with the solution. Plan and insure that the application users are trained and educated on the correct use of the application. This training and education must be connected to the users' workflows as well as to application functionality. Finally, connect the vision with the reality of what is planned – this will simultaneously set realistic expectations and connect the user's perceived losses with the reasons for the loss, fostering acceptance.

Recognize basic implementation requirements. First examination of core work processes. Break them into elemental steps and understand how migration to the electronic workflow will affect the user. Be willing to start with a clean slate with a bottom up approach within the context of the clinical practice. Determine the actual workflows by interviewing the staff with a process focus instead of an individual user focus. Understand and map information flow, information handoffs, patient flow and patient handoffs. Recognize that you may identify process issues that require correction before you can move forward.

Next, examine your users. Identify baseline skills such as use of email, familiarity with mouse use, typing skills, existing computer skill sets. Some users will be quite advance where other may be interacting with a computer for the first time. Use this information to define and plan the training strategy.

Recognize that user acceptance is important, but physician acceptance is critical. Implement during a slow season or with a reduced clinical work load when possible. Define time recovery strategies to reduce the burden on both physician and non-physician users. Increased staffing, reduced schedules during the implementation enhance the likelihood of implementation success. Most importantly, recognize the effect on workflow and proactively compensate where possible. Insure there are enough computers available for the physicians and other users to perform their tasks with minimal workflow disruption. Use wireless computers and devices when possible if workflow is benefited.

To accomplish physician acceptance, create a Steering Committee or Advisory Committee. Recruit champions from within the clinic ranks. This will enhance process ownership and provide a platform for appropriate policy generation. It will allow for academic integration and most importantly will reduce political push-back.

When configuring (setting the application up for use), a common error is an ancillary or silo centric workflow inadvertently inculcated into the configuration. For CPOE and other direct care provider applications that address workflows across the clinical continuum, it is very common to have difficulty recruiting the time of both doctors and nurses. When an implementation project team populated with ancillary clinical departments (lab, pharmacy, radiology, etc.) as the subject matter experts (SME's), they bring a clinical ancillary centered perspective or bias. What occurs is an unintentional emphasis on the needs and issues of prominent concern to these ancillary silos – often creating a more difficult, time consuming, electronic workflow for the direct care providers, as many ancillary workflow problems are now solved and the issues of direct care providers are neglected or exacerbated, resulting in a more time consuming front end workflow for the direct care providers. This reduces buy in and can cause an implementation to fail. Avoid silo centric configuration teams and recognize the key role of both physician and nurse direct care providers in the clinical workflows.

Leadership is key to a successful implementation. Recognize that leadership is ***actions*** and not a *position* and leadership must be focused on producing the needed change. Again, leadership must be present, must communicate and define both the potential as well as the reality of the project. This will link vision to process and connect the visionaries to the implementation.

Compensate for user issues related to the use of computers. *Cyberphobia* is an irrational fear and dislike of electronic and internet communications and technology [9]. *Itphobia* [10] is the fear of appearing incompetent, the fear of loss of autonomy, prestige, organizational position that creates resistance to standards, guidelines, outside scrutiny.

To overcome ITphobia, communicate, educate and train. Recognize that there is never enough communication, education or training. Train the leaders (even if they are never doers). Attitudes and culture are top down. When the leaders get trained, resistance to training is decreased. Before deployment, plan and implement direct communications to applications users as often as possible. In addition, send indirect communications via newsletters, email and flyers even though some will never be read. Add incentives such as time cost recovery, recognition and performance rewards. Publically recognize and praise examples of success in overcoming ITphobia. Utilize your *Clinical Leadership* to forge a shared vision, mission, values and goals to drive the process forward.

To further enhance user buy in and training, remove the fear factor in learning. It is recognized that 40–60% of future users may have little to no Microsoft Windows experience. Use *just-in-time training* plus ongoing incremental training to accomplish a sound learning foundation. This requires commitment from department management to make staff available for training. This commitment is critical to the project success. Implement education by both instructor lead and Computer-Based-Training (CBT) when possible. Train by cohorts – get the whole department together. For physician, one-on-one training works best and should be utilized if resources permit. Recognize that users need a **protected** training time. Finally, computer system competency should be part of performance review – skills only become valued when the organization values them.

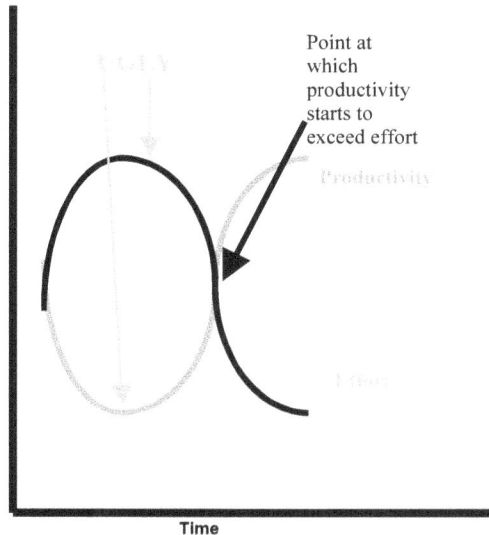

Point at which productivity starts to exceed effort

Figure 2. Effort and productivity transitions during the project life cycle.

Recognize that change is not a small transition. Initial resistance is normal, people are resistant to change. But also recognize that over 12–18 months there is a process typified by first, a fear of letting go, followed by resistance, transitioning into a period of indecision and culminating with getting started on the new [11] (see Fig. 2).

During the change transition, initially effort increases and productivity decreases, creating a difficult moment in the implementation. By focusing on the aforementioned implementation strategies, this difficult period can be abbreviated. Productivity will increase, effort will decrease moving to the project success crossover point.

Vision, skills, incentives, resources and cooperative action are all required for implementation success. Without vision there will be confusion, without skills there will be panic, without incentives there will be insurrection, without resources there is often blame storming as the project slows or fails and without cooperative action, we see the prisoners' dilemma where stake holders and users fail to work together towards a beneficial outcome.

To overcome resistance to change, insure participation in information systems steering groups or committees, and insure there is stakeholder evaluation of proposals. Also, populate a multidisciplinary implementation team with a champion in each clinical area if possible. Finally find a mechanism to supplement physician time to enhance physician participation.

Recognize that there are seven imperatives for success:

1. Strong Commitment from Administration to change. The project teams require frequent and conspicuous support from upper leadership.
2. Ownership by end user of system design, implementation and standardization. This insures process and workflow issues are considers as well as improving buy in.
3. Establish and communicate realistic goals and expectations.
4. Clinician's involvement: their role is pivotal in success of the implementation.

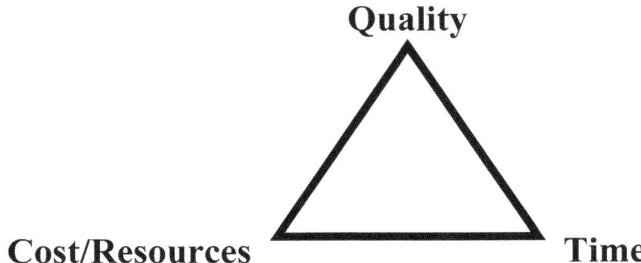

Figure 3. The triple constraint.

5. Internal Marketing by physician champions: it is a powerful and a beneficial success driver.
6. Process redesign requires more effort than system design – to paraphrase James Carville – "it's the workflow stupid" [12].
7. Recognition that learning is a continuous experience. Insure repeated and continuing education resourcing and opportunity.

The ugly reality is that 64% of IT implementations fail. Success requires planning, investment, time, communication, commitment and coordination. Success requires effective resourcing. It is recognized that for every dollar invested in acquiring (or developing) the system, successful rollout requires an investment of two to three dollars in implementation support (staff devoted to implementation, costs and time devoted to training, change management activities) [13].

In all projects, there is a triple constraint (time, quality & cost) or three variables from which you can manipulate not more than two of these three variables. Your selection should be based on the values of the organization. In clinical settings, quality should never be negotiable; hence the organization and project leader can choose cost or time, but not both. Here, as in all areas of life, there is no free lunch (see Fig. 3).

The project life cycle is accompanied by a clinical stakeholder emotional progression from enthusiasm and optimism at project kickoff, to concern, to distraction to other priorities, to the onset of pessimism and confusion of the stakeholder. Here can occur a loss of resolve and a risk of the group abandoning the project. To address this danger point and stay the course, it is import to return to and communicate the original vision; because that vision will drive the culture forward and renew the commitment to the project and changes it represents. This will enable perseverance, permit acceptance of the changes and ultimately result in enhanced adoption (see Fig. 4).

Successful Change Implementation requires an understanding of the desirable future state – the state where the paper free workflow and its benefits exists along with the resultant desirable outcomes. In order for the outcome to be present, there must be a change in the structure of the work and its processes. Process change can only occur as the result of culture change.

Though the vision will drive culture change, culture must be addressed and understood. This understanding is one of the unique values of clinical champions. Culture has both exposed and hidden layers. Though the exposed layers of culture: values and beliefs, actions and processes will be accessible to the organization's administrative and technical project team members. The hidden layer of culture – the hidden and unspoken basic assumptions that drive both attitude and behavior must be understood and

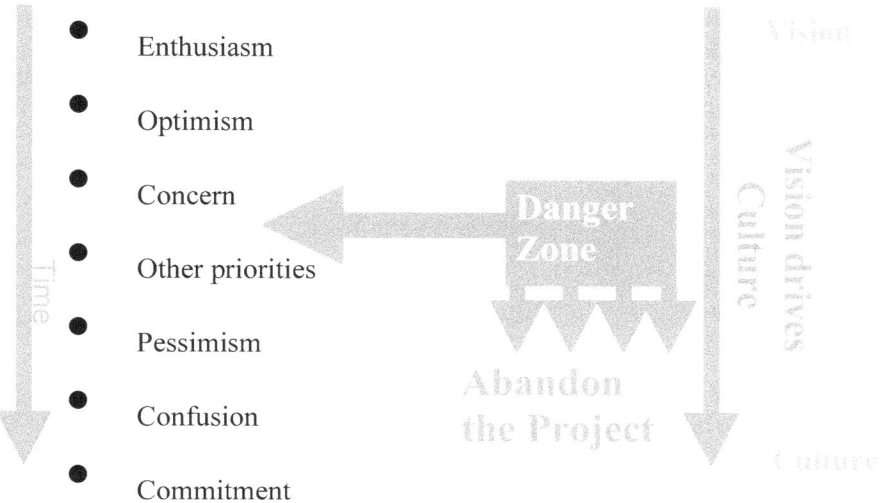

- Enthusiasm
- Optimism
- Concern
- Other priorities
- Pessimism
- Confusion
- Commitment

Figure 4. Emotions during the project lifecycle.

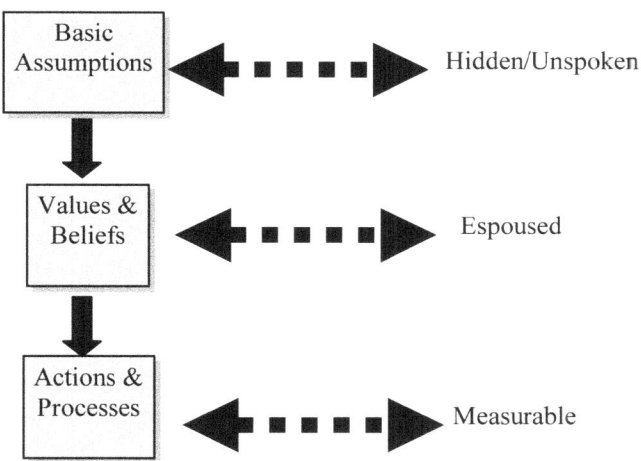

Figure 5. Layers of Culture.

accommodated in order to be successful in implementation and managing change (see Fig. 5). To best address this hidden layer, recruit clinicians to the project team. Not infrequently, a project team will assume that using of a subject matter expert as an occasional resource is an adequate substitute for clinical champion participation and leadership. This error can undermine otherwise excellent efforts.

User buy in is a key ingredient for success. In academic medical centers, bypassing house staff buy in and instead dictating or imposing a new electronic workflow on them will cause a significant push back and undermine the project. It is a common misjudgment to assume that because house staff are on the bottom of an academic hierarchy that they can be commanded and will respond to dictates. Their buy in is critical to deployment success. They need to be treated with the same respect as any group of affected stakeholders.

The vendor of the software product, as well as the software product itself being implemented, is an essential ingredient for project success, whether that is a 3rd party vendor or an internal software development team.

It is important to recognize what is required of the application:

- Functionality
- Usability
- Reliability
- Performance
- Scalability

1.2. Vendor and Application Issues

Functionality: The application functionality must meet the organizations and workflow's needs (also known as requirements). The only way to insure this occurs is to collect, understand and validate your requirements. It is a common error to select a solution only to find out it does not solve your problem. Product selection driven by correct requirements is essential to avoid this problem. When this problem occurs, it is difficult to resolve. Examples of specific requirements that may not be possible in a computerized physician order entry application commonly include:

- Alternating IV's fluid orders.
- Allow for ordering of tapering drug doses.
- Ability to change doctor name on orders mistakenly attributed to the wrong physician as a result of incorrectly entering verbal orders.
- Character limit on orders – limits sliding scale orders and relevant information in radiology orders.
- Twice-a-day Monday-Wednesday-Friday drugs can be difficult or impossible to enter.

When functional deficiencies are recognized after product acquisition, the alternatives become creative workarounds and requesting the vendor to enhance the product.

Usability is critical. One vendor has adopted the mantra: "If the doctors don't use it, not else matters." To be useable, the application should transactionalize the clinical workflow, providing a more intuitive workflow pathway. Vendors who don't understand workflows will have less usable applications that can increase the front end workflow burden of the clinical staff [14]. The user interface should be intuitive. If an application requires a significant amount of training in order to permit safe and effective use, then there are significant usability issues. Ideally, these issues should be exposed during product selection.

Reliability is the single most important aspect of an application. Application reliability issues can cause project failure.

Performance is an important but often unmet expectation. Clinician time is an important resource and should not be wasted. Application screens transition should ideally be second to sub-second. This standard is frequently unmet. Thick chart patients can be especially problematic – slowing or application timeouts due to performance issues will be regarded as unacceptable by physicians and nurses. To avoid this difficulty, site visits to assess performance of the application is an essential part of product selections. To simply trust vendor claims without validation is inadequate and an abrogation of the responsibility to perform due diligence in product selection.

Scalability is the ability to add users, patients, hospital units or additional hospital units to the application. It is important to understand if the application can grow to support the organization's growth needs.

Failure to proactively identify and address the organizations functional requirements may result in the adoption of a software product that does not meet the organizations needs. When this occurs, the organization can request the vendor enhance or modify its software. This may require substantial time and effort from the vendor. Their response may be that the product was working as designed and could not or would not admit to defective design [15].

Recognizing and accommodating workflow is the key to success. Often, the migration to from paper to an electronic chart alters the workflow paradigm. Where nurses once reviewed and initialed a paper chart to denote a daily chart check had occurred, initialing the electronic application workflow may not be an option. Communication of new or urgent orders is altered from the paper workflow. In the paper workflow, a visible indicator on a chart may be all that is required. In the corresponding electronic workflow, a completely different strategy will be needed because there will need to be a trigger to log into the electronic application to view the new orders. Such strategies include status boards and electronic alerts that trigger pagers. These strategies become part of the new workflow paradigm.

1.3. IT Department Issues

The IT department is the third significant success ingredient.

Conflicting goals – deployment vs. patient care: IT departmental issues include the natural tension between expediency (time) and safety (quality) as depicted by the triple constraint. By clarifying and communicating goals early in the project, the tension between expedient deployment and patient safety can be proacted.

Competition for resources – not matching capital resource delegation with project resources is a common problem. Software acquisition is only part of the cost. Failure to resource the project team with adequate people is a common problem. A deployment done on the cheap is more likely to fail.

In addition, failure to recognize that support needs of deployment persist long after initial rollout to users is a common problem. The organization must recognize and resource the project well after deployment in order for the vision of the project to be realized.

Connected to this issue, if there is poor vendor support, the application support burden is transferred to hospital IT department. This has the effect of causing properly planned project team resource delegation to be insufficient.

In summary, deployment is about getting the software into use. This will enable the organization to realize the goals of the project through a three step process: *Substituting* an electronic workflow for a paper workflow, followed by a period of *innovation*, culminating in *process transformation*. Ineffective deployments often stop at the first step.

Deployment can be approached incrementally or all at once. All at once deployments or big bang deployments have the advantage of getting the rapid completion. To be successful, big bang deployments require ample resources, both educational and support. Incremental deployments take more time, but can be less disruptive, allow a smaller team to provide training and support to fewer target users. In addition, incremental change creates less resistance to change [16].

2. Barriers and Overcoming Barriers or Lessons Learned in Migrating from Paper Workflows to Paperless Workflows

- **Lesson 1**: Staff will often ask why do we have to use the application, directing energy and scarce resource towards adopting and optimizing the application. Recognize that success requires departmental leadership becoming strong advocates of the change. Connect the reason for the change with the change being required.
- **Lesson 2**: staff doesn't make a serious effort to complete the activities that are necessary to effectively deploy the application. Needed steps get treated as optional or receive a low priority. This manifests as very poor attendance at scheduled training classes (ironically – when the staff member is untrained, their life is so much harder). Recognize that the deployment will be better, be less painful, require fewer resources, if there is active participation. Attitudes in every department are top down. If the leaders of each area prioritize and make CPOE important, the staff will as well. To demonstrate the importance of the application is for the leadership to become trained on the application.
- **Lesson 3**: Address the "It's not my job – it's your (IT department's) job to do it for me or to me," the passive recipient instead of one of active participation issue. Recognize that only the departmental leadership can effectively tell the staff what their job is – this requires leadership buy in. The IT dept can provide assistance regarding the roles and responsibilities, but it is only really credible coming from the leadership.
- **Lesson 4**: The "application is one more thing they make me do that I don't have time for" response is another buy in issue. To address this issue, forge a shared vision. The hospital decided to adopt the application to achieve a variety of benefits to the organization. Leadership's role is to insure everyone shares in the vision. Recognize that only leadership can effectively set and communicate organizational priorities.
- **Lesson 5**: "The application is hard to use (because I don't know how to use it)." Adequate training makes a major difference in perceived pain and suffering.
- **Lesson 6**: Address the attitude "I can't ask my staff to go to CPOE class on *their* own time." Leader buy in is important. If it's important to leadership, it will be important to our staff. Compensate for time. This training should be no different than other skills to be mastered in order to function at the hospital. If treated the same, it will enjoy the same level of proficiency that the other clinical skills do.
- **Lesson 7**: address the "It's not my job to check to see if my staff is using the application correctly" issue. "If IT wants my staff to use the application, they should monitor my staff." Again, another buy in issue – leadership should not be allowed to abdicate management responsibility. The deployment team can provide the tools, but the clinical experts must manage how those tools are being used. Once the clinical department incorporates the application into the set

of processes that they use to perform the departments function, then they will start to benefit from process automation.

- **Lesson 8**: Manage Workflow to address the "It's not my job; it's his/her job!" Or "She/he is not doing their job, so I will call the deployment project team." Again leadership buy in means leadership accepts the managerial responsibilities for the new workflow. In advance of the deployment, define the scope of the support role. Leadership should articulate clear policies and manage those policies to insure that scarce resources are usefully directed.

- **Lesson 9**: Address the Safety Myth: "It's a waste of time to put all that time, money and energy into the application. My clinical practices are safe and excellent." The Institute of Medicine has reported that each year, more Americans die as a result of medical errors made in hospitals than as a result of injuries from automobile accidents. Tragically, as reported in the literature [17], though "substantial proportions of the public and practicing physicians report that they have had personal experience with medical errors, neither group has a sense of urgency."

- **Lesson 10**: Address the "If I just resist long enough, the application will go away" attitude. Engage leadership to help to staff understand the reasons for change and its necessity. Connect the change process to the core values, harness the energy and professionalism that makes the doctors, nurses and other staff members so special. Articulate the vision and strong commitment to the application to help overcome resistance to change. Recognize that people go through a process where they are afraid of letting go; they become resistant, then indecisive. Following these stages, they get on with the new and recognize that resistance can be prolonged or abbreviated based on the attitudes and guidance offered by an area's leadership.

- **Lesson 11**: That's another reason why we shouldn't have to use the application, it makes us have to stop and fix all those processes that are partly broken. This speaks for itself. This is one of the immeasurable benefits of application deployment. It causes process correction and benefits the hospital. Stated another way: You can not repair a broken process with automation.

- **Lesson 12**: There's not enough time to comply with the schedule – can the schedule be delayed? There is never enough time. Recognize that if we do it now, it can be done now. If we delay the work, it may never be done. Delay begets delay. Address with resources instead when possible.

- **Lesson 13**: Recognize your assumptions about your organization and about your vendor: Don't assume the vendor understands health care and your workflow and don't assume you don't understand health care and your workflow. Don't abdicate responsibility to your vendor any more than you want your end users to abdicate to your IT department – understand relative roles and act accordingly.

- **Lesson 14**: Vendor support: Don't assume your vendor will be there when you need them. Don't assume the product is stabile – test and monitor. Don't assume your vendor would warn you about known defects. Don't assume your vendor will fix defects – test the product against your workflows before you move the application to patient care (production) use.

- **Lesson 15**: Don't buy a product and hope it meets your needs – know your needs (have good requirements) BEFORE you buy and be certain the product addresses your needs! "You're writing a contract for a product that's impossible to describe, that will change over time and needs to be renegotiated, that will make you dependent on the provider and for which termination is not an option [18]."

3. Future

In the future, the worthiness of the goal will be well understood and embraced more universally. Modern information tools will be used in partnership to enable possibilities that the unaided human mind cannot do. When we use such tools we may see a picture of medicine we have not seen before [19]. Public awareness of medical errors will be one driving force towards change.

Today, of the physicians, nurses, and administrators surveyed, 80% believe that "fundamental" changes are needed to ensure patient safety, 78% feel that their organization should take responsibility for developing solutions to the quality challenge, 95% of physicians, 89% of nurses, and 82% of administrators report having witnessed a serious medical mistake [20], yet there is no organized effort or sense of urgency for change.

When surveyed, most healthcare leaders believe that patient safety is a major issue in the United States – but not at their facility. If you can imagine an error occurring when reflecting on how your organization delivers care, it can, probably will or even has already happened [21]. The myth that *everyone has a safety problem but us*, will be exposed and overcome. National groups and government will become a force for change [22].

The cost of entry into electronic workflows will be reduced as information system standards occur and evolve enabling data sharing between systems to occur, vendors offer true workflow integration and a proven migration pathway.

In addition, the software itself must evolve so reliability improves, costs reduce and solutions become cost effective. Today, a representative cost model [23] for implementing CPOE at a single, 500-bed hospital. "This model estimates total one-time capital plus operating costs of $7.9 million and annual ongoing costs of $1.35 million. The model assumes that the hospital organization already has the high-capacity network capabilities required for CPOE, and some level of clinical information system capability that would require moderate upgrades. Hospitals without such capabilities would incur higher costs."

The transition from paper to electronic will be marked by new errors as electronic workflows replace paper workflows, computer errors will replace paper based errors [24] until experience with the new electronic paradigm occurs and software solutions evolve.

As these changes occur, we will see an increase in adoption of electronic ordering solutions from the minority of hospitals to becoming a standard of care. Organizations that embrace change will receive competitive advantages in patient safety, financial performance with demonstrable returns on investment and increased patient satisfaction.

4. Conclusion

To be successful in migrating from a paper to a paperless workflow, one must

- Achieve buy in of all affected stakeholders and users.
- Understand and accommodate workflow.
- Provide leadership.
- Provide adequate resources.
- Recognize that CPOE can be more front end intensive to physicians – invest heavily in clinical champions and optimize the application configuration to address and accommodate direct care provider workflows.
- Begin the configuration with the multidisciplinary clinical team lead by clinical champions – this will identify the clinical use cases and the configuration validation testing.
- Plan: Planning is the essential ingredient – those who fail to plan, plan to fail.

5. Tables

Table 1. Example of connected silos: Lab Pharmacy Linkages

	Relationship	Example	Computer role
Drug selection	Lab contraindicates drug	• + pregnancy test◊ ACE inhibitor • Azotemia→ Metformin	Prevents drug ordering
	Lab suggests drug indication	• ↑ TSH→Synthroid • ↑ lipids→ statins et al • ↑ Troponin or CK → β-blocker	Generates reminder of need for pharmacologic intervention
Dosing	Lab affects drug dose	Azotemia → Digoxin, aminoglycosides	Performs dose calculations based on age, gender, weight, height & lab results
	Lab indicates need for drug dose titration	• Coumadin→ PT/INR • Anticonvulsants◊ drug level	Dose adjustment suggested based on chart or other resource
Monitoring	Abnormal lab result indicates toxicity	• LFT's→ INH, Actos, Avandia, NSAID's • Anemia, leucopenia→ chloramphenicol	Generates alert to assess
	Drug warrants lab monitoring for toxicity	• Clozapine→ WBC • Amphotericin→ creatinine	Insures scheduling of baseline & serial monitoring tests
Lab Interpretation	Drug influencing or interfering with lab	• Carbamazepine → thyroxine • NTG◊ urine VMA	Computer warns against false –/+
	Drug impacts response to lab	• Insulin → ↑ or ↓ glucose • Penicillin→ +RPR	Reset response for treated patients to prevent unneeded alerting
Improvement	Drug toxicity/ Effects Surveillance	Detects signals of previously undocumented/infrequent reactions (i.e. hepatotoxity, event clusters)	Data mining lab and drug data
	Quality oversight	Treatment delay following abnormal result (↑ TSH) and therapy (Synthroid initiate or dose adjustment upward)	Monitor time intervals between result requiring intervention and the therapeutic intervention

References

[1] Kohn LT, Corrigan JM, Donaldson MS (eds). To Err Is Human: Building a Safer Health System. Institute of Medicine, Committee on Quality of Health Care in America. Washington, DC: National Academy Press, 2000.
[2] Institute of Medicine and the Centers for Disease Control and Prevention.
[3] Source: Reducing the Preventing Adverse Drug Events to Decrease Hospital Costs. Agency for Healthcare Research and Quality. www.ahrq.gov/qual/aderia/aderia.htm.
[4] Private conversation: Tom Handler, MD; Research Director Gartner Healthcare Industry Research & Advisory Services.
[5] Thomas EJ, Studdert DM, Newhouse JP et al. Costs of medical injuries in Utah and Colorado. Inquiry. 1999;36:255-64.
[6] Attributed to Yogi Berra.
[7] Ahmad A, Teater P, Bentley TD, et al. Key Attributes of a Successful Physician Order Entry System Implementation in a Multi-Hospital Environment. JAMIA 2002;9:16-24.
[8] Schiff GD, Klass D, Peterson J, Shah G, Bates DW Archives of Internal Medicine. 2003;163(8): 893-900.
[9] Webster's New Millennium™ Dictionary of English, Preview Edition (v 0.9.6) Copyright © 2003-2005 Lexico Publishing Group, LLC.
[10] Not an actual word (yet).
[11] Human Side of Change – Peg Neuhauser.
[12] 1992 Presidential Election Campaign.
[13] Metzger J, and Slye D. Inpatient e-ordering. Healthcare Informatics May 2001: 63-67, 2001.
[14] Some applications purposefully impose structure to enforce a preferred workflow to deliberately address a clinical problem. This may be perceived as reduced usability – but in fact is an enforced modification of an undesirable workflow.
[15] CPOE vendor response to numerous issues submitted by University Medical Center, Tucson Arizona.
[16] Peter Senge: The Fifth Discipline: The Art and Practice of the Learning Organization. New York, Doubleday Currency 1990: pg 22- The parable of the Boiled Frog.
[17] N Engl J Med 2002;347:1933-40.
[18] Paul Roy, a partner at Mayer, Brown, Rowe & Maw LLP.
[19] Paraphrased from Larry Weed.
[20] Robert Wood Johnson Foundation, Pursuing Perfection, 2001.
[21] Dr. Brian Shea, Patient Safety Leader, Cap Gemini Ernst & Young Health.
[22] N Engl J Med 2002;347:1933-40.
[23] Costs, Benefits and Challenges of CPOE, a Case Study Approach, First Consulting Group, January 2003.
[24] Some Unintended Consequences of Information Technology in Health Care: The Nature of Patient Care Information System-related Errors, JOAN S. ASH et al, J Am Med Inform Assoc. 2004;11: 104–112.

III. Special Applications of Telemedicine

Current Principles and Practices of Telemedicine and e-Health
R. Latifi (Ed.)
IOS Press, 2008

Telemedicine in Extreme Conditions: Disasters, War, Remote Sites

Ronald C. MERRELL, MD, Stephen W. CONE, MD and Azhar RAFIQ, MD
Medical Informatics and Technology Applications Consortium,
Virginia Commonwealth University, Richmond, VA

Abstract. Telemedicine has developed around certain assumptions about connectivity and format. From the pioneer work of Kenneth Bird in the 1970's medical events separated by distance were connected for videoconference interaction [1]. The connection implied well developed telecommunications tools at both ends of the interaction. Telemedicine in its most common manifestations relies upon electronic and professional familiarity plus training with proper technical support. This is true even with Internet telemedicine at the low end of bandwidth. A workable Internet service provider and intact telecommunication services are required at both ends. The assumption of intact, robust telecommunications fails when there is any significant disruption of services, power, or trained people to initiate a telemedicine request. The very nature of disasters whether made by nature, made by fellow humans or in war declarations implies a rupture of the social fabric, a failure of infrastructure. This loss of infrastructure and connection happens at a cruel time when the need for services in health matters is generally very much exacerbated. Extreme remote sites have never had infrastructure and therefore fit into this chapter. Is telemedicine incompatible with support and relief in disasters of remote places? Certainly not. However, telemedicine must adapt to the situation in ways not generally associated with standard telemedicine. New solutions can meet the expectation of being wherever services are need whenever the need arises. This chapter looks at the experiences, successes and failures of telemedicine in natural disaster, war, and extreme remote sites. The presentation is concluded with recommendations to make telemedicine integral to any disaster response and a natural tool for any human endeavor that requires sending people to remote and hostile environments.

Keywords. Disasters, wars, extreme conditions, hostile environments, earthquakes

Introduction

In telemedicine as with medicine in general patients seek out assistance from an intact system of care delivery, one with telephones, web sites, offices, convenient parking and a working appointment system. Such a system relies heavily upon infrastructure of power grids, intact telecommunications, transportation, fuel for cars and personnel arriving for a regular work day in a routine manner to do the work scheduled for that day. Even for emergency services in an intact health system, the only party not prepared for the medical crisis is the patient. The other elements of emergency response including telephony, ambulances, trained personnel, supplies, etc. are available with redundancy and assurance of timely response. However, when infrastructure has been left behind as in extreme environments or military expeditions, destroyed by war, natural disaster or sabotage or collapses from neglect as in civil disruption the delivery of routine medical care including telemedicine is severely compromised and does not come near the expectations of the public or the medical profession unless appropriate measures are taken. In this chapter military telemedicine refers to care by telemedicine for military personnel in battle or in camp. Telemedicine for war victims is different and will be covered separately. Telemedicine in natural disasters will refer to generalized disasters that rupture services on a large scale such as in hurricane, earthquake, volcano or tsunami. In these instances the disaster not only inflicts great harm that calls for medical assistance but also disrupts infrastructure and isolates those in need of services. These disasters also inflict harm by that very isolation of patients who rely upon regular care for disease management. Extreme environments are those where infrastructure never existed and transportation to definitive medical services is unlikely or untimely. Antarctica, ships at sea and outer space are examples.

Telemedicine has been applied for over 20 years to disaster events (Table 1) [2–6]. Many lessons have been learned but to date telemedicine frankly is not a routine part of the disaster response by humanitarian or international relief organizations.

In the examples in Table 1, telemedicine assistance arrived after initial relief and brought along appropriate telecommunications equipment. In Table 2 the modalities for telemedicine in various responses make it clear that disaster telemedicine must rely upon satellite telecommunications when the infrastructure of telecommunication in the locale is not available [7]. This is a very important point. When telecommunications are disrupted, only satellite telecommunications are reliable and must be promptly available if telemedicine is to be used in meaningful disaster relief.

Telemedicine by the military is an application early recognized and applied with vigor by visionary telemedicine figures such as Zajtchuk and Poropatich [8–11]. Military telemedicine is the first area of consideration in this chapter.

1. Military Telemedicine

Concern for the soldier in war is evident from earliest descriptions such as that of the Trojan War in Homer's *Iliad*. He records scores of injuries in detail and even describes some treatments although the mortality of the injuries was horrific. Medicine customarily makes great advances in war when the volume of otherwise rare injuries is very large and there is sense of urgent inquiry to find a better way to treat the soldier. Paré was overwhelmed by amputations in the siege of Turin (1536–1537) and ran out of the standard hot oil used to cauterize the severed stumps. He resorted to ligature of the vessels and was stunned to find the clinical outcome far superior to time-honored cautery results. Baron Larrey introduced the ambulance to swiftly take the Napoleonic casualty out of the battle and back to a hospital. Dr. Basil Pruitt catalogued the impact of war and civilian research following wars [12] (Table 3). The mortality for common wounds has dropped dramatically, even 10-fold in the case of colonic injuries, in the 20th century US wars up to Viet Nam. Data coming from Iraq suggest even further reduction in [downtime] (Fig. 1). Military telemedicine uses advanced information technology as in the BMIST system that records, processes, transmits medical information from the far forward medical person (Fig. 2) and informs that individual with massive amounts of timely and specific information to manage a situation [13]. Casualty data joins an information continuum connecting the injured soldier and caregiver to a huge network of assistance and function. Telemedicine can now be considered integral to the effort to

Table 1. Summary of military and civilian disaster-related telemedicine deployments

Year	Area or Project	Infrastructure	Usage
1985	Earthquake in Mexico (civilian)	ATS-3	Voice communication support
1989	U.S./U.S.S.R. Telemedicine Space Bridge (civilian)	INTEL-SAT, COMSAT	1-way video, 2-way audio, fax
1990	Hurricane Hugo (military)	INMARSAT, land lines	CT
1991	Gulf War (military)	INMARSAT, land lines	CT
1992	Somalia (military)	INMARSAT, land lines	CT, still image
1993	Primetime 1, Macedonia and Croatia (military)	Orion satellite	CT, still image
	Space Bridge, Moscow (civilian)	GTE Spacenet, G-Star II, WSDRN satellite (Russian)	2-way video, audio, telepathology
1994	Eruption of a volcano, Rabaul (Papua, New Guinea)	ETS-V	Voice communication between disaster sites and hospitals
1994	Haiti (military)	INMARSAT, ACTS satellite	CT, video, still image, digital acquisition devices
1995	Primetime II, Croatia (military)	Orion satellite, ATM technology	CT, still image, ultrasound, color Doppler
1996	Primetime II, Bosnia (military)	Orion satellite, ISDN	CT, still image, ultrasound, color Doppler, store-and-forward
	ACTS Montana Demonstration (civilian)	ACTS satellite	On-site acquisition devices (audio, video, cata)
2004	Tsunami, India (ESA, I-DISCARE)	GPS, Globalstar, INMARSAT, Eutelsat	To connect mobile teams of rescue workers with hospitals via satellite
2004	Tsunami, India (ISRO)	VSAT, INMARSAT	Has brought 3 hospitals in Andaman and Nicobar islands into ISRO telemedicine network. Connected to medical facilities on the subcontinent and received specialist services.
2004	Earthquake, Islamabad, Pakistan (ITU)	INMARSAT	ITU partnered with INMARSAT to provide 40 regional broadband global network satellite terminals (RBGAN) and 15 (GAN) from its own in-house stock, for deployment in Pakistan

Sources: J Am Med Inform Assoc. 1999 Jan-Feb; 6(1): 26-37; Int J Med Inform. 2001 May;61(2-3):87-96; Dinerman T. Telemedicine and distance learning after the tsunami. Monday, January 10, 2005; The Space Review, website: http://www.thespacereview.com/article/301/1; Indian Space Research Organization, website: http://isro.org/pressrelease/tsunami.htm; International Telecommunication Union, website: http://www.itu.int/ITU-D/CDS/newslog/index.asp?Article=775.

care for the wounded warfighter [14]. The management of information for seamless response, the use of robotics, the use of smart materials and standard teleconsultation all play an important role in military planning (Fig. 3). Even advanced consultation

Table 2. Telemedicine package configurations for various disaster cases

Disaster cases	Functions of medical equipment and medicines	Transportation	Communication devices	User interfaces
Typhoon/hurricane Floods/Tsunami	Relief from drown Prevention for infectious diseases	Boats, helicopters	Telephone, telemedicine equipment	Wireless, satellite
Earthquakes/fire	Relief from burn Relief from crash syndrome	Vehicles, helicopters	Telephone, telemedicine equipment	PSTN, mobile Wireless, satellite
Volcano eruptions	Relief from poisonous gas Relief from burn	Vehicles, helicopters	Telephone, telemedicine equipment	PSTN, mobile Wireless, satellite
Air crash/traffic accidents	Relief from crash syndrome Relief from fracture of bones and burn	Vehicles, helicopters	Telephone, telemedicine equipment	Wireless, satellite, mobile
Nuclear power station trouble	On site sampling of HLA type for bone marrow transplant	Vehicles, helicopters	Telephone, telemedicine equipment	PSTN, mobile Wireless, satellite
Terrorism by bombing	Burn, Barotrauma, Pulmonary injury	Vehicles, helicopters	Telephone, telemedicine equipment	PSTN, mobile Wireless, satellite
Terrorism by poisonous gas	Secured aspiration	Vehicles, helicopters	Telephone, telemedicine equipment	PSTN, mobile Wireless, satellite

Source: International Telecommunication, Union website: http://www.itu.int/md/d02-rgq14.1.2-c-0045/e. A proposal for telemedicine package standardization; PSTN = Public Switched Telephone Network.

Table 3. Mortality rates, U.S. Army Casualties in 20th Century Conflicts

Conflict	Colon Wounds (%)	Chest Wounds (%)
World War I	66.8	24.1
World War II	26.5	8.3
Korea	18.2	5.3
Vietnam	6.5	7.0

Source: 1992 Fitts Lecture. J Trauma. 1993 Jul;35(1):78-87.

such as ophthalmology can be pressed to far forward sites to support the care of the wounded [15]. Military casualties in most wars have only been attributable in a minority of instances to the battlefield since infectious disease, thermal injury and malnutrition all had their greatest impact where the armies were in camp away from customary services such as clean water and stable food supplies. Telemedicine in the military brings consultative services in epidemiology, radiology, dermatology [16–18], otolaryngology [19], etc., to the home bases of military personnel and their dependents where specialist medical staffing is impossible and also to the deployed forces not yet in battle but far from definitive medical services (Fig. 4). The immediate past surgeon general of the US, Vice Admiral Richard Carmona, emphasized the irrevocable

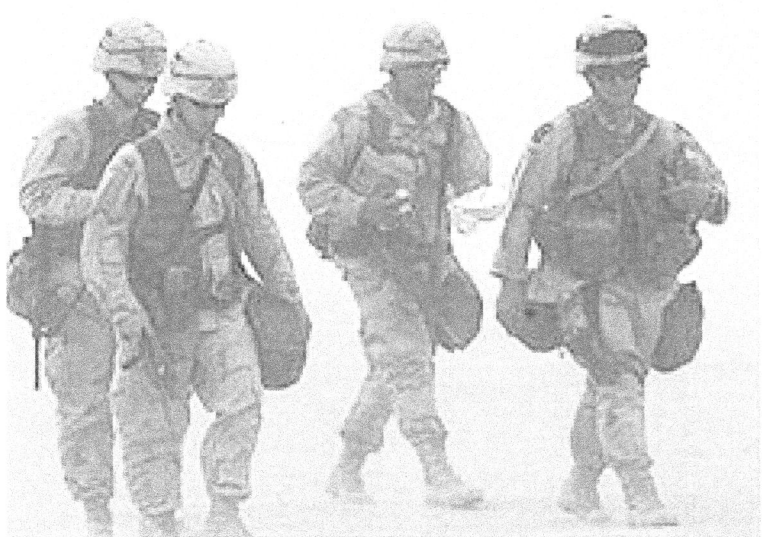

Figure 1.

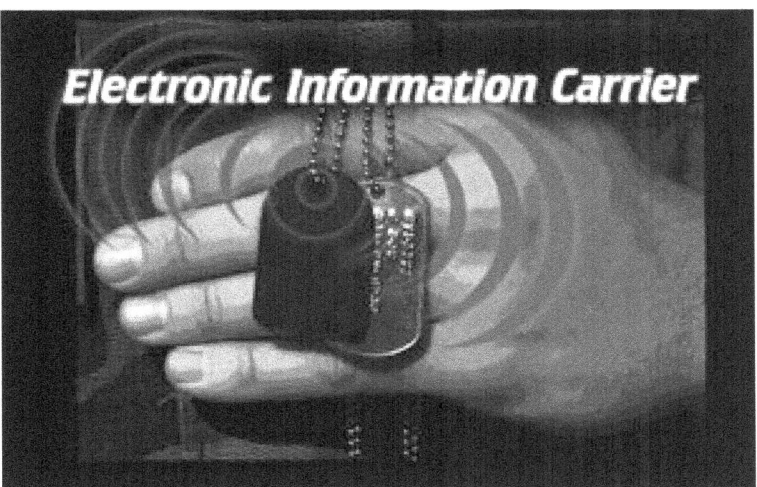

Figure 2.

inclusion of telemedicine in military medicine in a 2003 editorial [20]. Proper implementation of military telemedicine involves organizational as well as technological issues [21]. In addition to standard war wounds much has been learned about mental health [22] and support services such as radiology [23]. The Army is certainly not alone in its applications of telemedicine. The Navy has a very strong interest in telemedicine and has provided great leadership by sharing their experiences generously with the telemedicine community [24,25]. Telehealth, distance learning for medical

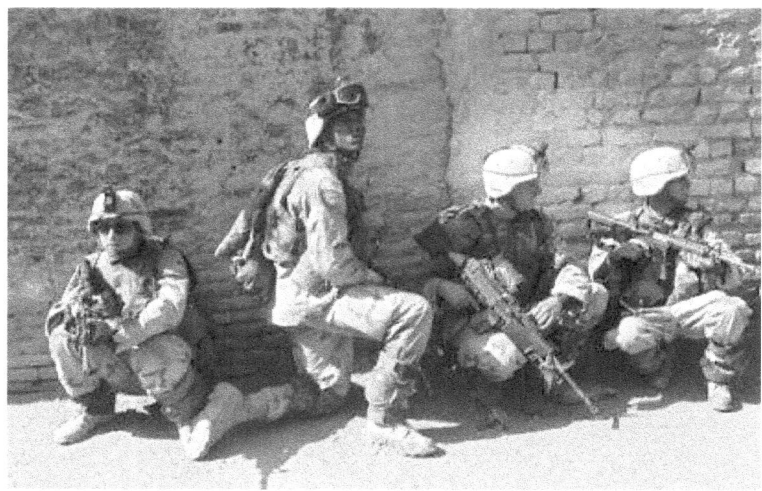

Figure 3.

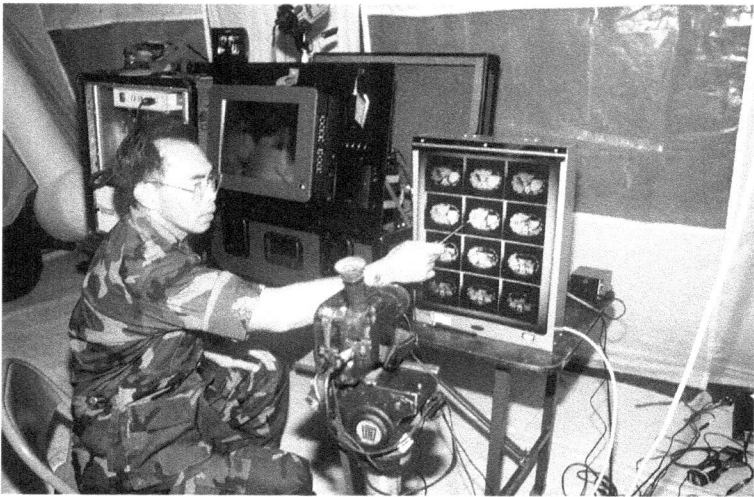

Figure 4.

personnel, electronic simulation for medical skills and a general use of advanced tele-communications strategy has put the military far ahead of the civilian sector in actual application of telemedicine principles of information science and telecommunications. The highly advanced state of military telemedicine is in response to special needs but the benefit to civilian telemedicine technology has been enormous. Not only has the US military been active in telemedicine but allies in NATO have been in strong collaboration for interactive seamless care of armies made of units from many countries [26]. The Greek army, serving a nation and myriad islands, has been especially keen on telemedicine innovation [27].

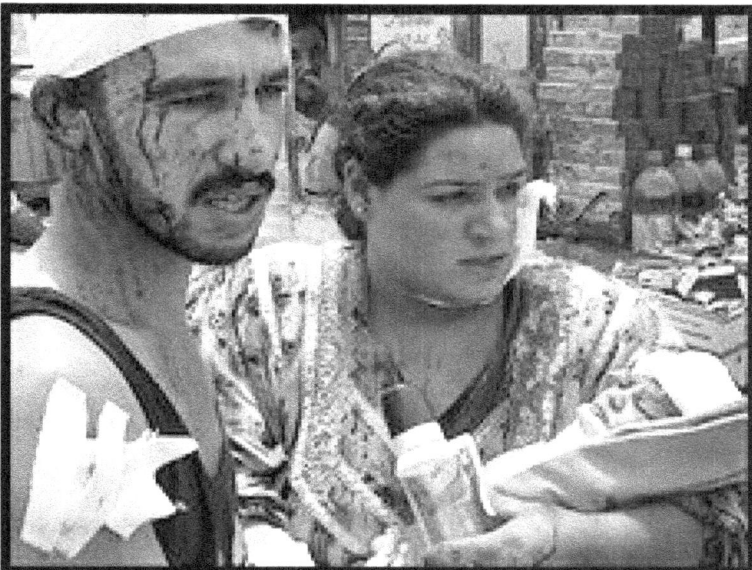

Figure 5.

2. Civilian Casualties

Civilians have never been mere spectators in the drama of combat. In modern conflicts the weaponry still lacks the precision to protect non-combatants and many times impacting the civilian populace seems to be a deliberate military tactic. The use of military weaponry in civilian areas can generate large numbers of casualties that can overwhelm an intact medical response infrastructure or the use of ordnance can destroy that infrastructure and isolate the population in need (Fig. 5). It is very difficult to get figures for the civilian wounded, even long after conflicts have ended. In Iraq, civilian injuries and deaths were not tallied at the outset and now widely disparate figures identify the political bias of the writer more than illuminate the truth about what is actually happening. Greater importance is placed on who is doing the injury than the plight of the injured (Fig. 6). However, it is beyond doubt that there have been hundreds of thousands of injuries in Iraq and in July and August 2006, 6599 civilians were killed [28]. It is important to note the news reports when available emphasize the deaths. For those who die of the immediate injuries there is no medical response, telemedicine or otherwise. However, it is reasonable to assume that the injured requiring medical aid are at least equal in number to the dead. Of course that is not the case for a crashed airliner but rather close for exploding ordnance. Telemedicine could be a powerful tool to assist the humanitarian efforts and to introduce corrective measures into refugee situations [29,30]. However; the application has certainly not been pervasive in practice or even in preparations. Usually, by the time camps for displaced persons are established, medical efforts can be amplified and supported with telemedicine. Unfortunately, the opportunity just does not seem to have been seized and civilian casualties are generally outside military coverage. In the telemedicine effort in Iraq, some 11% of all consultation has involved Iraqi civilians and personnel. In reconstruction, on the other hand, the

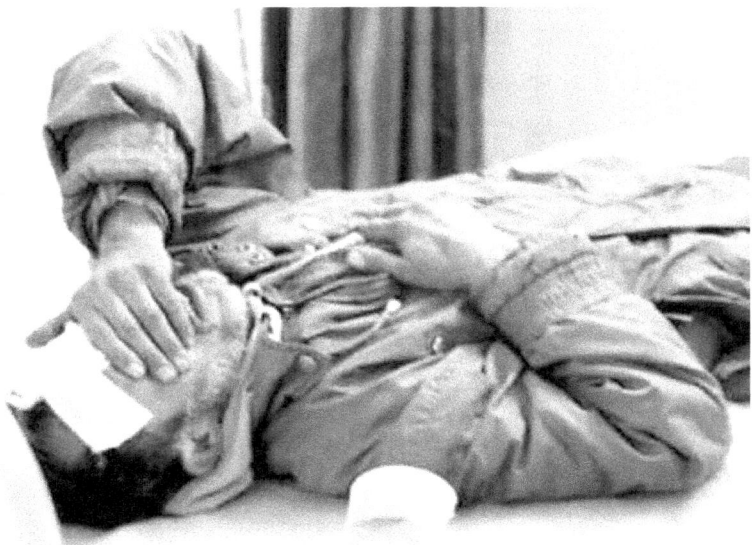

Figure 6.

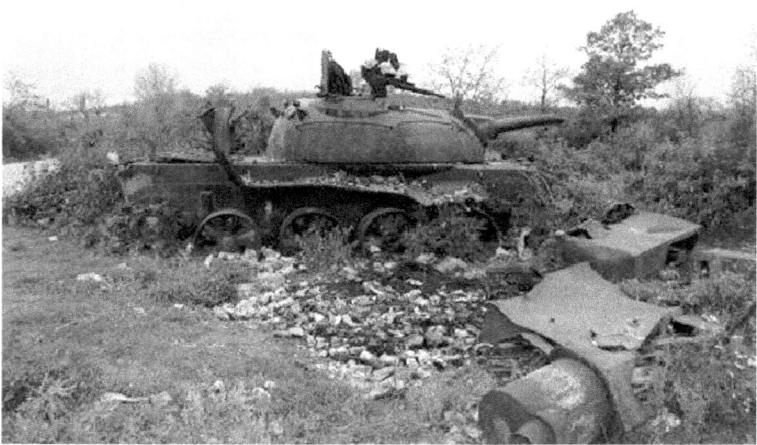

Figure 7.

experience in Kosova has been highly instructive and favorable [31]. When infrastructure was restored for communications and service delivery, telemedicine was a powerful tool for rapid resumption of care (Fig. 7). The urgent situation of civilian casualty
and infrastructure damage benefited in great ways by thoughtful planning and application of battlefield lessons.

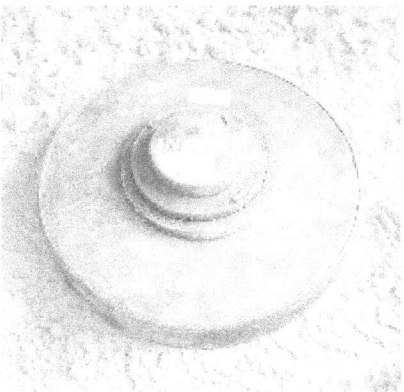

Figure 8.

Telemedicine has also been useful in resolving some of the residua of war such as landmine injuries [32] (Fig. 8). With perhaps 50,000,000 landmines in the field and casualty reports from over 50 countries per year, landmine management and elimination could benefit from telemedicine consultation and data management. The Committee for International Rehabilitation has been particularly strong, led by Dr. William Kennedy Smith, adapting distance learning to empower those struggling with landmine injuries [33].

3. Natural Disaster

Despite the ghastly predictability of natural disaster there has been little creative response supported by telemedicine in the acute phase of the event. The Tsunami of 2004 was a fine opportunity for telemedicine assistance but there is little evidence that the resource was applied until rather late after other services had been brought to bear late application of telemedicine. India responded very early with a robust system already in place coordinated by the Indian Space Research Organization. However, as Dinerman reports, US telemedicine response arrived with the USNS *Mercy* 4–6 weeks after the disaster [4].

The late application of telemedicine was true for the 2005 hurricane season as well (Fig. 9). One lesson learned in the Katrina situation was that the medical needs of the isolated population are related only in a minority of instances to injury. The population at risk included large numbers engaged in disease management regimens for diabetes, anticoagulation, congestive heart failure, immunosuppression, mental illness and Alzheimer's. The victims were older as one would expect from the general demographic of the US. Their management relied heavily upon medical systems, pharmacies, transportation and stable living circumstances. These medical conditions do not customarily rank high in planning for disaster and their management cannot be expected in the skill set of emergency workers including physicians.

Within 4 days of Hurricane Katrina, a NASA team had established satellite teleconsultation, planning and coordinating at Stennis Space Center in Mississippi near the site of land fall. However, the response required sending every element to the site since

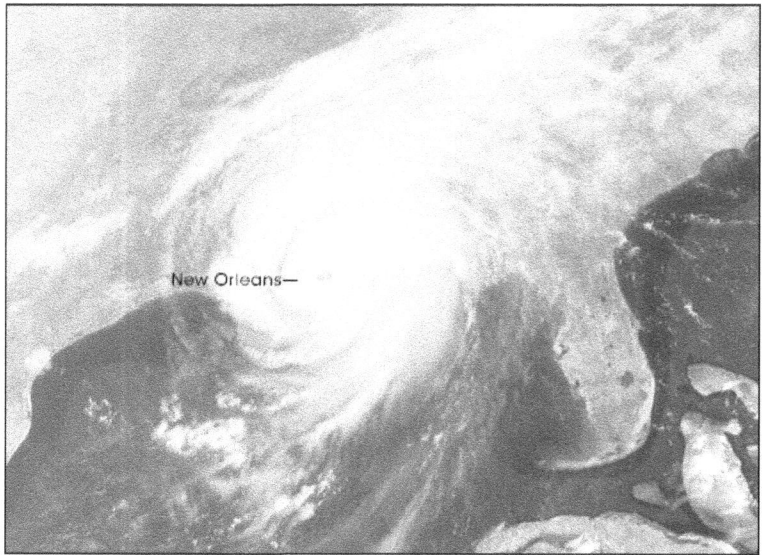

Figure 9.

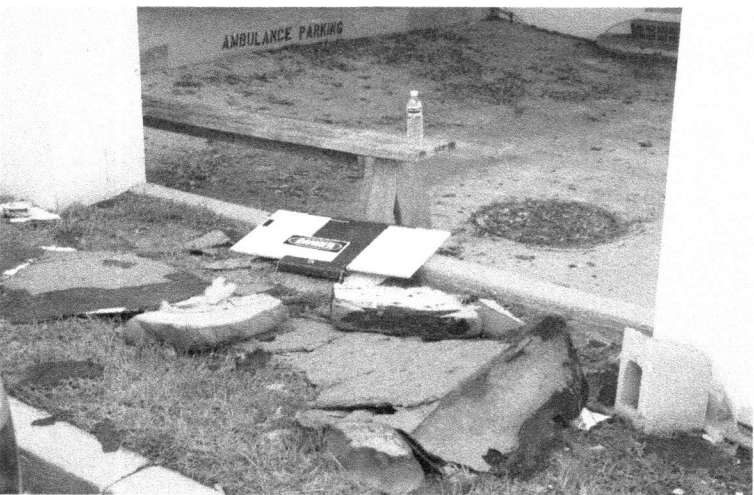

Figure 10.

there were no prepositioned assets for telemedicine (Figs 10 and 11) Telemedicine could be an invaluable tool to restore some kind of continuity of management to people isolated by disaster from their medical systems.

In 2005, an estimated 91,900 people were killed by natural disaster and an uncounted number injured requiring urgent medical assistance [34]. It is unclear how many of those who perished might have been saved had there been early, coordinated medical care supported by telemedicine. An exception to this sad tale is the relief effort

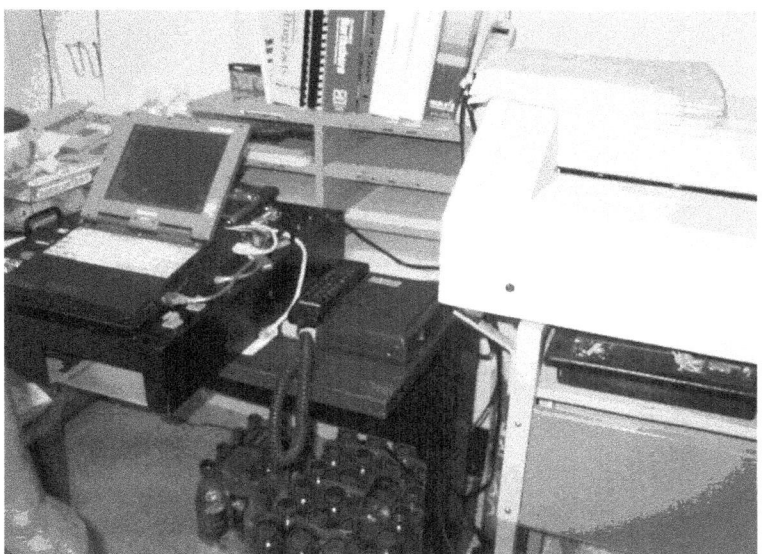

Figure 11.

in Pakistan after the earthquake of October, 2005. In this instance telemedicine was extensively used for triage, coordination, consultation and follow-up [35]. The explanation is very important later in this chapter when recommendations are made. In Pakistan there had been a vigorous telemedicine program with international classes prior to the disaster. When the earthquake struck, there was at hand a critical mass of people with equipment and training including a courageous group of medical students who put a laptop, a camera and a satellite phone into a rucksack and headed into the mountains. They were tireless and highly effective in coordinating unconnected relief agencies and moving patients down from triage to the hospitals in Rawalpindi. They set up telemedicine facilities to serve the surgical patients who returned to refugee facilities in the mountains after surgical care (Fig. 12). This program organized by Dr. Asif Zafar serves as a clear example of potential at least partially realized for telemedicine in natural disaster.

4. Terrorism

By its very intent, terrorism is a disruption of normalcy striking when least expected at nebulous targets. Therefore, prior arrangements at the site of the event are unlikely. However, in planning terrorism responses telehealth plays a very strong theoretical role in various models [36,37]. In the acute phase of terror response, the greatest role of telemedicine may be information gathering, management and distribution, rather than specific medical interventions [38–40]. However, the first responder can clearly be equipped to gather information and to benefit from information to integrate their work into a more comprehensive data driven effort (Fig. 13).

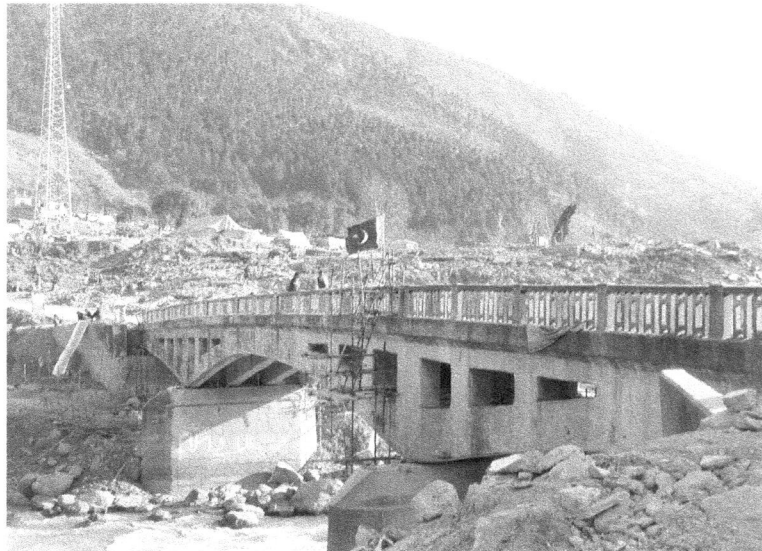

Figure 12.

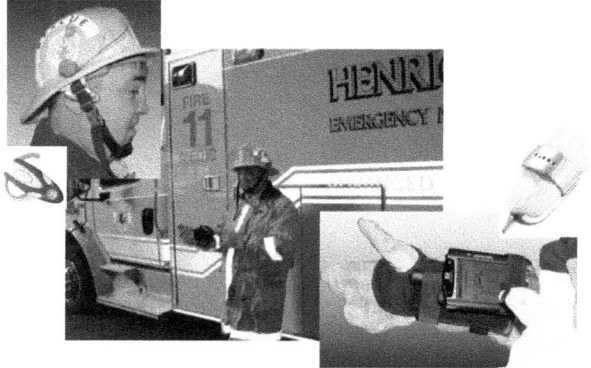

Figure 13.

5. Telemedicine in Extreme Environments

Telemedicine has shown real worth in expeditions to extreme environments where medical problems cannot receive the kind of prompt intervention expected back home. Early work on Mt Everest [41–43] provided in depth telemedicine consultation for climbers at base camp in 1997 and 1998. The unit there diagnosed gallstones, retinal hemorrhage due to altitude and the consultants provided some psychiatric interventions and crisis management (Figs 14 and 15). The scientific program in Antarctica has excellent support with telemedicine in all the national stations [44,45]. Perhaps the story of Dr. Jeri Nielson is the most dramatic instance of telemedicine in that remote place inaccessible for many winter months to even air relief. Dr. Nielson found a breast mass during self examination and, with advice and instruction from colleagues, diagnosed

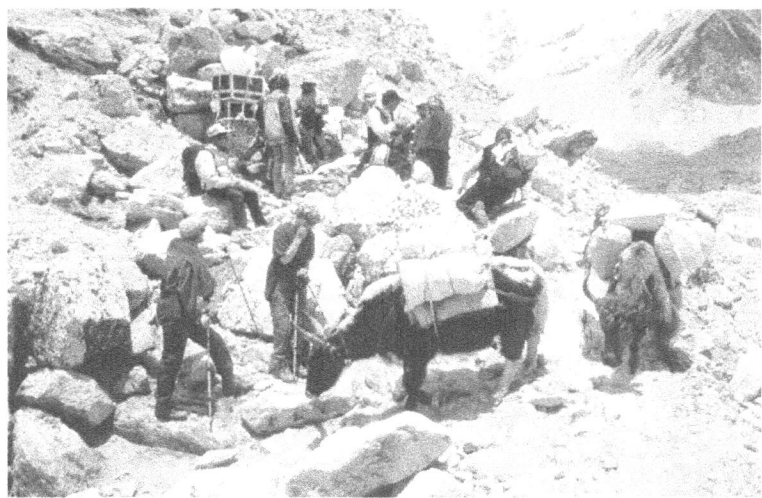

Figure 14.

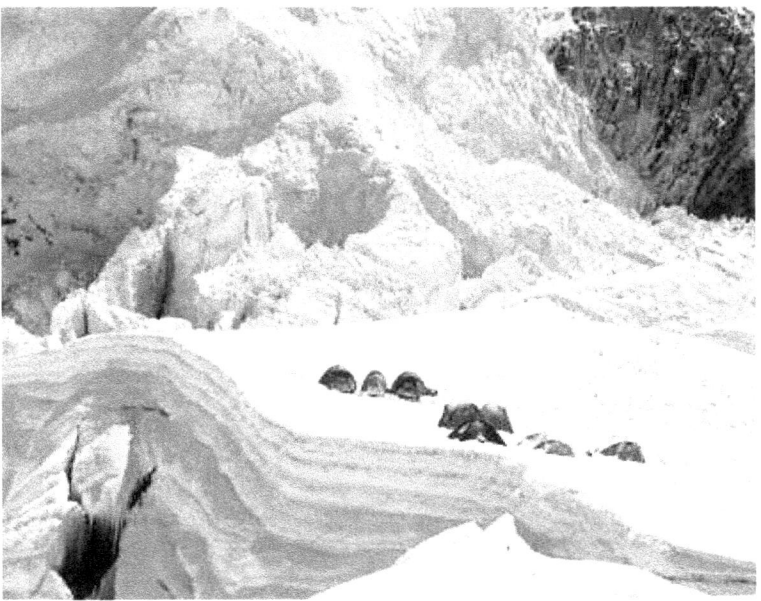

Figure 15.

carcinoma and planned a treatment course to temporize the situation until she returned home [46,47]. It is rare in medical work that a tale becomes a movie of courage empowered by technology but this story became a movie for television on CBS [48]!

Telemedicine has been applied in remote parts of Africa [49–51], the Amazon [52,53] and the Gobi desert [54]. However, perhaps the most underrated use of telemedicine is in one of its earliest application for astronauts and cosmonauts. Telemetry and telemedicine were in use from 1962 onwards [55–57]. The remarkable safety record of the space programs is in no small part due to the enablement of distant management by telemedicine. NASA was a leading force in telemedicine technology and global implementation [58,59].

NASA continues to foster progress in telemedicine with such astounding efforts as the NASA Extreme Environment Mission Operation (NEEMO). Using microwave transmission to a habitat off Key West, surgeons in Canada were able to perform and instruct surgical tasks to the underwater team in a seamless continuum of telecommunications [60,61]. This program is ongoing in collaboration with the US Army.

Extreme environments must include the voyages of mariners transporting much of the world's goods and natural resource needs in their cavernous holds. Excellent support programs are described for Scandinavian programs [62,63]. Marine telemedicine where evacuation is not possible has set a very high standard as to what can be done when alternatives are not available.

6. Recommendations

1. *Telemedicine should be vigorously applied to solve medical needs in extreme and disrupted environments.* The data available in demonstrations and those examples of broad involvement as in the military confirm that early use of telemedicine can be a cost effective and clinically valuable adjunct to other medical efforts. The telemedicine community should move forward with all haste to join relief and expeditionary medical efforts with their experience and technology. The data are even better with regard to reconstruction after war and other disasters. There is no easy argument *against* rebuilding a health system on a foundation of electronic information, data driven programs, open communication among health workers and ready access to databases. In fact, to rebuild with paper, professional isolation and anecdote is expensive, outdated and patently less effective. Rebuilding a model of health care predicated on labor intensive paper is simply illogical. The high cost of information systems and telecommunications was accepted in the advanced medical systems of the world not because the systems had money to waste but because the cost of the old methods was prohibitive.

2. Beyond economics, all health workers should have access to useful information and all patients are entitled to a well informed health care worked. This ideal can only be realized by e-health and telemedicine.

3. *The lessons learned in extreme situations by telemedicine should be fully reported in peer reviewed publications.* Perhaps some efforts are hastily applied with little time to structure statistics, comparisons and the usual scientific metrics. Indeed much of the information that could be gathered may be negative in that telemedicine did not meet the higher expectations of those involved. However, even negative results could be very useful to planners. Experiments should not always support the hypothesis!! However; much of the information presented in this chapter came from unedited web sources and press reports. Many disaster telemedicine efforts have the character of technology demonstrations. No criticism is intended. However, planners could work much better from carefully prepared, scholarly reports that inform the reader as to the methods and results of an effort. The reports need not and should not be only in the telemedicine journals but in specialty journals for disaster medicine,

military medicine and clinical specialties that have a readership that is likely to include decision makers for those specialties.

4. The telemedicine community should engage all planning agencies to include WHO, ICRC, military, FEMA, NGO'S, ministries of health and others responsible for medical care in urgent and disruptive situations. The message to these planners must be factual and based upon careful analysis of clinical, technical and financial data applicable to the matter the agency is addressing.

5. *Telemedicine should be embedded in programs of relief and rebuilding.* Protocols and plans should not isolate telemedicine or make it an appendage. Rather, the relief effort should have a foundation of information gathering and sharing using the best in information science and telecommunications to support health workers.

6. The telemedicine community should develop and validate telemedicine systems for a broad range of medical needs in any part of the world. Beyond concepts and plans, the response needs proven products and practices. Kits of equipment, procedures, and training should be among the tools available to the planners for emergency and rebuilding response. There are many kinds of telemedicine units and the planners may be confounded by the number of choices. Therefore, the telemedicine community should make a priority of vetting a series of telemedicine units applicable to any expected topology of telecommunications and power situation. For early response it is absolutely clear that the telecommunications connection must be satellite based and all units should be of course easily portable. The units should tolerate a palette drop from a relief aircraft and should work as soon as activated. The power needs should be minimal and readily supported by solar panels. The software should be open access and highly intuitive to minimize computer support and training. The training modules should be highly detailed for the support personnel who might be back at a command unit; however, for the forward or first responders, the training should be just in time employing the best in educational principles. The telemedicine unit should be dispatched with the first medical relief materials and personnel.

7. Telemedicine systems and programs for disaster response should be heavily employed in all training exercises and be thoroughly familiar to the early responders.

8. There should be an urgent effort to broaden the telemedicine community to include colleagues already working in areas at risk for disruption. Virtual communities of medical workers connected by telemedicine should be in place so that the nearest area of intact services after a disaster could provide the first telemedicine support rather than all support coming form another continent. If telemedicine systems are in place in an area of disaster they could be activated to contact colleagues with appropriate expertise and familiar working relationships very early while the medical workers in a disrupted region are waiting for relief supplies. Some level of telemedicine access should be prepositioned in daily clinical practice such that the people in the challenged area can immediately report their needs and telemedicine can respond with information and consultation. The widely dispersed units cannot be as sophisticated as those kits prepared for relief efforts. The power needs and telecom needs should be simple and achievable even very early in the response. This may include satellite phones for a large medical facility and generator power.

Battery or solar backup should be available at every clinic with a laptop, camera and phone. The knapsack example from Pakistan is quite instructive. Furthermore, in that case the establishment of an extended telemedicine community made it very much more likely that contact with the outside world would happen early in the process. In order for the telemedicine community to grow as an inclusive and personal asset for health workers around the world community should work aggressively to make itself available by e-mail and any other means to collaborate as a part of our daily lives. Then in the event of a disaster established professional contacts are immediately available for support.

9. *For reconstruction of medical systems, the telemedicine community should be prepared to share distance learning, curriculum, advice, collegiality, consultation, conferences, webcasts and cognitive material appropriate to the region and situation.* Surely someone will be there on the ground but they should be the representatives of a huge community of individuals and programs with the telecommunications and information capability to help in substantive ways to electronically embrace a disabled system with the competence and compassion of colleagues anywhere in the world. In order to do this the telemedicine community should be informed of the issue of reconstruction and ready to provide electronic solutions where applicable. White papers written by the telemedicine community reflecting experience and consensus conferences would be an excellent start.

Nine simple recommendations are easy to write. They represent a huge effort not yet initiated by either the telemedicine community or the organizations responsible for relief of misery associated with war, natural disaster, isolation or civil breakdown. There are a lot of data and many experiences, positive and negative. Convergence of interests in this area could lead to a very quick formulation of a structural inclusion and thereby quantum improvement in the medical response to service disruption and massive injury.

Acknowledgements

We would like to thank Ms. Chasity Roberts for her editorial work with this chapter.

References

[1] Murphy RL, Bird KT. Telediagnosis: a new community health resource; observations on the feasibility of telediagnosis based on 1000 patient transactions. Am J Public Health. 1974 Feb;64(2):113-9.
[2] Garshnek V, Burkle FM Jr. Applications of telemedicine and telecommunications to disaster medicine: historical and future perspectives. J Am Med Inform Assoc. 1999 Jan-Feb;6(1):26-37.
[3] Nakajima I, Juzoji H, Wijarnpreecha S, Pichith K. The final report of the project 'AMINE' the Asia Pacific Medical Information Network using with ETS-V. Int J Med Inform. 2001 May;61(2-3):87-96.
[4] Dinerman T. Telemedicine and distance learning after the tsunami. Monday, January 10, 2005 The Space Review. http://www.thespacereview.com/article/301/1. Last accessed September 22, 2006.
[5] Indian Space Research Organization website http://isro.org/pressrelease/tsunami.htm. Last accessed September 22, 2006.
[6] International Telecommunication Union website. http://www.itu.int/ITU-D/CDS/newslog/index.asp? Article=775. Last accessed September 22, 2006.

[7] International Telecommunication Union website. http://www.itu.int/md/d02-rgq14.1.2-c-0045/e. A proposal for telemedicine package standardization. Last accessed September 22, 2006.

[8] Gomez E, Poropatich R, Karinch MA, Zajtchuk J. Tertiary telemedicine support during global military humanitarian missions. Telemed J. 1996 Fall;2(3):201-10.

[9] Morris TJ, Gilbert G, Patterson JM, Poropatich RK, Clerici DR, Hendricks CE, Calcagni D, Roller J. "SMART" technologies for anti-terrorism and homeland security. Telemed J E Health. 2003 Summer;9(2):223-6.

[10] Eliasson AH, Poropatich RK. Performance improvement in telemedicine: the essential elements. Mil Med. 1998 Aug;163(8):530-5.

[11] Poropatich CR, Detreville R, Lappan C, Barrigan CR. The u.s. Army telemedicine program: general overview and current status in southwest Asia. Telemed J E Health. 2006 Aug;12(4):396-408.

[12] Pruitt BA Jr. Trauma care in war and peace: the Army/AAST synergism: 1992 Fitts Lecture. J Trauma. 1993 Jul;35(1):78-87.

[13] Morris TJ, Pajak J, Havlik F, Kenyon J, Calcagni D. Battlefield Medical Information System-Tactical (BMIST): The Application of Mobile Computing Technologies to Support Health Surveillance in the Department of Defense. Telemed J E Health. 2006 Aug;12(4):409-16.

[14] Romano JA, Lam DM, Moses GR, Gilbert GR, Marchessault R. The future of military medicine has not arrived yet, but we can see it from here. Telemed J E Health. 2006 Aug;12(4):417-25.

[15] Simon DP, Thach AB, Bower KS. Teleophthalmology in the evaluation of ocular trauma. Mil Med. 2003 Mar;168(3):205-11.

[16] Pak HS, Harden D, Cruess D, Welch ML, Poropatich R; National Capital Area Teledermatology Consortium. Teledermatology: an intraobserver diagnostic correlation study, Part I. Cutis. 2003 May;71(5): 399-403.

[17] Pak HS, Harden D, Cruess D, Welch ML, Poropatich R; National Capital Area Teledermatology Consortium. Teledermatology: an intraobserver diagnostic correlation study, Part II. Cutis. 2003 Jun;71(6): 476-80.

[18] Pak HS. Implementing a teledermatology programme. J Telemed Telecare. 2005:11(6):285-93.

[19] Haegen TW, Cupp CC, Hunsaker DH. Teleotolaryngology: a retrospective review at a military tertiary treatment facility. Otolaryngol Head Neck Surg. 2004 May;130(5):511-8.

[20] Carmona RH. Military health care and telemedicine. Telemed J E Health. 2003 Summer;9(2):125-7.

[21] Lam DM, Mackenzie C. Human and organizational factors affecting telemedicine utilization within U.S. military forces in Europe. Telemed J E Health. 2005 Feb;11(1):70-8.

[22] Grady BJ, Melcer T. A retrospective evaluation of TeleMental Healthcare services for remote military populations. Telemed J E Health. 2005 Oct;11(5):551-8.

[23] Harcke HT, Statler JD, Montilla J. Radiology in a hostile environment: experience in Afghanistan. Mil Med. 2006 Mar;171(3):194-9.

[24] Melcer T, Crann B, Hunsaker D, Deniston W, Caola L. A retrospective evaluation of the development of a telemedicine network in a military setting. Mil Med. 2002 Jun;167(6):510-5

[25] Reed C, Burr R, Melcer T. Navy telemedicine: a review of current and emerging research models. Telemed J E Health. 2004 Fall;10(3):343-56.

[26] Lam DM, Poropatich RK, Gilbert GR. Telemedicine standardization in the NATO environment. Telemed J E Health. 2004 Winter;10(4):459-65.

[27] Labiris G, Tsitlakidis C, Niakas D. Retrospective economic evaluation of the Hellenic Air Force Teleconsultation Project. J Med Syst. 2005 Oct;29(5):493-500.

[28] Wadhams, N. U.N.: Iraq Civilian Deaths Hit a Record. http://abcnews.go.com/International/wireStory? id=2472447. Last accessed October 4, 2006.

[29] Benner T, Schachinger U, Nerlich M. Telemedicine in trauma and disasters–from war to earthquake: are we ready? Stud Health Technol Inform. 2004;104:106-15.

[30] The UN Refugee Agency website. http://www.unhcr.org/cgi-bin/texis/vtx/research. Last accessed September 21, 2006.

[31] Latifi R, Muja S, Bekteshi F, Merrell RC. The role of telemedicine and information technology in the redevelopment of medical systems: The case of Kosova. Telemed J E Health. 2006 Jun;12(3):332-40.

[32] Adopt-A-Minefield website. http://www.landmines.org/crisis/landmine_fact_sheet.cfm. Last accessed October 4, 2006.

[33] Center for International Rehabilitation website. http://www.cirnetwork.org. Last accessed October 4, 2006.

[34] Terra Daily website. http://www.terradaily.com/reports/Natural_Disasters_Killed_91_900_In_2005.html. Last accessed October 4, 2006.

[35] Patoli A. Role of Telemedicine in Disaster Management. eHealth International website. http://www.ehealthinternational.net/vol2num2/Vol2Num2p34.pdf. Last accessed October 4, 2006.

[36] Belard JL. Meeting Medical Challenges in a Changing World: The International Program of the U.S. Army Telemedicine and Advanced Technology Research Center (TATRC). Telemed J E Health. 2006 Aug;12(4):426-31.

[37] Simmons SC, Murphy TA, Blanarovich A, Workman FT, Rosenthal DA, Carbone M. Telehealth tech-nologies and applications for terrorism response: a report of the 2002 coastal North Carolina domestic preparedness training exercise. J Am Med Inform Assoc. 2003 Mar-Apr;10(2):166-76.

[38] Douglas B, Rafiq A, Merrell R, Hummel R. Integration of Information Technology and PDA for TACIT. Telemed J E Health. 2006;12(4):466-474.

[39] Teich JM, Wagner MM, Mackenzie CF, Schafer KO. The informatics response in disaster, terrorism, and war. J Am Med Inform Assoc. 2002 Mar-Apr;9(2):97-104.

[40] Yellowlees P, MacKenzie J. Telehealth responses to bio-terrorism and emerging infections. J Telemed Telecare. 2003;9 Suppl 2:S80-2.

[41] Harnett BM, Satava R, Angood P, Merriam NR, Doarn CR, Merrell RC. The benefits of integrating Internet technology with standard communications for telemedicine in extreme environments. Aviat Space Environ Med. 2001 Dec;72(12):1132-7.

[42] Angood PB, Satava R, Doarn C, Merrell R; E3 Group. Telemedicine at the top of the world: the 1998 and 1999 Everest extreme expeditions. Telemed J E Health. 2000 Fall;6(3):315-25.

[43] Satava R, Angood PB, Harnett B, Macedonia C, Merrell R. The physiologic cipher at altitude: tele-medicine and real-time monitoring of climbers on Mount Everest. Telemed J E Health. 2000 Fall;6(3): 303-13.

[44] Pillon S, Todini AR. eHealth in Antarctica: a model ready to be transferred to every-day life. Int J Cir-cumpolar Health. 2004 Dec;63(4):436-42.

[45] Grant IC. Telemedicine in the British Antarctic survey. Int J Circumpolar Health. 2004 Dec;63(4): 356-64.

[46] Williams J. Doctor battled for her life at the South Pole. USA Today.com http://www.usatoday.com/ weather/resources/coldscience/adrop0.htm.

[47] Nielson J, Vollers M. Ice Bound: A doctor's incredible Battle for Survival. Miramax Books, 2001.

[48] CBS Television movie, Ice Bound: A woman's survival at the South Pole. http://www.cbs.com/ specials/ice_bound/.

[49] Telemedicine gets mobile. Science in Africa, September 2004. http://www.scienceinafrica.co.za/2004/ september/telemedicine.htm. Last accessed October 4, 2006.

[50] Merrell RC, Merriam N, Doarn C. Information support for the ambulant health worker. Telemed J E Health. 2004 Winter;10(4):432-6.

[51] Lee S, Broderick TJ, Haynes J, Bagwell C, Doarn CR, Merrell RC. The role of low-bandwidth tele-medicine in surgical prescreening. J Pediatr Surg. 2003 Sep;38(9):1281-3.

[52] Mora F, Cone S, Rodas E, Merrell RC. Telemedicine and electronic health information for clinical con-tinuity in a mobile surgery program. World J Surg. 2006 Jun;30(6):1128-34.

[53] Cone SW, Gehr L, Hummel R, Merrell RC. Remote anesthetic monitoring using satellite telecommuni-cations and the Internet. Anesth Analg. 2006 May;102(5):1463-7.

[54] Rafiq A, Harnett B, Merrell G, Doarn C, Merrell R. Telemedicine Application during a search for Gen-ghis Khan in Mongolia. 9th Annual Meeting & Exposition of the American Telemedicine Association. Tampa, FL, May 2004. Telemed J E Health 10(Supp 1):S112, 2004.

[55] Cermack M. Monitoring and telemedicine support in remote environments and in human space flight. Br J Anaesth. 2006 Jul;97(1):107-14. Epub 2006 May 26.

[56] Grigoriev AI, Orlov OI. Telemedicine and spaceflight. Aviat Space Environ Med. 2002 Jul;73(7): 688-93.

[57] Feliciani F. Medical care from space: Telemedicine. ESA Bull. 2003 May;114:54-9.

[58] Kozlovskaya IB, Egorov AD. Some approaches to medical support for Martian expedition. Acta Astro-naut. 2003 Aug-Nov;53(4-10):269-75.

[59] Houtchens BA, Clemmer TP, Holloway HC, Kiselev AA, Logan JS, Merrell RC. Telemedicine and in-ternational disaster response: medical consultation to Armenia and Russia via a Telemedicine Space-bridge. Prehospital Disaster Med. 1993 Jan-Mar;8(1):57-66.

[60] NASA Extreme Environment Mission Operations (NEEMO) website. http://spaceflight.nasa.gov/ shuttle/support/training/neemo/neemo7.

[61] Schirber M. NEEMO's Undersea Operations: Making Telemedicine a Long Distance Reality. http://www.space.com/scienceastronomy/neemo_surgery_041019.html.

[62] Norum J, Moksness SG, Larsen E. A Norwegian study of seafarers' and rescuers' recommendations for maritime telemedicine services. J Telemed Telecare. 2002;8(5):264-9.

[63] Westlund K, Svard H. Radiomedical services for seafarers in Sweden. Int Marit Health. 2002; 53(1-4):59-66.

Current Principles and Practices of Telemedicine and e-Health
R. Latifi (Ed.)
IOS Press, 2008

Technologies for Complex and Critical Care Telemedicine

Laurence S. WILSON
CSIRO ICT Centre, Sydney, Australia

Abstract. While telemedicine is now well established in many areas of medical practice, it is only beginning to create impact in some of the more complex medical applications such as critical care. New systems based on advanced technologies such as the Virtual Critical Care Unit and the eICU have recently successfully demonstrated the provision of critical care services from a distance in emergency and intensive care respectively. These specialties make particular demands on a telemedicine system, and studies in computer supported collaborative work as well as studies of work practices suggest that there is a minimum threshold of technology complexity for supporting such applications. The eICU relies mainly on transmitting a rich data space to a remotely located specialist, while ViCCU® relies on creating a sense of presence. Other systems rely on complex physiological models. These approaches exemplify two trends in telemedicine systems of the future, with enhanced immersiveness creating a high sense of presence, and ready access to structured patient-specific data providing assistance to decision support. The future of telemedicine technology may see a convergence of these two trends.

Keywords. Broadband, critical care, telemedicine, telepresence

Introduction

Telemedicine (defined broadly as the provision of health care when not participants are co-located) is well established into many forms of medical practice in the early years of the 21st century [1]. But most applications continue to lag behind the possibilities being created by recent developments in communications and human computer interface [2] and two paradigms still dominate the majority of clinical telemedicine applications:

- Store and forward methods are extensively used for asynchronous, mainly image-based diagnosis such as radiology or pathology;
- Synchronous telemedicine consultations most frequently use industry-standard videoconferencing equipment as used extensively outside medicine (especially in business).

Consequently, these consultations often take place away from the point-of-care, and are conducted in a telemedicine 'suite' separate from the parts of a hospital where clinical care is delivered. Communication typically relies on readily-available infrastructure, and user interfaces (especially hardware) are not often tailored for their application, but are similar to those used already used in computer-based medicine (e.g. PACS) or for videoconferencing. The reliance on existing communications and interface infrastructure has contained costs, but has also constrained development of new technologies for delivering health care over a distance. A useful summary of realtime (mostly point-of-care) telemedicine was recently provided by Wootton [3].

A categorization of existing and emerging applications of telemedicine has been provided by Krupinski [4]. That paper identifies Radiology, Pathology, Psychiatry and Dermatology as mature telemedicine applications, while Surgery, Pediatrics, Emergency Medicine and Rare Diseases are seen as emerging application areas. From this list, the mature applications are seen to be mainly image-based techniques, with diagnosis based on inspection of one or more images together with some patient records, and occasionally involving consultation among physicians. The emerging application domains are generally more complex and multimodal in the information space they occupy, and may involve multiple medical workers working at the point of care in a time-critical environment.

This paper explores recent advances in the types of technology required to supply telemedicine services in complex medical care situations, especially critical care. *Critical care* refers to the treatment of patients in life-threatening situations, and conventionally includes the specialties of emergency medicine, intensive care medicine and anesthesiology. Telemedicine has often been used in emergency [5–9] and intensive care [10–12] applications, but few of these applications have been shown to be both sustainable and to substitute fully for the need for on-site expertise. Mostly, the technology has been based closely on that already used for less critical applications, rather than being built for purpose. Recently, several operational and commercial telemedicine systems have begun to address the special needs of the two sub-specialties of emergency medicine and intensive care medicine, using technology specifically designed for the application. There is considerable overlap in the needs of these two sub-specialties, and the similarities reflect the complexity of the clinical situations they address.

This paper describes the design, implementation, trialling and evaluation of the Virtual Critical Care Unit (ViCCU®) [13,14], which was designed by Australia's Commonwealth Scientific and Industrial Research Organisation (CSIRO) in close collaboration with Sydney West Area Health Service. This is compared with some other complex care technologies, notably the eICU [15], developed by the Visicu Corporation, and the Virtual Center for Regional Support [16,17], developed by the University of Seville. These special-purpose units have brought to complex and critical care, levels of technology commensurate with the complexity of the application domain.

While they share the characteristics of being more complex in their technology than many existing telemedicine systems, they are also representative of two classes of emerging systems which represent the next generation of such systems. An investigation of the similarities and difference between the approaches taken by these examples of new-generation technology gives considerable insight into the directions in which advanced telemedicine is evolving.

1. Current Developments

Critical care has unique characteristics that differentiate it from many other clinical domains of telehealth, and which make the achievement of remote diagnosis and care even more challenging:

- Critical care's work patterns and patient loads are variable and unpredictable, and clinicians work in a busy and sometimes noisy environment [11]. Telemedicine consultations can rarely be scheduled.
- Emergency medical care is delivered by highly trained and motivated teams working simultaneously on different aspects of treatment, although multitasking is also often necessary [18].
- Observations in Emergency Departments have shown that 80% of the time, team members are engaged in communications events, some of which might be overlapping conversations or involve multitasking. 90% of information transactions between team members involve informal communication and communication problems among roles are a significant source of inefficiency [19,20]. About 30% of verbal interactions take the form of interruptions.

For a specialist to correctly assess and treat a patient they require information from multiple sources in a timely manner; these sources include:

- Direct observation of the patient.
- The patient's medical record.
- Physiological monitoring data.
- Medical images.
- Reports and written notes.
- On-going observation in changes to the patient's condition by nursing staff caring for the patient.

Telemedicine has rarely been called on to support the form of team interaction encountered in critical care, especially emergency care. It has also rarely been called upon to support the generation and transmission to an entire care team, in real time, of information in as many forms as in emergency or intensive care; nor has it been required to support decision-making in a data space as complex as that encountered in critical care, especially intensive care. This is a direct consequence of the paradigms of "conventional" telemedicine, favoring simple person-to-person interaction or asynchronous access to structured electronic patient information.

A common desired outcome of telemedicine systems is an improvement in safety and quality in the health care provided, due to the ability to engage expertise located over a wider geographical area than the immediate facility. A measure of safety and quality is the incidence of medical errors, and medical errors in critical care have been the subject of a number of studies. For example, the National Academy of Sciences' Institute of Medicine noted that an ICU patient is more likely to experience an adverse event than a patients in other parts of the hospital [21]. Specific findings include a report of an average medical error incidence rate of two per patient per day in ICU [22], a 14% preventable death rate for three of the commonest conditions encountered in the ICU (cerebrovascular accident, pneumonia, or myocardial infarction) [23]; and an adverse drug event rate double that of non-ICU patients [24]. There are many possible technological solutions to the improvement of safety and quality, and access to expertise via telemedicine is regarded as an important component in reducing errors [25].

Telemedicine has been used in a number of projects to support critical care, although most have used general-purpose telemedicine systems and have actually been able to support only limited aspects of the complex process of critical care support [5,7,8,11,26]. However, these applications have not, in the main, been aimed at completely and transparently overcoming the distance between members of the support team. Rather, the philosophy has been to fill specific gaps in the information space which can be readily filled by the types of communication channel and user interface provided by commercially-available telemedicine systems.

Critical care telemedicine is characterized by a rich data space (heart rate and rhythm, blood pressure, central venous pressure, intracranial pressure, respiratory rate, oxygen saturation are routinely recorded continuously over periods of many hours), a need for constant interaction, and a need for constant decision-making with severe penalties for incorrect decisions. There is a level of incorrect decision-making which is already higher than in some other areas addressed by telemedicine. Support for decision making has been the subject of considerable research inside and outside the realm of telemedicine [27,28]. Advanced telemedicine systems offer the possibility of delivering clinical decision support by two independent means: automatic generation of advice or alarms based on access to electronic information, and access to human expertise located remotely.

2. Learnings from Telecollaboration Research

In the 1980s, telecollaboration in complex work situations was addressed by the theory of *media richness* [29,30]. This theory recognized that communication in organisational structures characterized by complexity and uncertainty required richer media channels for communicating the information required for those decisions. Richness in this case can be interpreted as supporting information flow which is both greater in magnitude (i.e. higher bandwidth) and supporting heterogeneity of media. Current studies in Computer Supported Collaborative Work point to the relationship between the media complexity and the type and extent of interaction required for a team to work successfully over multiple sites [31].

In recent years, the fields of Computer Supported Collaborative Work (CSCW) and Human Computer Interaction (HCI) have deepened our understanding of how humans collaborate over a distance, and with complex media. Surprisingly, this research has had little impact on telemedicine, and most applications of these technologies have been in such areas as surgery and surgical training [32–34]. As new technologies become available, telehealth has begun to look to the CSCW world for guidance on meeting new challenges [35].

At a very broad level, the requirements of a telemedicine system unique to the critical care environment can be summarized as supporting

- A level of personal interaction which supports the unique team dynamics of critical care.
- Access to data and information which is both timely and complete, in order to support decision-making.

While both requirements are important to the field of critical care telemedicine, emergency medicine relies more strongly on personal interactions, while the intensive care environment involves less team interaction, but the participants need to make decisions based on access to a very rich data space. We can interpret the CSCW literature as telling us that in order for a clinician to function in these environments in a way which is closely analogous to face-to-face, the technology for transmitting and presenting information needs to have a level of complexity well in excess of that employed in most current telemedicine applications. Such technology is now becoming available to telemedicine.

3. The Virtual Critical Care Unit (ViCCU®)

3.1. The Need

Australia's large distances and relatively small population have prompted many developments in telemedicine [36,37], and most States have extensive telemedicine networks based on bandwidths up to a few hundred kilobits per second. However, the delivery of more complex health care services has been limited by the available technology, and there has been minimal impact on, for example, Critical Care services. In 2001, Australia's Commonwealth Scientific and Industrial Research Organisation (CSIRO) commenced the CeNTIE (Centre for Networking Technologies for the Information Economy) project, supported by the Australian Department of Communications, Information Technology and the Arts. Members of a Focus Group set up as part of the CeNTIE process were asked to identify medical applications suited to the use of broad band networks, and not addressed by current telemedicine technologies. Provision of specialist services in Critical Care, especially in Emergency Departments in smaller hospitals, emerged as a need unmet by current technologies, and the CSIRO team worked with clinicians from Sydney West Area Health Service to develop the technology.

3.2. Design Process

The principal design objective was to create an environment in which a specialist at a major referral hospital could interact with and guide a team caring for a patient in an Emergency Department, in a manner which was as near as possible to actual physical presence. The stressful, time-critical nature of the work of the Emergency Department team demanded a system which satisfied the following requirements:

- Minimal impact on the usual work practices of the clinicians, particularly at the peripheral hospital.
- Easy to use and technologically transparent to doctors and nurses so that they able to focus on patient care, rather than dealing with technology.
- Robust, reliable continuous consultative services during the treatment.
- The use of a mobile trolley at the peripheral hospital allows the system to be shared among beds/departments.
- Low latency (time delay) for natural and immediate responses to questions and answers at both sides.
- Minimum on-site technical support to satisfy the unscheduled consultation requirement.

A highly user-centred design philosophy was adopted, and the system technical requirements were based closely on current work practices with a view to minimal impact on those practices; this was seen as a particular requirement of emergency telemedicine. The design was iterated using simulated scenarios to characterise the interactions among team members [38]. In order to facilitate the communication between sites, four cameras at the peripheral node were required, comprising:

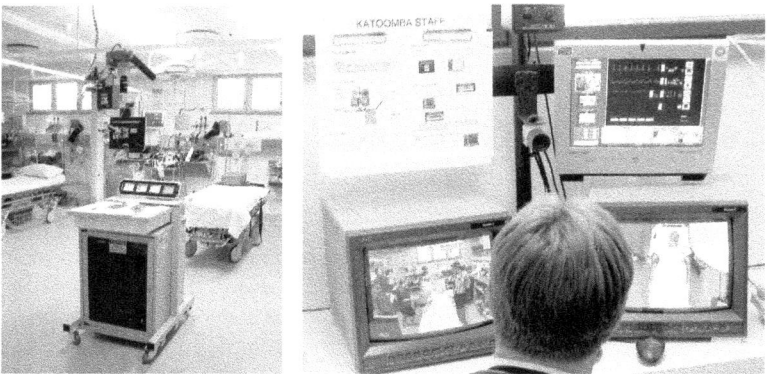

Figure 1. Virtual Critical Care Unit peripheral (left) and specialist (right) nodes.

- A room overview camera, giving the view the specialist would have if standing at the end of the patient's bed, and including the patient and attending team;
- A patient view camera, showing the patient's upper body seen from above;
- A mobile camera which can be moved into position for close-up views;
- A document camera, for medical images and paper-based records.

Additionally, the team at the peripheral node have a near life-size head-and-shoulders view of the specialist. High quality audio is provided by a single shotgun microphone at each end. The peripheral and specialist nodes are shown in Fig. 1.

Communications between the sites is provided by a dedicated optical-fibre connection supporting 100 Mbit/s communications. Thus video and audio are near-broadcast quality with imperceptible latency. The above technical specifications contribute to a high level of "presence" achieved with the system.

The system is designed to operate without any technical support, since all uses are unscheduled, and an "always-on" mode was adopted early in the project. This means that technical faults are usually detected before the system is required for clinical use, and this also promotes a sense of "one team over two sites," since staff at the two sites can interact casually as well as during episodes of critical care.

3.3. Implementation

In December 2003, a clinical trial using a prototype system commenced between two hospitals on the outskirts of Sydney: Nepean Hospital (a major tertiary referral Hospital located on the western edge of the Sydney metropolitan area) and Blue Mountains Anzac Memorial Hospital, located at Katoomba in the Blue Mountains a further 60km west of Nepean Hospital. The Katoomba Hospital is an 85-bed facility with minimal specialist coverage for its emergency department, and patients are often transferred to Nepean Hospital. During the two-year trial, over 500 uses of the system were logged. The trial was evaluated for clinical and technical effectiveness. In the technical evaluation [39], users of the system expressed high levels of satisfaction with its ability to engage specialists as if they were co-located with the patient (in the evaluation, only 6% of users expressed dissatisfaction with the design). A commercial version of the system is being developed.

3.4. Presence Studies

One of the main design principles was to create a high level of "presence" with ViCCU®, and during its evaluation, several users commented on this aspect of its use. The technical evaluation of ViCCU® included a quantification the degree of presence it achieved, and the role it played. Presence is the subject of a number of studies outside telemedicine, and several definitions exist. For example, Heeter [40] recognizes three aspects/dimensions of presence:

- Physical presence: the sense of being in one place or environment.
- Social presence: the feeling of being connected to other people in the place or environment.
- Environmental presence: the extend to which the environment itself appears to know that you are there and reacts to you.

Since ViCCU® aims to create a system that gave clinicians located in a rural hospital the feeling that the specialist located in a major hospital was physically present at the end of the bed, we focused our initial study on the physical aspect of presence.

Following the decision to focus on physical presence, we chose to adopt an extension of Witmer & Singer's definition of presence for this study [41]. That is: 'the subjective experience of being, or someone else who is remotely located being, in a place or environment, even when they are physically situated in another.' The instrument used was the SUS Presence measure [42], administered to 50 system users comprising nursing and medical staff from the two hospitals. This study was incorporated into an overall study of the design success of ViCCU®, which indicated a high level of satisfaction with the design (see above) [39]. There was evidence in this study that the high level of satisfaction experienced by users of ViCCU® was related to its ability to create a sense of presence. Physical presence is usually regarded as the "gold standard" for collaborating over a distance, but surprisingly, a significant proportion of users of ViCCU®, especially those in the peripheral hospital, expressed a preference for virtual presence of the specialist over actual physical presence. This confirms that the level of presence achieved in ViCCU® is an important factor in its apparent success with users.

From this study, the Virtual Critical Care Unit appears to have achieved its aim of effectively substituting for the physical presence of a specialist in a wide range of situations encountered in the Emergency Department of a small hospital. It has achieved this through using technology which provides not only rich diagnostic information, but also a sense of presence which facilitates collaborative work in this difficult environment.

4. Complex Data Systems

4.1. The eICU

The eICU [15] was developed during the 1990s in response to a perceived shortage of intensivists with the skills required to provide to provide care with the highest standards of safety and quality in all locations. It is designed to relieve the on-site attending physician of major decision-making responsibilities by providing a specialist intensivist located remotely with sufficient information to make these decisions. Information transmitted to the intensivist includes real-time invasive and non-invasive vital signs (exactly as they appear on the bedside monitoring screen), a complete electronic medical record, a clinical decision support tool, high-resolution radiographic images, and teleconferencing into the ICU.

Cameras in the patient room provide multiple views of the patient and the room, and may be programmed to view instrumentation such ventilator screens or infusion pumps. They also provide the intensivist with the ability to make diagnoses based on patient appearance, including neurologic function, respiratory efforts, facial expression and skin colour. There is also the option of assisting bedside staff with procedures, although the intention is not to create a sense of presence, but to augment the data flow with views of the patient and the patient's environment.

Interaction with the data flow from the patient's bedside is one of the most important distinguishing features of the eICU. The system maintains a dynamic, structured electronic record of vital signs by capturing data from a variety of bedside instruments. This allows the intensivist to use data manipulation tools to review trends and exceptional events in the patient's vital signs. The system incorporates decision support tools which may be programmed to alert the intensivist or the physician attending the patient of a range of situations requiring intervention, based on combinations of vital signs falling outside acceptable ranges.

The eICU has proven its value in augmenting local expertise with specialist intensivist expertise located in a small number of central locations. For example, Leong et al noted a significantly reduced mortality rate (from 12.9% to 9.4%) after the introduction of the eICU, as well as a reduction in hospital costs [43,44]. It has been successfully used for providing care over intercontinental distances using a base station located in the Tripler hospital in Honolulu, Hawaii connected to a clinic in Guam, 5300 km distant [45].

4.2. The Virtual Center for Renal Support

Systems which monitor well-defined, complex physical processes may do more than visualise or even analyse complex, multiparameter data. A physical model (anatomical or physiological) can form the basis on which data is represented to the distant physician. Such a situation occurs in renal dialysis, where complex physiological processes need to be monitored against patient-specific hemodynamic and pharmacokinetic models. The Virtual Center for Renal Support (VCRS) has been developed to provide monitoring from a distance of the complex physiology underlying renal dialysis [16,17]. In particular, a specialist using this system will be able to monitor patients receiving dialysis away from major centres, or even in their own homes. The usual vital signs measurements are supplemented by frequent biochemical analyses. This information becomes the input for a physics-based model of the patient's urea kinetic and water flows between major human pools (vascular, interstitial and cellular) and can be used in a decision support mode to predict and prevent adverse events such a hypovolemia. The system reduces the complex array of data to a simple visual display which illustrates the patient's physiological state, using physics-based mathematical models. The bandwidth requirements of such systems are small (telephone lines are adequate), and there is seen to be no need for human-human interaction. But the data space is sufficiently complex that sophisticated algorithms and visualisation techniques are employed in order to produce a representation of this space which supports decision-making by a remote physician.

5. Comparison of ViCCU® and Data-Rich Systems

5.1. Design Philosophies

The systems described in this paper are technically advanced systems for providing telemedicine support in complex and Critical Care. They take advantage of recent advances in information and communications technologies to provide a richer information space than previously considered necessary for telemedicine, and this is commensurate with the relatively complex medical environment they support.

Each system has chosen to extend the information available to clinicians in a different form, and it is instructive to consider the complementarities of the two approaches. The eICU does not attempt to create a sense of presence for the physicians as its video system is comparable to existing telemedicine, and most installed systems do not even include a view of the specialist, since such a view does not convey any diagnostic information. The VCRS focuses entirely on physiological parameters. By contrast, ViCCU® has been designed almost entirely around creating a sense of telepresence, with multiple cameras and two-way video communication. The media quality of ViCCU® is well beyond that previously reported as being essential for diagnostic purposes [46], and contributes to the ability of the specialist and the other workers to form a team. There is not usually time for the specialist to consider large amounts of information, and this is restricted to that which reaches the specialist verbally from team members or via a direct view of patient or instruments. Thus the ViCCU® is a transparent window into the world of the emergency department, and there is no facility for storing or analyzing information.

The eICU and VCRS have taken advantage of the ability of medical information systems to record, analyze and visualize complex medical information using structured databases. Intensive care is characterized by a large quantity of data, much of which is generated automatically as continuous records and therefore containing information which might not necessarily be brought to the attention of the intensivist. These systems make a complex data space available to a remotely located specialist, as well at to the local physicians and have some capabilities to analyze and filter this data and provide alerts or decision support.

In order to meet the challenges of these two varieties of critical care, these two systems can be thought of as advancing telehealth in two orthogonal directions. ViCCU® is "presence-rich" but relatively data-poor, while eICU and VCRS are data-rich, but does little to advance physical presence beyond current practice. A clinician dealing with a patient in Critical Care has to be aware information which is presented in two forms:

- Information closely associated with physical presence; this includes the appearance and demeanor of the patient, their physically apparent signs, the way they speak and response to stimuli including palpation; the information conveyed verbally by other carers.
- Information converted into electronic form related to the patient's electronic record; this can include notes and previous observations, as well as continuous records of vital signs related to physiology, including body chemistry. This "electronic space" is sometimes processed in a complex form in order to create a virtual space constructed from patient data. In the case of the VCRS, this takes the form of a graphical representation of a physiological model, inferred through mathematical modeling from physiological data. The data visualisa-

Table 1. Classification of advanced telemedicine systems

	Physical Telepresence	Data space	Virtual Data Presence
ViCCU®	**		
eICU	*	*	*
VCRS		*	**

tion can also be anatomical rather than physical, in which case the data consists of medical images, which construct a virtual physical space used for computer-guided surgery [47]. The distinction between physical and data spaces can become blurred, especially when they are combined in applications of augmented reality [48].

A clinician dealing with a patient face-to-face needs to be highly aware of events occurring in both the physical space (inspection, palpation, interview etc) and the data space (medical records and measurements). The medical world is not unique, and this is a common situation explored in the CSCW world. If the clinician is to perform the same function from a remote location, the system needs to reproduce his/her access to those two spaces.

This is summarized in Table 1, in which the interaction with modeled data is referred to as *virtual data presence*, suggesting that such a rich visualisation of a data space corresponds in some ways to physical presence. Its closest analogy in the telepresence literature [40] is *environmental presence* (see Section 3.4 above).

6. Future Telemedicine Systems

6.1. Advanced Telepresence in Medicine

A device such as ViCCU®, while relying on telepresence for its impact on health care delivery, is in many ways an extension of the videoconferencing paradigm. The main extension of that paradigm is in the use of high media quality and multiple video channels. The expansion of broadband networks, spurred by initiatives such as Internet2 [49], is permitting the transmission of more complex information types between two collaborating sites, leading to enhanced telepresence. User interfaces which interact more fully with the body's sensory space are creating a heightened sense of immersion; this can occur through occupying a greater proportion of a particular sensory space, such as 360 degree visual fields [50], or interacting simultaneously with several senses. In the latter case, visual and audio interaction can be supplemented by "haptic," or force-feedback interaction with a non-collocated object [51]. Manipulation of the remote environment by robotic means is already in use in some areas of surgery [52]. Where they contribute to the efficacy of treatment and diagnosis, these technologies are certain to find their way into routine telemedicine, provided the technology is matched to the task and is cost-effective for that task.

6.2. Data-Rich Environments

The healthcare environment is becoming increasingly rich in data and knowledge deliverable in electronic form. Much of this information is patient-specific (as manifested in Electronic Medical Records), but clinicians also rely on such information as established best-practice criteria evidence-based guidelines or contra-indications for drug administration. Optimum diagnosis and treatment of patients demands that both types of information are available to clinicians when they make their decisions. This is especially important in critical care, because of the time-criticality of decision-making. The availability of this information to the clinician at the point of care is limited mainly by the ability to provide access to the information using advanced computer-human interfaces [53], but it is likely to become increasingly difficult to practice many forms of medicine at an acceptably high standard without such ubiquitous, secure access to electronic information.

Historically, while telemedicine and informatics are together regarded as constituting "e-Health," their development and communities of interest have been separate, and their convergence is long overdue.

6.3. Convergence

The ICT infrastructure which can provide telemedicine support at the point of care is also ideally suited to providing access to electronic information. The challenges of mobility and human computer interface are common to both types of application, and the desired outcomes of both types are common, i.e. to provide access at the point of care to information which will positively influence the course of treatment for a patient. If some of this information is machine-generated, it creates an environment in which human expertise is used only for those higher-level judgments which cannot be generated by machine.

It is highly likely that information and communication systems will continue to converge, and future telemedicine systems will incorporate shared access to highly tailored information. The research challenges exist in such areas as creating an environment in which information from many disparate sources can be brought together seamlessly, and creating means for human interaction with a complex data space, and creating systems which are "smart" enough to bring to the attention of the local physician only that information which complements his/her capabilities. In future systems, physicians will be able to engage and interact with remote physical spaces, as well as virtual spaces composed of visualizations of patient-specific data. Medical knowledge will be automatically embedded in these virtual data spaces, facilitating rapid and accurate decision-making while reducing the likelihood of medical errors. The ViCCU® and other systems referred to in this paper are glimpses into different aspects of this future.

7. Conclusions

Telemedicine has proven its capabilities in applications requiring asynchronous applications or synchronous applications in relatively non-complex treatment settings. The expansion into more complex applications, especially critical care, has begun with the availability of new network architectures and interface technologies. The successful applications described above have shown that it is possible for the specialists who will make vital decisions in critical care to be located at some distance from the point of care. An analysis of the key enabling technologies for these applications is enlightening in pointing the way to telemedicine addressing more complex application domains. Enhanced sense of presence enables teams to function over more than one site in a seamless fashion with a high sense of trust, while access to a rich data space reduces the chance of human error. Further enhancement and convergence of these technologies will enable even more complex medical services to be delivered independent of the location of specialist and patient.

8. Acknowledgements

The Virtual Critical Care Unit was the result of a major team effort between staff of the CSIRO ICT Centre and Sydney West Area Health Service.

Members of the CSIRO team included Tony Adriaansen, Leila Alem, Keith Bengston, Steve Broadhurst, Michael Hogan, Susan Hansen, Rosemary Hollowell, Alex Krumm-Heller, Jane Li, Alija Kajan, Neil Killeen, Alex Murdoch, Terry Percival, Rong-Yu Qiao, Bob Shields and Bob Tyler.

The Sydney West Area Health Service team included Patrick Cregan, Stuart Stapleton and Monique Murphy.

CeNTIE (the Centre for Networking Technologies for the Information Economy) is supported by the CSIRO and the Australian Department of Communications, Information Technology and the Arts.

Development of the Virtual Critical Care Unit was supported by a grant from New South Wales Health.

References

[1] W. Grigsby, *2004 TRC Report on US Telemedicine Activity*. Kingston, NJ: Civic Research Institute, 2006.

[2] H. Tanriverdi and C.S. Iacono, "Diffusion of telemedicine: a knowledge barrier perspective," *Telemed J.*, vol. 5, no. 3, pp. 223-244, 1999.

[3] R. Wootton, "Realtime telemedicine," *J Telemed Telecare.*, vol. 12, no. 7, pp. 328-336, 2006.

[4] E. Krupinski, M. Nypaver, R. Poropatich, D. Ellis, R. Safwat, and H. Sapci, "Telemedicine/telehealth: an international perspective. Clinical applications in telemedicine/telehealth," *Telemed. J. E. Health.*, vol. 8, no. 1, pp. 13-34, 2002.

[5] J.A. Brennan, J.A. Kealy, L.H. Gerardi, R. Shih, J. Allegra, L. Sannipoli, and D. Lutz, "Telemedicine in the emergency department: a randomized controlled trial," *J. Telemed. Telecare.*, vol. 5, no. 1, pp. 18-22, 1999.

[6] R. Latifi, K. Peck, J.M. Porter, R. Poropatich, T. Geare, III, and R.B. Nassi, "Telepresence and telemedicine in trauma and emergency care management," *Stud Health Technol Inform*, vol. 104, pp. 193-199, 2004.

[7] F.B. Rogers, M. Ricci, M. Caputo, S. Shackford, K. Sartorelli, P. Callas, J. Dewell, and S. Daye, "The use of telemedicine for real-time video consultation between trauma center and community hospital in a rural setting improves early trauma care: preliminary results," *J. Trauma*, vol. 51, no. 6, pp. 1037-1041, Dec. 2001.

[8] E.M. Brebner, J.A. Brebner, H. Ruddick-Bracken, R. Wootton, and J. Ferguson, "Evaluation of a pilot telemedicine network for accident and emergency work," *J. Telemed. Telecare.*, vol. 8 Suppl 2, pp. 5-6, 2002.

[9] J.P. Marcin, D.E. Schepps, K.A. Page, S.N. Struve, E. Nagrampa, and R.J. Dimand, "The use of telemedicine to provide pediatric critical care consultations to pediatric trauma patients admitted to a remote trauma intensive care unit: a preliminary report," *Pediatr. Crit Care Med.*, vol. 5, no. 3, pp. 251-256, May 2004.

[10] B.L. Grundy, P. Crawford, P.K. Jones, M.L. Kiley, A. Reisman, Y. H. Pao, E.L. Wilkerson, and J.S. Gravenstein, "Telemedicine in critical care: an experiment in health care delivery," *JACEP*, vol. 6, no. 10, pp. 439-444, Oct. 1977.

[11] S. Kaplan and G. Fitzpatrick, "Designing support for remote intensive-care telehealth using the locales framework," in *Proceedings of the conference on Designing interactive systems: processes, practices, methods, and techniques* Amsterdam, The Netherlands: ACM Press, 1997, pp. 173-184.

[12] P.E. Shile, H.L. Kundel, S.B. Seshadri, B. Carey, S. Kishore, I. Brikman, E. Feingold, P.N. Lanken, and J.A. Purcell, "Factors affecting the electronic communication of radiological information to an intensive-care unit," *J Telemed Telecare.*, vol. 2, no. 4, pp. 199-204, 1996.

[13] P. Cregan, S. Stapleton, L. Wilson, R.Y. Qiao, J. Li, and T. Percival, "The ViCCU Project – achieving virtual presence using Ultrabroadband internet in a Critical Clinical application – initial results," *Stud Health Technol Inform*, vol. 111, pp. 94-98, 2005.

[14] J. Li, L.S. Wilson, R.Y. Qiao, T. Percival, A. Krumm-Heller, S. Stapleton, and P. Cregan, "Development of a broadband telehealth system for critical care: process and lessons learned," *Telemed J E. Health.*, vol. 12, no. 5, pp. 552-560, Oct. 2006.

[15] L.A. Celi, E. Hassan, C. Marquardt, M. Breslow, and B. Rosenfeld, "The eICU: it's not just telemedicine," *Crit Care Med.*, vol. 29, no. 8 Suppl, p. N183-N189, Aug. 2001.

[16] M. Prado, L. Roa, J. Reina-Tosina, A. Palma, and J.A. Milan, "Virtual center for renal support: technological approach to patient physiological image," *IEEE Trans. Biomed. Eng.*, vol. 49, no. 12, pp. 1420-1430, Dec. 2002.

[17] M. Prado, L. Roa, J. Reina-Tosina, A. Palma, and J.A. Milan, "Renal telehealthcare system based on a patient physiological image: a novel hybrid approach in telemedicine," *Telemed J E. Health.*, vol. 9, no. 2, pp. 149-165, 2003.

[18] K. Williams, W. Rose, and R. Simon, "Team work in Emergency Medical Services," *Air Med J*, vol. 18, pp. 149-153, 1999.

[19] E.W. Coiera, R.A. Jayasuriya, J. Hardy, A. Bannan, and M.E. Thorpe, "Communication loads on clinical staff in the emergency department," *Med J Aust.*, vol. 176, no. 9, pp. 415-418, May 2002.

[20] E. Coiera and V. Tombs, "Communication behaviours in a hospital setting: an observational study," *BMJ*, vol. 316, no. 7132, pp. 673-676, Feb. 1998.

[21] *To Err is Human: Building a Safer Health System.* Washington, DC: National Academy Press, 1999.

[22] Y. Donchin, D. Gopher, M. Olin, Y. Badihi, M. Biesky, C.L. Sprung, R. Pizov, and S. Cotev, "A look into the nature and causes of human errors in the intensive care unit," *Crit Care Med.*, vol. 23, no. 2, pp. 294-300, Feb. 1995.

[23] R.W. Dubois and R.H. Brook, "Preventable deaths: Who, how often, and why?," *Ann Intern Med*, vol. 109, pp. 582-589, 1988.

[24] D. Cullen, B. Sweitzer, and et al., "Preventable adverse drug events in hospitalized patients: A comparative study of intensive care and general care units," *Crit Care Med*, vol. 25, pp. 1289-1297, 1997.

[25] K.S. Rheuban, "The role of telemedicine in fostering health-care innovations to address problems of access, specialty shortages and changing patient care needs," *J Telemed Telecare.*, vol. 12 Suppl 2, pp. 45-50, 2006.

[26] S. Tachakra, U.C. Uko, and A. Stinson, "Four years' experience of telemedicine support of a minor accident and treatment service," *J. Telemed. Telecare.*, vol. 8 Suppl 2, pp. 87-89, 2002.

[27] B. Nannings and A. bu-Hanna, "Characterizing decision support telemedicine systems," *Methods Inf. Med.*, vol. 45, no. 5, pp. 523-527, 2006.

[28] K. Kawamoto, C.A. Houlihan, E.A. Balas, and D.F. Lobach, "Improving clinical practice using clinical decision support systems: a systematic review of trials to identify features critical to success," *BMJ*, vol. 330, no. 7494, p. 765, Apr. 2005.

[29] A.R. Dennis and S.T. Kinney, "Testing Media Richness Theory in the New Media: the Effects of Cues, Feedback, and Task Equivocality," *Information Systems Research*, vol. 9, no. 3, pp. 256-274, 1998.

[30] R.L. Daft and R.H. Lengel, "Organizational Information Requirements, Media Richness and Structural Design," *Management Science*, vol. 32, no. 5, pp. 554-571, 1986.

[31] B.A. Nardi, "Beyond Bandwidth: Dimensions of Connection in Interpersonal Communication," *Comput Supported Coop Work*, vol. 14, pp. 91-130, 2005.

[32] B.M. Cameron and R.A. Robb, "Virtual-reality-assisted interventional procedures," *Clin. Orthop. Relat Res.*, vol. 442, pp. 63-73, Jan. 2006.

[33] R.M. Satava, "Accomplishments and challenges of surgical simulation," *Surg. Endosc.*, vol. 15, no. 3, pp. 232-241, Mar. 2001.

[34] B.K. Wiederhold and M.D. Wiederhold, "The future of cybertherapy: improved options with advanced technologies," *Stud Health Technol Inform.*, vol. 99, pp. 263-270, 2004.

[35] W. Pratt, M.C. Reddy, D.W. McDonald, P. Tarczy-Hornoch, and J.H. Gennari, "Incorporating ideas from computer-supported cooperative work," *J Biomed. Inform.*, vol. 37, no. 2, pp. 128-137, Apr. 2004.

[36] G.K. van, M.R. Haas, and R. Viney, "From flying doctor to virtual doctor: an economic perspective on Australia's telemedicine experience," *J Telemed. Telecare.*, vol. 8, no. 5, pp. 249-254, 2002.

[37] P.M. Yellowlees, "Intelligent health systems and third millennium medicine in Australia," *Telemed J*, no. 2, pp. 197-200, 2000.

[38] G. Weerakkody and P. Ray, "CSCW-based system development methodology for health-care information systems," *Telemed. J E. Health.*, vol. 9, no. 3, pp. 273-282, 2003.

[39] J. Li, L.S. Wilson, S. Hansen, R.-Y. Qiao, A. Krumm-Heller, S. Stapleton, P. Cregan, and M. Murphy, "Meeting user needs for quality – design and technical evaluation of a telehealth system for critical care," in *The Second IASTED Conference on Telehealth*. F. Pinciroli, Ed. Anaheim: ACTA Press, 2006, pp. 44-48.

[40] C. Heeter, "Being there: the subjective experience of presence," *Presence: Teleoperators and Virtual environments*, vol. 1(2), pp. 262-271, 2006.

[41] B.G. Witmer and M.J. Singer, "Measuring Presence in Virtual Environments: A Presence Questionnaire," *Presence: Teleoperators & Virtual Environments*, vol. 7, no. 3, pp. 225-240, 1998.

[42] M. Slater, M. Usoh, and A. Steed, "Depth of presence in virtual environments," *Presence: Teleoperators in Virtual Environments*, vol. 3, pp. 130-144, 1994.

[43] M.J. Breslow, B.A. Rosenfeld, M. Doerfler, G. Burke, G. Yates, D.J. Stone, P. Tomaszewicz, R. Hochman, and D.W. Plocher, "Effect of a multiple-site intensive care unit telemedicine program on clinical and economic outcomes: an alternative paradigm for intensivist staffing," *Crit Care Med.*, vol. 32, no. 1, pp. 31-38, Jan. 2004.

[44] J.R. Leong, C.A. Sirio, and A.J. Rotondi, "eICU program favorably affects clinical and economic outcomes," *Crit Care.*, vol. 9, no. 5, p. E22, Sept. 2005.

[45] B.W. Berg, D.S. Vincent, and D.A. Hudson, "Remote critical care consultation: telehealth projection of clinical specialty expertise," *J. Telemed. Telecare.*, vol. 9 Suppl 2, pp. S9-11, 2003.

[46] D.G. Ellis, J. Mayrose, and M. Phelan, "Consultation times in emergency telemedicine using realtime videoconferencing," *J Telemed Telecare.*, vol. 12, no. 6, pp. 303-305, 2006.

[47] D.T. Gering, A. Nabavi, R. Kikinis, N. Hata, L.J. O'Donnell, W.E. Grimson, F.A. Jolesz, P.M. Black, and W.M. Wells, III, "An integrated visualization system for surgical planning and guidance using image fusion and an open MR," *J Magn Reson. Imaging.*, vol. 13, no. 6, pp. 967-975, June 2001.

[48] T.M. Peters, "Image-guidance for surgical procedures," *Phys. Med Biol.*, vol. 51, no. 14, p. R505-R540, July 2006.

[49] M. Kratz, M. Ackerman, T. Hanss, and S. Corbato, "Ngi and Internet2: accelerating the creation of tomorrow's internet," *Medinfo.*, vol. 10, no. Pt 1, pp. 28-32, 2001.

[50] C. Demiralp, C.D. Jackson, D.B. Karelitz, S. Zhang, and D.H. Laidlaw, "CAVE and fishtank virtual-reality displays: a qualitative and quantitative comparison," *IEEE Trans. Vis. Comput Graph.*, vol. 12, no. 3, pp. 323-330, May 2006.

[51] M. Hutchins, S. O'Leary, D. Stevenson, C. Gunn, and A. Krumpholz, "A networked haptic virtual environment for teaching temporal bone surgery," *Stud Health Technol Inform.*, vol. 111, pp. 204-207, 2005.

[52] M. Anvari, C. McKinley, and H. Stein, "Establishment of the world's first telerobotic remote surgical service: for provision of advanced laparoscopic surgery in a rural community," *Ann Surg.*, vol. 241, no. 3, pp. 460-464, Mar. 2005.

[53] R. Gururajan, C. Moloney, and J. Soar, "Challenges for implementing wireless hand-held technology in health care: views from selected Queensland nurses," *J Telemed Telecare.*, vol. 11 Suppl 2, p. S37-S38, 2005.

Current Principles and Practices of Telemedicine and e-Health
R. Latifi (Ed.)
IOS Press, 2008
131

Intensive Care Telemedicine: Evaluating a Model for Proactive Remote Monitoring and Intervention in the Critical Care Setting

Robert H. GROVES Jr., MD, FCCP, Barry W. HOLCOMB Jr., MD, FCCP, and Marshall L. SMITH, MD, PhD, FACOG
Banner Health, Phoenix, Arizona

Abstract. Historically, telemedicine has focused on the application of traditional physician-to-patient (and physician-to-physician) interactions enhanced by two-way video and audio capability. This "one-on-one" interaction via a telemedicine link can dramatically extend a physician's or other caregiver's geographic range and availability. However, this same telemedicine model is most often implemented "on-demand" for a specified time-limited encounter. The remote Intensive Care Unit (ICU) model to be described similarly expands the geographic range of ICU physicians, but also allows a single specialist to simultaneously monitor multiple patients on a continuous basis by leveraging computerized "intelligent" algorithms and an electronic medical record interface. This new application of telemedicine wedded to computer technology facilitates maximum leveraging of specialists' cognitive skills but also mandates significant process changes in how ICU services are provided. In short, the remote ICU represents a "re-engineering" of how ICU care is delivered and establishes a new paradigm for the field of telemedicine, expanding the reach, scope and availability of intensivist specialty expertise.

The re-engineering occurs through a number of ways. First, the telemedicine connection is continuously available in a pro-active fashion that can be provided 24 hours a day, 7 days a week (24/7). Secondly, the system utilizes computerized clinical intelligence algorithms with direct electronic links to physiologic, laboratory and lab/pharmacy data as well as patient diagnoses to focus attention on potential adverse outcomes or trends in individual patients and notify caregivers before trends manifest as adverse outcomes. Third, the traditional physician, nurse, and patient relationship is substantially augmented when there is an ICU physician immediately available to address issues in patient care, particularly at night when physicians are less likely to be present at the bedside. The current preliminary data suggest that this system can be quite effective in improving ICU quality of care, thus leading to reductions in the cost of ICU care, ICU patient mortality, ICU patient outliers, and ICU length of stay (LOS).

Given the extensive data showing improved ICU outcomes with daily ICU physician participation in care of critically ill patients, and the national shortage of ICU physicians, nurses, and ancillary staff; the electronic ICU system is gaining popularity as an alternative paradigm for the expansion of an ICU team's expertise in the care of the severely ill. Interestingly, internal Quality Improvement (QI) data from several healthcare systems have shown that improved outcomes occur even when remote ICU telemedicine is applied to a pre-existing 24/7 in-house intensivist care model. The reasons for this remain speculative at this point, but pro-active and hourly remote "virtual rounds" on the most critically-ill patients, and use of computerized algorithms in triaging ICU physicians' attention may contribute to the success of this system. Also, we will show how the system supports key elements of error reduction theory even in well-staffed critical care units.

Multiple challenges remain before remote ICU systems become more broadly accepted and applied. These include cost of implementation of the system, resistance to the system by ICU physicians and nurses, and integration of data systems and clinical information into the remote electronic ICU model. In this chapter, we will provide background information on error reduction theory and the role of the remote ICU model, review current data supporting use of the remote ICU system, address the current obstacles to effective implementation, and look to the future of the field for solutions to these challenges.

Keywords. Telemedicine, ICU, remote critical care, aging population, physician shortage, mortality rate reduction

1. Current Problems in Critical Care

1.1. Shortage of ICU Staffing and the Role of the Remote ICU

In the past decade there has been a dramatic rise in the demand for ICU services. Average life expectancy has increased, and estimates predict that by the year 2020 the population in the United States age 65 and older will increase by 50%. Additionally, estimates predict that this same population will increase by 100% by the year 2030 [1]. As the average age of the population continues to increase, the demand for critical care services is expected to rise rapidly. Technologic advances in the field of ICU medicine have allowed opportunities for health care professionals to prolong life and reduce morbidity even in the advanced stages of many diseases, including COPD, coronary artery disease, renal failure, and cancer. Furthermore, conditions such as severe pneumonia, sepsis, gastrointestinal hemorrhage and multi-organ failure are far more common in an elderly population and often require intensive care services.

The shortage of trained intensivists is now broadly recognized and is expected to worsen significantly in the coming years as recently reported through an analysis from the Health Resources and Services Administration (HRSA). Durbin et al. reported this data regarding the severity of the shortage of ICU physicians and staff at the Critical Care Workforce Partnership in 2006. This HRSA data reports that the current full-time ICU physician workforce in the United States is made up of approximately 2000 full-time intensivist physicians, and this number is expected to increase to about 2,800 by the year 2020, still falling far below the HRSA benchmark number of 4,800 full-time ICU physicians. These numbers along with other compounding factors reinforce a continuing overall shortage of full-time ICU-trained physicians in the US [1]. In 2000 the Committee on Manpower for Pulmonary and Critical Care Societies (COMPACCS) reported that demand for ICU physicians will grow rapidly while supply either remains near constant or declines, leading to a shortfall of ICU physician hours equal to 22% of demand by 2020 and 35% by 2030 [2]. Some in the field believe that we ought to have on-site intensivists in every ICU 24/7. If we apply this higher standard, an estimated 30,000 full-time intensivists would be required. Given these present and anticipated shortages in ICU health care professionals, it is apparent that alternative methods to provide high-quality care for critically ill patients are necessary.

The emergence of telemedicine technology, specifically remote, computer-based ICU monitoring, involving round-the-clock coverage by ICU physicians and nurses, is a potentially valuable resource to alleviate the staffing constraints we currently encounter in the care of ICU patients.

1.2. Unacceptable Frequency of Adverse Events

It is clear that there are pressing reasons based on shortages alone to consider alternative ways to leverage the cognitive expertise of ICU physicians and nurses across an expanding underserved population of critically ill patients. There are also cogent arguments to support the remote ICU concept as a means to reduce errors in medicine and improve the reliability of ICU care independent of the issues surrounding the caregiver shortage. Medical errors are now widely recognized as a major cause of morbidity and mortality, and the reliability of medical care has come under increasing scrutiny from all parties with a stake in the care delivery process. When optimally implemented, the remote ICU concept can play a significant role in supporting key elements of error reduction theory.

In 1994 Leape et al. published an article analyzing and discussing the nature and prevention of errors in the delivery of medical care, including the care of critically-ill ICU patients [3]. He postulated that medical errors are largely preventable if systems are implemented to detect and treat potential errors in management early in the patient's care. Dr. Leape's review of existing literature at the time found that most errors in the care of patients fortunately do not result in serious complications.

However, due to the sheer number of errors on a daily basis, the occurrence of grave harm as a result of medical errors is still quite substantial. This was made clear recently in the Institute of Medicine's report *To Err is Human* where they estimated that somewhere between 44,000 to 98,000 patients per year in the United States die related to medical errors [4].

The ICU is an area of particular interest in medicine because of the complexity of care required. More complex processes required by the critically ill are more prone to error. The complexity of managing ICU patients often requires "multi-tasking," which potentiates the chances for errors and variations in the care of critically ill patients that could lead to serious complications and unintended outcomes, such as increased morbidity and mortality [3]. Because physicians and nurses are trained to achieve error free care of patients, mistakes are generally regarded to be unacceptable in the field of medicine. This has lead to the concept that error does not occur in the absence of negligence. When error does occur without serious injury to the patient, the event is perceived as an anomaly or unusual event, also termed as an "outlier." This attitude among healthcare workers leads to under-reporting of medical errors and also impairs efforts to focus on process improvement rather than on blame.

Other industries that routinely encounter complex non-linear problems have implemented processes and systems that effectively minimize the impact of inevitable human error. The goal is to prevent errors before they occur and to minimize the impact when they do occur by using smart systems and standardized "best evidence" processes. Strategies which can be applied to medical care delivery include:

- standardized processes across complex systems to minimize mistakes caused by variation [5]
- error proofing to disallow the implementation of actions that are outside standard safety margins
- tightening of feed-back and control loops to minimize errors of communication
- redundancy to catch events that slip through other buffers

- empowerment of every team member to contribute to the safety effort with meaningful authority to interrupt or challenge any process if problems are identified [3].

Unfortunately, such error reduction practices in the medical industry are in their infancy in the United States. We still have largely non-standardized care processes in our ICUs that rely on human memory and domain expertise for their effectiveness, and the unreliability of these systems has been repeatedly demonstrated. Further compounding the problem is the national shortage of critical care providers necessary to provide appropriate care. In this current scenario, costs will continue to escalate (an issue of particular importance in the ICU where 10% of the inpatient beds account for 30% of inpatient costs) [6–8] and quality will continue to suffer.

There is now accumulating evidence that the remote provision of intensivist domain expertise via ICU telemedicine, when coupled with proactive physician surveillance and intelligent computerized algorithms, can effectively help to address many of the current process problems in the delivery of ICU care. As a re-engineering system, the ideal remote telemedicine unit effectively addresses multiple aspects of error reduction theory including standardization across a system of critical care units, redundancy of observation and monitoring of critically ill patients, tightened feedback control loops, buffers against "slips" and errors, and error proofing via computerized physician order entry. And importantly, when the remote (telemedicine) team is given sufficient authority to intervene, the remote ICU supports the concept that all members of the team are empowered to protect patient safety. Such a system ultimately leads to improved patient outcomes and lower cost of care.

2. Evidence-Based Data Supporting Remote ICU Concept

There is an abundance of data in traditional ICU care models that standardization of ICU care can significantly reduce unintentional human error and lead to measurable and significant improvement in patient outcomes. Care is often standardized around process measures from the evidence-based peer-reviewed literature. Such interventions have included reduction of tidal volumes in mechanically ventilated patients with Acute Lung Injury (ALI) or Acute Respiratory Distress Syndrome (ARDS), intensive glucose control, standardized sedation protocols with scheduled daily interruptions, early recognition and treatment of relative adrenal insufficiency (RAI), and early goal directed therapy in patients with severe sepsis or septic shock, to name a few. It is also clear that the model of care delivery is important. Literature from numerous sources shows that intensivist-led multidisciplinary teams can dramatically reduce mortality, length of stay and, by most estimates, cost of care for the critically ill [6,8–11].

Despite these data pointing undeniably to improved outcomes in ICU care, most ICUs are unable to reliably apply evidence-based protocols and bundles to their ICU patients and few have adequate intensivist staffing to meet state-of-the-art care model requirements.

In 1998, a consortium of U.S. health care purchasers representing over 50 million insured lives in all 50 states initiated a program to promote the safety and overall value of healthcare to consumers. Termed the "Leapfrog Group" the initiative was based on concerns that healthcare, including ICU care, had fallen into a state of economic and quality "gridlock." One of the three primary "Leapfrog" mandates is that trained intensivists should manage patients requiring ICU care. Such intensivists should be dedicated, without competing concerns, and active participants in the daily management of all critically ill patients. Should a problem or trend be identified, 24/7 coverage should be assured with rapid availability of intensivist-led intervention [9]. In support of this concept, Pronovost et al. published a systematic review in JAMA in 2002 showing that "high-intensity" ICU physician staffing, meaning an ICU physician was either the attending physician or was a mandatory consultation in every ICU patient's care, resulted in a significant reduction in ICU and hospital mortality and LOS [10]. These findings were the culmination of more than a decade of studies across multiple disparate ICU populations, and the vast majority was in agreement. For example, Manthous et al. in the Mayo Clinic Proceedings in 1997 showed that the addition of an ICU physician to the care of ICU patients decreased ICU mortality from 20.9% to 14.9%, and in-house mortality from 34.0% to 24.6%, regardless of APACHE II scores [11]. How then do we as ICU health care professionals effectively manage an ever-growing population of ICU patients as staffing growth remains stagnant?

According to the Leapfrog Group and the current preliminary data the answer is, in part, found in the evolution of ICU telemedicine [1,9]. Current advances in ICU telemedicine have provided caregivers the ability to communicate directly with on-site caregivers and to directly visualize the patient via remote high-resolution camera technology 24/7. Continuous off-site hemodynamic monitoring with the addition of data links and computer technology facilitates intelligent monitoring algorithms that allow early detection of physiologic derangements or new laboratory results that may prompt early intervention in a patient's care and improve overall outcome. This model for ICU telemedicine allows for 24/7 proactive care of ICU patients using a remote system linked to the electronic medical record (EMR) and real-time physiologic data, with an ICU physician-led multidisciplinary team providing oversight, redundancy, and tight feedback control to the bedside care team. Most remote ICU teams include a board certified or eligible ICU physician, one to two experienced or certified critical care nurses, a healthcare administrator in charge of clerical functions, and an information technology service available 24/7 for trouble-shooting issues with the computerized monitoring systems being utilized at the central monitoring station (CMS). The CMS team, with the help of computerized algorithms and close communication with the bedside caregivers, is able to monitor multiple ICU beds at multiple facilities simultaneously thereby helping to alleviate the difficulties with the shortage in ICU physicians and staff. The availability of on-site physicians and staff help determine the degree of involvement of the telemedicine ICU staff. Some rural healthcare centers may require 24/7 telemedicine ICU support, while more urban tertiary referral centers may require telemedicine ICU support only part of the day, such as at night when physician and staffing are reduced or less available.

Most remote ICU systems currently being utilized have a similar design ergonomically within the CMS. All remote ICU telemedicine team members, including physicians, nurses, and clerical assistants, have their own workstation made up of multiple computer monitors and computer processors. Ideally, there are dedicated screens used to provide continuous, essentially real-time telemetric, hemodynamic and physiologic data through direct interfaces to bedside monitors. These physiologic data are also delivered to the EMR and an intelligent alert system to populate the EMR trending data and drive pre-programmed alarm algorithms. Another screen is dedicated to the patient's EMR with "dashboard" options displaying critical data in an easily accessible and digestible format for rapid reference. Further detail and trending data may be accessed as needed by drilling down into the electronic medical record for additional or specific displays of vital sign trends, physician and nursing notes, current medication lists or more comprehensive laboratory data for example. Usually at least one monitor is used to access bedside high-resolution pan/zoom cameras that are able to visualize the patient, bedside monitors, ventilator parameters and intravenous fluid and medication administration in situations where data links to these parameters are incomplete. The camera and microphone system also facilitates direct communication with bedside staff, the patients and/or their family members. There is often a multi-use monitor that allows for review of digitalized radiographic studies as well as access to internet or intranet literature-based best practices or reference data. A separate screen to display real-time critical alerts leverages the computerized intelligence system to focus attention on those patients most in need. This triage function allows a single caregiver to provide oversight to many more patients than would be practical otherwise. Most systems are designed to assign an acuity level to each monitored patient based on diagnosis, how recently they have been admitted to the ICU, hemodynamic and physiologic stability, and severity prediction scores. Such severity ranking also serves to focus attention on those patients most in need. Virtual rounds may be conducted on the sickest patients every hour to review critical "dashboard" data. These virtual rounds serve to keep intensivist care proactive and ensure compliance with the existing plan of care, as directed by the bedside team, as well as document consistent uninterrupted delivery of evidence based practices. Less acute patients may be seen less frequently but acuity designations remain fluid and flexible, should circumstances for the patient change. Alarms or alerts are also ranked by severity and can be promptly investigated by the tele-clinicians and addressed as they occur, often leading to early recognition of an event that may require intervention by the telemedicine ICU team or by a bedside caregiver. If bedside care is required, the telemedicine ICU team can contact the appropriate caregiver to attend to the patient's issues. The high-resolution camera systems are extremely useful in assessing the patient, including respiratory patterns, skin color or turgor, presence of drains, catheters, IVs, compression devices, etc. [12].

Because ICU physicians, nurses, and clerical assistants in the CMS work side by side throughout the course of the shift, a multidisciplinary approach to care is facilitated. This intimacy leads to sharing of information and enhanced communication between team members, encouraging mutual education and a teamwork approach to the care of the ICU patient. The CMS environment is also significantly more calm and controlled than the ICU bedside setting. Many ICUs can become quite hectic and stressful, leading to distractions and unintentional errors. The remote ICU telemedicine environment in the CMS allows the care providers to concentrate and make more careful decisions regarding a patient's management in support of the bedside team.

The remote ICU care team is not meant to replace bedside care, but to serve as an added layer of protection that can ideally provide back-up, enhance communication and error prevention, recognize early potentially negative trends in a patient's clinical course, and provide a proactive and prompt system of intervention to minimize human error and adverse outcomes. It can also serve as a more efficient conduit for bedside staff to communicate with on-call but off-site bedside physicians. It is not unusual for remote ICU care providers to contact off-site, on-call caregivers to assist in management of a developing problem in a patient, leading to a more prompt response to the problem by the bedside physician.

3. Data on Critical Care Telemedicine

In 2000, Rosenfeld et al. published the first study using 24/7, full-time ICU telemedicine physician monitoring in a ten-bed surgical ICU in an academic-affiliated community hospital. The study involved two 16-week baseline periods adjusting for time of year and level of acuity in the ICU related to anticipated seasonal variations.

Following the two baseline periods, a 16 week "interventional period" was performed employing ICU telemedicine technologies via a Baltimore-based company called VISICU®. Data collection included APACHE III scores of all patients enrolled at the time of admission to the ICU with comparison of these scores to the national APACHE III database. Endpoints included risk-adjusted ICU and hospital mortality, ICU and hospital LOS, and complication rates sustained while patients were in the ICU. These results were compared to predicted risk of ICU or hospital mortality and ICU and hospital LOS based on the national APACHE III database. Results of the study revealed that severity adjusted mortality was reduced 30% in the intervention group compared to the two baseline period groups. Complication rates were also significantly reduced in the intervention group, with rates of 15.1%, 18.8%, and 9.5% in the first baseline, second baseline, and intervention groups, respectively. ICU LOS was significantly reduced in the intervention group by 26%. Total hospital LOS did not significantly change. ICU outliers, accounting for 45% of additional ICU costs, were significantly reduced from 8.2% to 4.5%. Also, total ICU costs were significantly reduced in the intervention group by 31%. Total hospital costs were not significantly affected. The authors concluded that through a proactive, 24/7 ICU telemedicine monitoring service, ICU mortality, LOS, cost, and complication rates can be significantly reduced, likely due to more vigilant monitoring leading to earlier detection of potential adverse events [13].

Though limited, further peer-reviewed data has been published regarding the development of this specific model of ICU telemedicine. Breslow et al. published a significant study in Critical Care Medicine in 2004 evaluating the utility of a now commercially available remote ICU telemedicine system (VISICU Inc. Baltimore, Maryland). The study involved two ICUs of a large tertiary care, teaching hospital integrated system (Sentara Healthcare), with 2,140 ICU patients included in the study.

Patients were risk adjusted per APACHE III criteria prior to enrollment in the study. Of note, one important feature of the study was that the bedside attending physicians were given the opportunity to determine the remote ICU physician's level of autonomy. Autonomy was designated by categories. Category 1 attending physicians elected to retain all decision-making authority, except in emergency situations (where the electronic ICU team was allowed to make decisions in patient care). Otherwise, the remote intensivist was required to contact the on-call attending physician for all patient management issues requiring physician intervention. Category 2–4 attending physicians delegated some or all of their decision-making authority to the remote ICU team.

Interestingly, though the majority of physicians initially elected to be Category 1 status, many of these attending physicians changed their status to Category 3 or 4 by the end of the study period. The remote ICU physician rounded on all high-acuity patients on an hourly basis, regardless of attending MD Category status, and rounded on more stable patients less frequently. The remote ICU nursing team also regularly evaluated patients and communicated with the bedside care team. Rounds included:

- review of vital signs
- laboratory results
- direct visualization of patients using a sophisticated pan-zoom-tilt camera system
- continuous hemodynamic monitoring
- review of care plans on patients
- including electrolyte repletion protocols
- glycemic control
- DVT and stress ulcer prophylaxis
- direct contact with bedside caregivers either through a microphone-based system at the bedside or by direct telephone contact.

Results of the study revealed 26.7% reduction in ICU mortality and a 26.4% reduction in hospital mortality in the intervention study population. ICU LOS decreased by 16% in the intervention group, though hospital LOS was not significantly different between the baseline group and the intervention group. ICU costs were reduced by 24.6% in the intervention population studied, resulting in a monthly contribution margin of $524,000 dollars, an increase of 66%. Overall, the study revealed a $3.14 million dollar benefit over the 6-month intervention period [14].

The authors concluded that improvement in mortality, LOS, and costs were likely due to earlier recognition and intervention for problems in patient care. They postulated that prompt intervention via the remote ICU telemedicine system resulted in decreased complications, reduced unintentional errors, and decreased ICU mortality and LOS. They also noted that because of the ability of the remote ICU care team to contact and communicate with the bedside caregivers and on-call physicians, information transfer regarding a patient's status was augmented. In other words, a "proactive" remote ICU model resulted in improved outcomes.

Other data regarding the effectiveness of ICU telemedicine is being produced, though still preliminary. An abstract submitted to the Society of Critical Care Medicine (SCCM) from Shaffer et al. in 2005 reviewed the effects of remote ICU assistance with patients experiencing cardio-pulmonary arrest in a large healthcare system on Florida's east coast. The odds ratio for a code per patient and code per patient day in the post remote ICU period, compared to the pre-remote ICU period, was 0.70 and 0.61 respectively. Both of these reductions in odds ratio reached statistical significance per the author's reports. Additionally, initial resuscitation in patients sustaining a code was successful in 65.6% of cases when remote ICU was involved, compared to 51.6% during the pre-remote ICU implementation [15].

Also in 2006, Cowboy et al. submitted an abstract of a study to SCCM reviewing the effectiveness of implementation of a remote ICU system in reduction of ventilator dependent days in a large ICU population involving three ICUs in Virginia. This retrospective analysis reviewed three different populations of mechanically-ventilated patients based on the degree of intervention that was allowed by the patients' admitting physicians. ICU A population allowed broad remote ICU autonomy for decision making in 94% of cases, including implementation of DVT, stress ulcer prophylaxis, and ventilator bundles. In ICU B only 56% of physicians allowed broad remote ICU autonomy, and in ICU C only 18% of physicians allowed remote intensivist decision-making autonomy. Data was collected for a 12-month period prior to remote ICU implementation and for nine months after remote ICU implementation. A dramatic reduction in ventilator-dependent days was noted in ICU A (8.0 vs. 6.0) compared to ICU B

(8.7 vs. 7.0) or ICU C (8.8 vs. 9.0). The variation in ventilator-dependent days was correlated with the percentage of remote ICU intervention, and this was statistically significant (p < 0.001) [16]. In essence, increased remote telemedicine physician autonomy was associated with improved outcomes.

A large multi-facility hospital system in the Pacific Northwest (Swedish Medical Center) has also been employing a remote ICU system since September 2004. Their system engaged two large tertiary care facilities and one smaller primary/secondary hospital. It included medical ICU beds, cardiovascular and surgical ICU beds, and neurological ICU beds. Compared to the baseline period from 2003–2004, the remote ICU intervention period from 2004–2005 was associated with an average monthly reduction in mortality rate of 13%. Ventilator bundle protocols were implemented in 95% of mechanically ventilated patients during the intervention period coincident with a dramatic reduction in ventilator-associated pneumonia (VAP) incidence per 1,000 device-use days. These interventions by the remote ICU system were further associated with a $920,000 dollar annualized cost saving in 2005 for this hospital system [17].

Not only has implementation of remote ICU telemedicine systems resulted in improved patient outcomes, it has also been shown to improve bedside nursing job satisfaction and ancillary staff satisfaction. Parkview Healthcare Systems, based in the Indiana, performed a survey of their hospital's bedside nursing staff regarding job satisfaction and evaluated nursing turnover and bedside nursing retention. They had a 75% overall response rate to the survey. Nurse satisfaction increased substantially subsequent to remote ICU implementation. Open positions for new employees in that ICU, reflecting the frequency of nursing turnover, was reduced by 75% after implementation of the remote ICU telemedicine system. There was also a 37% increase in nurses surveyed who strongly agreed that they would feel safe being treated in that particular ICU after the remote ICU system had been employed [18]. Chicago-based Advocate Healthcare submitted results of a nursing survey that revealed greater than a fifty percent increase in nurses' confidence that physician orders were being carried out correctly with the use of the remote ICU system and in their ability to reach an ICU physician in a timely manner. Bedside nursing vacancy rates were also reduced in five of six different hospitals in that healthcare system [19].

3.1. Obstacles to Overcome in Implementing Remote ICU Systems

VISICU® was the first company in the United States to promote and market the integrated remote ICU telemedicine system as described in this article, and is still the only national commercial provider of the system to date. Other health informatics organizations have been evaluating the field and "homegrown" solutions do exist which are similar in design and function to VISICU's eICU® technology solution, but these alternative systems are yet a tiny minority of the market share. The VISICU® version of remote ICU telemedicine has begun to have meaningful market penetration with now over 30 Central Monitoring Stations covering more than 150 hospitals with 4000 to 5000 hospital ICU beds, which comprises about 7% of the estimated total number of ICU beds in the US. This cumulative experience has revealed certain predictable patterns of resistance and common barriers to successful implementation. Among these, cost is certainly a substantial obstacle with implementation costs of $3 million to $5 million to get the system up and running commonly quoted by the vendor. There are also ongoing operating expenses which total tens of thousands of dollars per year for each ICU bed and this cost burden is borne exclusively by the health care delivery system, as there are currently no mechanisms in place to collect third party reimbursement for remote physician services. The Society of Critical Care Medicine is lobbying for a specific CPT code for remote intensivist services but it is unclear when or perhaps even if this will occur. The Sentara study referenced earlier did have an independent financial audit of their system implementation and at least in their hands, the implementation and operations costs were offset by shorter LOS, lower ancillary costs and increased ICU throughput, as well as a trend toward more favorable case mix adjustment. Breslow et al. reported a return on investment in the Sentara system in less than one year [14]. It is less clear that other systems have enjoyed the same financial benefits, as cost accounting in healthcare is notoriously difficult and regional variations in payor mix and staffing patterns compound the complexity. Most systems will need to have a long-term view of at least several years to document a direct positive impact on the bottom line. Implicit in this process is that systems which choose this route will need to assure political will and financial resources to persevere until benefit can be unequivocally established. There are also many potential indirect financial positives that are secondary to improved quality of care, better real-time data collection and, as reported by several systems, improved nursing satisfaction with reduced turnover which have not yet been effectively captured by cost-benefit analyses.

Quality-of-care improvements have been easier to demonstrate than financial benefits and are critical to the ongoing success of the model. Beyond the peer reviewed published data, the consistent finding of trends toward improved quality metrics for almost all systems which have undertaken formal evaluation of process and outcomes measures are hard to ignore. Nonetheless, many hospitals still will not have risk adjusted mortality and length-of-stay data prior to implementation, the lack of which will, for those systems, create difficulty in justifying the model to all stake-holders.

This is particularly true if the bedside model, staffing patterns and/or case-mix change independently during remote ICU telemedicine implementation. In such circumstances it may take several years to clearly document quality benefits. This creates a further obstacle to the long-term acceptance of remote ICU telemedicine. Clearly further peer reviewed studies are needed.

Physician and staff resistance to the model has been a significant issue at almost every program, and the author's program here at Banner Health® in Phoenix is no exception. Most often physician resistance centers on physician autonomy. Physicians like to believe that their care is exemplary and will often feel threatened by the perception that someone is looking over their shoulder and perhaps even putting them at liability risk if they disagree with the recommendations of the virtual intensivist.

Furthermore the historical hierarchy of care with physicians at the apex, and the general lack of understanding or endorsement of error reduction theory so integral to this reengineering process, creates barriers to a team approach implicit in this remote ICU telemedicine model that is difficult to overcome. This resistance is exacerbated in many instances by the bedside physician's lack of a personal relationship with the virtual intensivist who is seen as an "outsider" to the medical staff and interfering with the status quo. Finally, the history of misaligned incentives with respect to physician-hospital relations often fosters mistrust between the two groups and independent physicians may feel that the change is being forced upon them by the administration. The lack of trust in the motives of the health system further increases resistance to the program.

The experience with nurse resistance is that it is far less entrenched than physician resistance and that nurses do eventually embrace the concept and model. Initially, however, nurses' issues are similar to those of the physicians with autonomy and privacy topping the list. If physicians with whom the nurses personally work remain resistant, however, their loyalty to their bedside physician group may lengthen the acceptance period. Ultimately, as we have described, nurse satisfaction seems to improve and turn-over is reduced once the initial resistance fades.

Liability issues have also been raised, primarily by physicians, but also by nurses and other staff. Unclear delineation of roles and responsibilities and poor communication between bedside and remote caregivers leads to a level of mistrust that can promote increased medico-legal risk for all parties. This risk is not unique to the remote telemedicine model, but deficiencies in medical staff communication and delineation of roles and responsibilities may be accentuated in the re-engineering process, particularly where bedside clinician resistance is high. When communication and collegiality are present there is reason to believe that improved documentation, monitoring, identification of adverse trends and prompt rescue should reduce liability risks.

Incomplete integration of data between hospital and remote ICU systems can create inefficiencies and increase the burden on bedside caregivers that can significantly influence their receptiveness to remote ICU telemedicine implementation and limit the effectiveness of the entire re-engineering process. Unfortunately, for the vast majority of programs significant holes in seamless integration will likely persist for some time to come. For example, most innovative health systems (the very systems which are likely to be early adopters of the remote intensivist model) have made plans for an enterprise-wide clinical information system. Such enterprise systems are necessarily complex and must fit the needs of users across the enterprise including those in critical care units. The enterprise systems for the most part have not developed the sophistication specific to the ICU to deliver a "turn-key" suite with clinical intelligence and decision support similar to the VISICU® system. The end result is that often two parallel systems must be accessed in the remote ICU CMS and that much data for hospitals which rely on paper charts must be faxed or scanned and then manually entered into the VISICU® system to populate the data fields which drive clinical intelligence and decision support. Though system interfaces are conceivable for much of these data, the interfaces are often not made available. The failure to develop and implement such interfaces is multifactorial and includes in part the number and complexity of the needed interfaces. Moreover, though VISICU® has expressed a willingness to participate in interface development, health enterprises and medical information companies must make decisions about how to allocate scarce information technology resources with the additional cost and effort required to build, test and perfect complex interfaces. This is further complicated by "turf wars" for market share among the clinical information system companies, some of which have an eye on the market now dominated by VISICU® with whom they are therefore necessarily less likely to cooperate. While there is sufficient experience to show that "work-arounds" such as double data entry and parallel systems can be used to achieve improvements in patient outcomes, the cost will be hard to justify in the long term and clearly the maximum efficiency and effectiveness of the remote ICU telemedicine model are compromised.

4. Solutions

In order for the remote ICU telemedicine model to have enduring success, significant obstacles must be addressed. Perhaps first and foremost, further well designed studies of the impact of this care model on patient outcomes and hospital margins are needed to support the concept as a minimal acceptable standard for patient safety. Certainly with the staggering costs of care for the critically ill (estimated to be about 30% of total inpatient costs) and with the clear deficiencies in reliable and safe delivery models (estimated 54,000 preventable deaths per year in the ICU alone), this is an appropriate area in which to focus research dollars.

The cost issue is unlikely to go away soon as the market is dominated by a publicly traded, for-profit company (VISICU®) that has a broad and powerful method patent in place to protect its intellectual property. In fairness to VISICU®, it is entirely unclear that the homegrown models that have developed to date are any less expensive to develop and operate than VISICU®'s "turn-key" program. VISICU® seems to have been a good steward of its responsibilities to date with continuous refinements, effective nation-wide user groups and benchmarked reporting of process and outcome measures. These data that drive clinical and system improvement are not as readily accessed by the homegrown versions and the scale of VISICU®'s accumulating data base and therefore its power to answer clinical questions and drive improvement of the technology is increasingly impressive. The attractiveness of the VISICU® option has been that it is essentially a complete operation with well thought out and developed clinical intelligence, decision support and implementation design. However, the recent VISICU® public offering should at least raise concerns that the mission of the company will in the future be more slanted towards stockholders in a field where VISICU® has a virtual monopoly. Competitive cost reductions in any case would seem unlikely in the near future.

Overcoming the cost obstacle then is likely to be addressed indirectly on many fronts. For example, taking advantages of the economies of scale, smaller institutions can band together with other like institutions to create the necessary size and financial position to support the venture. Other institutions may choose to outsource remote ICU telemetry to existing programs on a per-bed fee basis. Also, new more accurate methods of financial accounting need to be developed such that the true cost of care and not simply revenue or length of stay data can be relied upon to assess the real financial impact of quality improvements associated with the system. Attempts should also be made to assess indirect financial benefits such as reduced nursing turnover and perhaps reduced physician burn-out as well as potential reductions in FTEs required to collect retrospective data which may now be prospectively collected during the course of care. Until these issues are addressed, however, successful implementation will continue to require a strong financial position and equally strong political will to sustain the program long enough to fairly assess the positive impact financially and clinically.

Physician resistance is arguably more of an obstacle than cost in terms of successful implementation and integration of remote ICU telemedicine. To some extent this resistance is unavoidable and most hospital systems will need to be prepared to deal with the issue to some degree. There are several factors that can reduce resistance and facilitate integration, and any health care delivery organization contemplating current ICU telemedicine models would be wise to spend adequate time and resources in this area. Clearly it is beneficial for remote physicians to have pre-existing relationships with bedside physicians. In some smaller to moderate-sized programs, the physicians or physician groups in the CMS are also the physicians providing care at the bedside. If the pre-remote ICU telemedicine model also includes routine intensivist involvement in all ICU patients then the transition will tend to flow very well.

Unfortunately, such a transition model will not be possible for larger programs such as Banner Health® and others which cross state lines or monitor multiple separate locations. Similarly, the absence of a model that routinely includes intensivists in the bedside model of care before implementation will increase the likelihood of resistance.

Substantial time needs to be devoted to consensus building and the development of local medical staff champions well before implementation begins. Ongoing communication with physicians through department meetings and scheduled reports of clinical outcomes, prompt response to any identified issues and informal visibility on the unit can significantly improve relationships. It is also wise for organizations with multiple options for sequential roll-out to choose units with established need, local champions and broad consensus in order to demonstrate early successes before expanding the program to other potentially more challenging units. Also, having good severity adjusted data prior to implementation is of paramount importance.

Improvements in patient outcomes should be widely shared to justify the program to both the medical staff and those with the financial purse strings. Setting up a unified plan with direct involvement of risk management, medical staff peer review and QI experts and leadership from all stakeholders will help build confidence in the new processes of care and alleviate many of the liability and quality concerns. Special attention should be paid to the development of care guidelines to clearly establish division of tasks, degrees of autonomy and work flows in routine and emergency situations with constant communication on "both sides of the camera" to ensure a clear understanding of roles and responsibilities. It is important to understand that mistakes will be made. Finally, there is no substitute for ongoing open communication between all concerned parties, and the response to all issues and concerns should be prompt and appropriate.

If physician resistance is dealt with fairly and consistently, nurse resistance is likely to be less of an issue. However, there are issues specific to nursing which should also be addressed before, during and after implementation. Relationship issues with nurses are similar to those of physicians in many ways and should be addressed accordingly; however, two issues more specific to nursing deserve special mention. First, if there are incomplete data interfaces (almost all programs); there will often be changes in nursing workflow and responsibilities that can interfere with patient care. Faxing paper documents, some dual data entry and more frequent "docking" of bedside lab tools (such as rapid glucose and ABG devices) to native computer systems are examples. If these workflow changes become too burdensome, and additional FTEs are not provided to help accomplish these tasks, then nurse resistance will increase or data completeness and ultimately patient quality will suffer. It is important to include nurses and all ancillary staff (secretarial, pharmacy, IT, RT, etc.) in the design process to ensure that workflow and required FTEs are realistic and that there is broad buy-in from the care team. Significantly changing physician workflow is much more difficult and has not yet been tackled in most programs as part of a remote ICU telemedicine project. The second important issue with nurses is their perception of being caught "in the middle." Ideally, the remote ICU telemedicine program should remove them from this position. When a bedside nurse recognizes a problem or issue, he or she should be able to contact the immediately available remote intensivist directly to discuss the problem and if bedside advice or attendance is warranted, the remote intensivist then has a direct physician-to-physician conversation with the bedside covering physician. This communication pattern puts two physicians together on the phone, one of whom often has personal longitudinal knowledge of the patients' course and care plan from direct bedside interaction and the other with first-hand real-time data. This creates the best opportunity for accurate and effective patient decision-making. However, if resistance is high in a particular unit or with a particular physician, the physician may not wish to communicate with the unwelcome "outside" intensivist. Therefore the nurse is back in an untenable position between two physicians who are communicating poorly, if at all.

In the first circumstance, nurse satisfaction is often dramatically improved; in the second, it is clearly not. Clear expectations about physician-to-physician communication need to be established early. Obviously, the best way to get the desired result is through the relationship building process already described. Reluctant participants may need to be convinced that such a communication flow is in the best interest of their patients and their nurses and certainly disruptive behavior on the part of any care team member should be dealt with promptly and appropriately.

Even though the preliminary data on improved patient outcomes are impressive, the long-term viability of the remote telemedicine model will require substantially improved integration of clinical information systems. For VISICU®, which currently dominates the market (and is admittedly an innovator in the development of this comprehensive re-engineering of ICU care delivery) this means that either they will invest substantially, possibly even unilaterally, in integrating their product into enterprise wide systems or eventually, patent issues aside, they will be surpassed by companies or homegrown solutions which provide the same service with effective integration. It is our view that we have only scratched the surface of what is possible with remote ICU telemedicine wedded to clinical information systems with real-time patient alerts and decision support. In order to truly leverage the potential of this model with regard to its efficiency and effectiveness in delivering the promise of improved patient outcomes and reduced cost, seamless integration with enterprise wide clinical information systems is mandatory.

An educational effort on improving patient safety and error reduction theory is increasingly a part of the broader healthcare delivery agenda. Specific education on how the remote ICU telemedicine model described addresses multiple components of error reduction theory will help administrators and clinicians understand the importance of this model for the future of care delivery on its own merits. The system as designed is intended to function as a redundant system with buffers, error proofing, tightened feedback loops, immediate availability of expert cognitive skills and facilitated outcomes data and process data collection to drive process improvement. For a large delivery system, the CMS can also serve as a base from which to drive clinical consensus teams and standardized best practices for ICU care across the organization.

Students of error reduction theory will recognize all of the key elements of error reduction embedded in this re-engineering process. Ongoing education on how the model ideally fulfills this role will facilitate implementation efforts. Independently, in an era of increasing demand for scarce ICU resources, the model is clearly the best care delivery option available to begin to meet the demand. The question is no longer whether remote ICU telemedicine is needed but when and how it is most effectively accomplished.

5. The Future of Remote ICU Telemedicine Systems

Care delivery is undergoing rapid change both domestically and internationally driven in part by increasing broadband availability, improvements in clinical information systems and increasing real-time rapid data transfer. Concerned physicians, nurses, consumer groups and now government agencies are increasingly recognizing that the science of health care delivery is as important as the science of medicine.

Payors and consumers are no longer willing to accept poor reliability, substandard effectiveness and shamefully poor outcomes associated with current care models. At the same time, fewer dollars and resources are available to drive change. These undeniable trends have brought a new kind of telemedicine to the forefront of healthcare delivery and remote ICU telemedicine is an example of what is possible in the field when telemedicine and clinical information systems are integrated with reengineering to achieve a common goal. This model is likely to expand to other areas of need such as emergency departments, post-anesthesia care units and acuity adjustable beds particularly in rural health facilities. Reimbursement policy will need to change substantially to keep pace with this transformation and facilitate broad adoption and further innovations. We believe that in the long run return on investment will be clear in lives and dollars saved. The sooner we develop credentialing and reimbursement policies to support the effort the sooner we will be able to realize the benefits.

In personal communication with academicians, a concern has been expressed that the advent of remote ICU telemedicine competes with a potential initiative within the academic community to promote a graded system of ICU triage, much as trauma centers are currently categorized as levels I-IV. These physicians feel that the most critically ill patients should be triaged to centers of excellence with reliable, skilled multi-specialty consultants and experienced intensivists in-house. The concern is that with ICU cognitive skills available via telemedicine, smaller and rural ICUs will be tempted to keep patients that might enjoy improved outcomes at more comprehensive facilities. We agree that the concept of formal ICU triage is likely in our future given the scarcity and urban concentration of critical care resources. However, we do not find the telemedicine and triage concepts mutually exclusive. In fact the experience with tele-trauma programs suggests that telemedicine in this setting improves the appropriateness of transfer allowing patients who can be handled locally to stay in their local facilities while identifying patients at particular risk or in need of specific services unavailable locally who should be transferred to another facility. We therefore believe that remote ICU telemedicine will facilitate the triage model rather than prevent it.

Finally, we see remote ICU telemedicine as an invaluable resource in times of local and eventually national disaster. Building collocated CMSs with redundant connectivity, power supply and data repositories seems wise in the future to facilitate "always on" capability and help direct critically ill or injured patients to available beds when portions of the care delivery system are either incapacitated or overwhelmed.

6. Conclusions

It is our conclusion based on evidence and experience that some iteration of the remote ICU telemedicine model will continue to grow nationally and internationally.

This growth is driven by the severe shortage of critical care providers. The preliminary evidence also suggests that the necessary re-engineering of care that attends implementation of this remote ICU telemedicine model leads to significant reductions in mortality, length of stay, ICU complications and (by most estimates) cost. We postulate that; because the new model supports several aspects of error reduction theory, and because of the proactive nature of the model (supported by sophisticated computer technology) similar positive outcomes will continue to be documented even in units that are well served by intensivists at the bedside.

There remain many roadblocks on the way to successful broad implementation of this remote ICU telemedicine model. The primary obstacles include cost, physician and nurse acceptance, information systems integration and (to date) the relative lack of well-designed peer-reviewed studies. We believe these obstacles will be overcome and that the theory behind this model and all the positive preliminary data are hard to ignore.

As an added layer of protection for existing care processes and staffing models, and with proper implementation, the future indeed looks bright for remote ICU telemedicine.

References

[1] Society of Critical Care Medicine: HRSA's Workforce Report Confirms Intensivist Shortage. Critical Connections 2006; 5:1,18. www.sccm.org/criticalconnections.
[2] Angus DC et al: Current and Projected Workforce Requirements for Care of the Critically Ill and Patients with Pulmonary Disease: Can We Meet the Requirements of an Aging Population? JAMA 2000; 284: 2762-2770.
[3] Leape LL: Error in Medicine. JAMA 1994; 272: 1851-1857.
[4] Kohn, LT et al (Eds): To Err is Human: Building a Safer Health System. Washington, DC, National Academy Press, 2000.
[5] Holcomb BW et al: New Ways to reduce Unnecessary Variation and Improve Outcomes in the Intensive Care Unit. Current Opinion in Critical Care 2001; 7: 304-311.
[6] Combs AH et al: Making the Business Case; Critical Care Summit: ICU Quality and Cost, SCCM, 2003.
[7] Critical Care Statistics. SCCM, 2006 www.sccm.org.
[8] Pronovost PJ et al: Intensive care Unit Physician Staffing: Financial modeling of the Leapfrog Standard. Critical Care Medicine 2004; 32: 1247-1253.
[9] ICU Physician Staffing, Fact Sheet: The Leapfrog Group; available at www.leapfroggroup.org accessed November 23, 2006.
[10] Pronovost PJ et al: Physician Staffing Patterns and Clinical Outcomes in Critically Ill Patients. JAMA 2002; 288: 2151-2162.
[11] Manthous CA et al: Effects of a Medical Intensivist on Patient Care in a Community Teaching Hospital. Mayo Clinic Proceedings 1997; 72: 391-399.
[12] Celi LA et al: The eICU: It's Not Just Telemedicine. Critical Care Medicine 2001; 29 (Suppl.): N183- N189.
[13] Rosenfeld BA et al: Intensive Care Unit Telemedicine: Alternate Paradigm for Providing Continuous Intensivist Care. Critical Care Medicine 2000; 28: 3925-3931.
[14] Breslow et al: Effect of a Multiple-site Intensive Care Unit Telemedicine Program on Clinical and Economic Outcomes: An Alternate Paradigm for Intensivist Staffing 2004; 32: 31-38.
[15] Shaffer JP et al: Remote ICU Management Improves Outcomes in Patients with Cardiopulmonary Arrest. Critical Care medicine 2005; 33: Abstract Supplement: A5, SCCM 35th Critical Care Congress, San Francisco, CA Jan. 7-11 2006.
[16] Cowboy EN et al: Impact of Remote ICU Management on Ventilator Days. Critical Care Medicine 2005; 33: Abstract Supplement: A1, SCCM 35th Critical Care Congress, San Francisco, CA Jan. 7-11 2006.
[17] VISICU® Annual User's Group Meeting November 2005, Baltimore, Maryland Swedish Medical Center presentation.
[18] VISICU® Annual User's Group Meeting November 2005, Baltimore, Maryland Parkview Health presentation.
[19] VISICU® Annual User's Group Meeting November 2005, Baltimore, Maryland Advocate Healthcare presentation.

IV. Clinical Telemedicine

Current Principles and Practices of Telemedicine and e-Health
R. Latifi (Ed.)
IOS Press, 2008

Telemedicine in Neurosciences

K. GANAPATHY [a,b,*] and Aditi RAVINDRA [b]
[a] *Department of Neurosurgery Apollo Hospitals, Chennai, India*
[b] *Department of Telemedicine, Apollo Hospitals, Chennai, India*

Abstract. It is well known that in most countries, there is a perennial shortage of specialists in neurosciences. Even the few available neurologists and neurosurgeons are clustered in the metros and urban areas. Those living in suburban and rural areas have limited or no access to neurological care. At the same time there has been an unprecedented growth in *ICT* (Information and Communication Technology). In this article, the authors review the increasing use of telemedicine in neurosciences.

Keywords. Telemedicine in neurosciences

Introduction

"Watson, come here I want you" said Alexander Graham Bell on March 20, 1876 when he inadvertently spilled battery acid on himself, while making the world's first telephone call. Little did Bell realize that this was also the world's first telemedical consultation [1]. We, have come a long way since then. In 1910, Brown had demonstrated the first electrical stethoscope and telephone relay of heart sounds. In 1924, on the cover of a popular magazine, *Radio News* was a picture of a live, interactive telemedical consultation between a child and his pediatrician. In 1959, the University of Nebraska College of Medicine used video communications to accomplish a telemedical consultation. Subsequently the Telemedical Emergency Neurosurgical Network (TENNS) in northern California was created to facilitate neurosurgical decision making before patient transport. This reduced transportation of patients who would not benefit from neurosurgical intervention.

Image acquisition, image storage, display, processing, and transfer form the basis of telemedicine [2,3]. While telemedicine has been developing in the last two decades, in the last five years the growth has indeed been exponential [4].

1. Teleneurology: Introduction to the Global Scenario

Neurological expertise is not available in several areas of the world [3,5–11]. 20% of the US population is without any neurological services. Establishing telemedicine would in part resolve the "man power" shortage problem. Worldwide there is difficulty in retaining specialists in non-urban areas as professional isolation would lead to mediocrity. Quite often, many patients are sent to far off places at considerable expense. In

* Corresponding Author: Prof. K. Ganapathy, Department of Telemedicine, #21, Greams Road, Apollo Hospitals, Chennai 600006, India. Telefax: 91 44 24364150, Email: drkganapathy@gmail.com.

many of these cases, treatment could have been carried out by the local doctor with advise from a specialist. This also results in considerable (and sometimes avoidable) overwork at these centers. Suboptimal management of difficult neurosurgical/neurological cases may sometimes occur due to the limited neurosurgical/neurological resources being utilized for management of cases that could have been managed in smaller (non existent!) centers. Using a Personal Computer, a scanner, a digital camera, networking, appropriate software and telecommunications it is possible to transfer clinical data and even carry out a reasonable clinical examination. Offering medical advice remotely, using state of the art telecommunication tools is now a regular feature in many parts of the world.

Studies have shown telemedicine to be practical, safe and cost effective. Telemedicine hinges on transfer of text, reports, voice, images and video, between geographically separated locations Success relates to the efficiency and effectiveness of the transfer of information. Telemedicine covers a wide range of activities. In the past it was primarily teleradiology – the transfer of high resolution medical images, X ray pictures, ultrasound, CT, MRl pictures, live transmission of ECG's and echocardiograms. Today even a detailed clinical examination can be conducted remotely [2].

Telemedicine is becoming an integral part of health care services in several countries including the UK, USA, Canada, Italy, Germany, Japan, Greece, and Norway. Most of the publications on teleneurology have been in the last five years [12]. Today, Telemedicine has been used in various sub-specialities of neurosciences. These include among others, neuroophthalmology [13], and pediatric neurology [14–16].

Neurological teleconsultations have benefited general practitioners by giving advice on patient medication and diagnosis. Unnecessary specialist consultations and laboratory examinations are avoided. Doctor-doctor teleconsultation allows the rapid resolution of queries which otherwise cause stress to patients and increase the cost and complexity of care [17]. Maulden stressed that the Internet is changing neurologists relationships to other professionals in the health care industry, including stroke management, movement disorders and epilepsy. The advantages and disadvantages of e-mail in teleneurology have been discussed [18]. The attitudes of general practitioners towards teleneurology, have also been documented in several reports [19–21].

Steven has discussed the role of telemedicine in developing countries as well [22]. Once the "virtual" presence of a specialist is acknowledged, a patient can access resources in a tertiary referral centre without the constraints of distance. Telemedicine allows patients to stay at home ensuring much needed family support. Geographic isolation contributes to inequity in health care. Theoretically, it is easier to set up a telecommunication infrastructure in suburban and rural areas and increase the reach of the limited number of urban neurosurgeons and neurologists, Telemedicine therefore, is the answer. In Utopia, every citizen has immediate access to the appropriate specialist. In the real world this cannot even be a dream. Incentives to entice specialists to practice in suburban and rural areas have failed. Traditionally it has been believed that communities most likely to benefit from telemedicine are those least likely to afford it or have the requisite communication infrastructure. This is no longer true. Computer literacy is fast developing and computer prices are falling. Health care providers are now looking at Telemedicine to bridge the gap.

In a large Telemedicine project in the USA 83% of patients who would have been transferred to an urban hospital remained in their community reducing the cost by at least 40 to 50%. This also ensures maximal utilization of suburban hospitals. It may be argued that body language is vital in any interpersonal relationship. Today's video conferencing systems are sophisticated, that several groups of people can be viewed simultaneously on a screen. Minute facial expressions can be discerned with unbelievable clarity. Participants remain in view at all times making it literally a face-to-face meeting. The spontaneity, naturalness, and interactivity of a conventional person-to-person meeting are all there – excepting that the patient and doctor are hundreds or even thousands of miles away. Acquiring high-quality video and transferring it with minimal loss of data, is crucial in the assessment of gait and movement disorders. In a study using several types of cameras in different settings, Schoffer et al., demonstrated that low cost cameras and email was sufficient [23].

Issues can be addressed and multiple opinions can be obtained from all around the globe. High-speed networks and multimedia servers allow medical professionals to exchange many types of health care information. Eventually, standard of health care in rural areas will increase, and costs will be reduced. Preliminary trials with telemedicine have revealed high levels of satisfaction among patients, general practitioners, specialists and technologists.

Interactive videoconference (IVC) units allows a patient at a distant site to be "seen and heard" by a hospital-based physician; simultaneously, the patient can "see and hear" the doctor [24]. An evaluation of the first year's experience with a low-cost telemedicine link in Bangladesh has been reported [25]. A simple digital camera was used to capture still images, which were then transmitted by email. During the first year, 12 neurological cases were referred. Referral was beneficial in 89%. The benefits included establishment of the diagnosis, reassuring the patient and the referring doctor, and a change in management. An email account with an Internet service provider and the local-rate telephone call charges sufficed. This successful telemedicine system has been suggested as a model for further telemedicine projects in the developing world. Studies are now available which emphasize the core principles to be employed for the successful development of telemedicine systems [26]. Telecommunications have been found useful in rural emergencies. An article with a provocative title "Brain surgery by fax" [27] illustrates this point.

2. Cost

A major advantage in using telemedicine is the savings from avoiding unnecessary transportation. Seriously ill neurological patients have to be accompanied by able bodied attenders. If the total man hours lost is added to transportation, boarding and lodging, the expenses are considerable. The cost-effectiveness of teleneurology consultations [28–31] and teleneuro radiological consultations [32,33] telepsychiatriy consults [34] have been worked out in western countries. Even in an advanced country a wide area computer network for neurosurgical consultation is used to reduce costs. Reviewing 100 consecutive telemedicine neurosurgical consultations from 20 western Pennsylvania community hospitals participating in the NeuroLink network and taking into account patient bed costs, and transportation charges, savings of more than half a million dollars was documented [28].

3. Legal Questions

Application of telemedicine has raised several legal questions [35]. Data security is crucial. Accidental loss of data must be avoided Artefacts must be recognized. Special encryption mechanisms that secure data against unauthorized access and even modifications are therefore necessary. Patients' rights to confidentiality are paramount. Unless regulations for special situations has been agreed to by both sides, the liability is on the side of the consulting rather than advising physician. Procedures for reimbursement of professional charges is in the process of being fine tuned.

4. Telemedicine in India

India, though considered a third world developing country, is a paradox. We now produce and launch our own satellites. Plans are under way to send an unmanned mission to the moon. Preliminary information is being gathered regarding the feasibility of launching a HEALTHSAT – a satellite exclusively for providing health care. There has been an unprecedented growth and development in Information Technology in India. Satellite transmission, fiber optic cables, increasing band width, fall in computer prices, licensing of private internet service providers, internet thro' cable etc have become the buzz words even in suburban and rural India. India no longer has to *follow* the advanced countries, they do not even have to *piggy back*, they can *leap frog*! Today there are about 120 telemedicine units located in suburban and rural India and about nine telemedicine units functioning in tertiary care hospitals. The Indian neurological community is in the process of viewing telemedicine as an additional and useful tool.

Using ISDN lines, broadband connectivity and VSAT satellites the author has helped family physicians in distant parts of India to manage simple and not so simple neurological and neurosurgical problems. Using appropriate need based technology many head injuries have been managed remotely. Telemedicine is also an excellent CME medium educating the non specialist in managing neurological problems. The knowledge that a specialist is only a mouse click away, does wonders for a rural physician's morale.

5. Telemedicine in Neurosciences In India

Detailed "tele neurological examination" is possible. An opthalmoscope can be connected directly to a PC and the fundus seen by a teleconsultant remotely. A para medical worker at the remote end elicits the reflexes and the response is seen by the specialist. All teleneurological examinations are recorded live. Replaying of the video enables one to study clinical signs in great detail. A movement disorder specialist for example will be able to give an accurate diagnosis even if he has not seen the patient live.

The successful use of telemedicine in the remote management of head trauma in India has been reported [36,37]. Head injuries are universally a public health hazard. In India a fatality occurs every four minutes, making head injury the sixth commonest cause of death. Only about 1000 neurosurgeons are available for a population of 1200 million. Though 100 new neurosurgeons qualify every year from 50 teaching programmes this is not enough. Only 125 out of 250 medical colleges have neurosurgery departments. There are less than 15 state of the art neuro trauma critical care units and 700 million living in rural India with no direct access to neurological care. Obviously there is a role for telemedicine in neurotrauma.

The author has in the last 7 years evaluated remotely 235 patients with various types of head trauma. Several serious head injuries not requiring surgery were successfully managed in the rural hospital. Three cases of head injuries were operated by the general surgeon who felt confident, as there was immediate access to the neurosurgeon in Chennai. In almost all cases the author was able to give a definite opinion and guide the local physician. Some cases required management in a tertiary care hospital. Details of the treatment were discussed at length, with the patient and the family so that they were well informed and fully prepared. These tele discussions were of considerable help. Tele consultation was particularly useful in the follow up of already treated patients [38]. The acceptance of tele consultation by the rural patient, the suburban doctor and the suburban community was much better than expected. None of them were averse to a tele consultation. The tele consultants have also accepted this new method of interacting with a patient. Detailed evaluation of the socio economic benefits needs to be done.

Interestingly, there has been a drop in neurosurgical tele referrals from the rural centers which have access to telemedicine facilities. The doctor at the remote centre has acquired the confidence to manage most cases of head trauma. In a general, community hospital setting, less than 10% of head injuries require referral to highly specialized neuro intensive care units or surgery. Earlier, the family physician did not have the skills to manage head injuries or simple poly trauma cases. With immediate access to specialists in tertiary care centers through telemedicine, this is no longer true.

As a pilot project, a fully equipped secondary level hospital (with CT, ultrasound, Echocardiography and six MBBS level doctors, one general surgeon and one pediatrician) was set up in a village called Aragonda, about 200 km from the tertiary care center in Chennai. Starting from simple web cameras and ISDN telephone lines, today the hospital has a state of the art video conferencing system and has a VSAT donated by ISRO (Indian Space Research Organization). More than 500 tele consultations have been given in neurosciences alone, to this center. Video clippings are available of pseudo-seizures, involuntary movements, Parkinsonism, myopathy etc. In all cases the teleconsultant was able to carry out a neurological examination. This was sufficient to guide the local doctor. Quality of CT images received were enough to give an opinion.

Today, India has at least thirty five tertiary care hospitals with telemedicine facilities. There are about 10 active mobile telemedicine units, which go to different villages every day. The villager gets into the specially designed dedicated hospital-on-wheels, a para medical technician focuses an opthalmoscope and the fundus is evaluated, in a tertiary care center. A VSAT on the truck transmits the images thro satellite technology.

6. Neuro Traumatology

The subspecialty in neurosciences in which Telemedicine has proved to be the most useful is neurotraumatology. All over the world, the number of neurosurgeons available to manage head trauma, is sub optimal [39]. Using Telemedicine, unnecessary transfers are reduced, reducing the work load on increasingly stretched hospital and ambulance services. More therapeutic measures are implemented *before* transfer, when investigations can be seen and the patient examined. The transfer time is shortened [40,41]. A study in France, revealed that teleradiology had a positive impact on emergency neurosurgical care, reducing time to diagnosis, avoiding unnecessary transfers and initiating earlier pre-hospital management [42]. A study from the US provided evidence that telemedicine is comparable to face-to-face care in emergency medicine and is beneficial in surgical and neonatal intensive care units as well as patient transfer in neurosurgery [43]. Review of inter-hospital teleradiology service in a French administrative area, indicated that cerebral pathologies (88%) and traumatic spinal pathologies (8%) were the commonest. Transfer was avoided in 37% and hospitalization in 12%, confirming the effectiveness of an inter-hospital teleradiology network [44].

With increasing deployment of telemedicine facilities several questions are being raised. Is regionalization of trauma care using telemedicine feasible and desirable? [45]. Is telemedicine useful in an accident and emergency setting? [46] Can the quality of information provided in telephone head injury referrals be improved [40]. Follow up study of remote trauma teleconsultations has confirmed its usefulness [47]. The report by Gray [48–52] on a national neurosurgical teleradiology system in Ireland is an example of how teleconsultation can considerably extend the reach of a small number of neurosurgeons. The system connected six major referring hospitals to the only two neurosurgical departments serving the entire population of 3.5 million people. The system was based on personal computers interconnected by leased data circuits and ISDN lines. The network was operational 24 hours a day, was user friendly and reliable. Over 750 emergency computerized tomography scans were transmitted and transmission failures occurred in only 6%. The authors pointed out that because of the widespread installation of CT scanners in peripheral hospitals, scans were obtained before referral to a neurosurgical center. Making the decision to transfer a patient to a neurosurgical unit, based solely on a voice telephone call, had been shown to be inadequate. In most cases the CT and MRI scanners could not be "upgraded" to become DICOM compatible, necessitating the use of hard copies for scanning. Scanning was also found to be beneficial for the transmission of lateral cervical spine films and chest films for trauma patients. Goh, in studies from Hong Kong has discussed whether teleradiology would improve inter-hospital management of head-injury [53,54]. Poca has addressed similar issues [55]. Eljamel evaluated the use of a computer-based image link system to assist inter-hospital referrals [56]. Moulin et al. review two networks started for Diagnosing and Treating Neurological Emergencies (RAIDS-UN/FC & RAIDS-UN/AVC) to better the quality of in-patient management for traumatic brain injuries and stroke. These networks were primarily for training experts, advisors and supervisors [57].

7. Technical Aspects

Literature on technical issues in the practice of telemedicine in neurosciences is available. Unfortunately due to the rapid changes in technology most of the published material becomes obsolescent soon. Transmission time for a sequences of six MRI scans (40 MB) was 10 min, a 10-min recording of 64-channel EEG was about 12 min, a 3-min video of low quality (MPEG1) was 16 min and of good quality (MPEG2) more than 1 hour [58,59]. However, transmission time is progressively being reduced. Publications on "Video as data" and networking with reference to neurosurgery, throw light on the several technical issues that have to be addressed [60,61]. Telemedicine may occasionally be limited by the need for fixed connectivity. Wireless technologies can be used in such situations [62].

8. Clinical Studies

Clinical trials [63–66], have shown that teleneurological evaluation is as effective, as a face to face evaluation. In one study, the concordance was 96%. Tele neurological evaluation has been successfully used for a variety of conditions. They include assessment of childhood migraine by compressed interactive video [67] and cervical spinal cord compression [68,69]. Sleep-disordered breathing (SDB) syndromes such as obstructive sleep apnea (OSA) are now being managed through telemedicine [70]. Trials with automatic SDB analyzers (Night Watch and Alice 4) are investigating the use of home SDB testing via telephone circuits or the internet, Continuous Positive Airway Pressure (CPAP) titration at home via remote-control, and super remote poly somnographic monitoring [70] and remote continuous physiological monitoring at home is now available. These have been called "Electronic House calls" [71]. Remote Video Surveillance (RVS) was used to assess whether a relationship existed between lip position and drooling in children with cerebral palsy [72]. This was compared with direct clinical assessment of lip position by determination of intra and inter-examiner agreement. It was felt that RVS offers a more unobtrusive approach. Telemedicine is being increasingly used in the evaluation and management of children with special needs [73].

Teleneuroradiology is the most developed branch of teleneurology. There are a large number of publications which discuss in depth, the pros and cons of different methods of transfer of data, maintaining cost effectiveness without compromising on quality [74–79].

9. Pediatric Neurology

There are not enough pediatric neurologists even in advanced countries. Members of the Child Neurology Society reported that the mean wait for a new patient clinic visit in the United States is 49 days, and 12% of patients must wait 3 or more months to be seen The Hospital for Sick Children in Toronto is using a telephone nursing line, to expand its services. To respond to calls, a nurse is trained in effective telephone triage. Long telephone calls (> 10 minutes) were strongly associated with a diagnosis of epilepsy [14].

Dedicated, planned telephonic consultations in child neurology practice, were available as early as 1999 [16]. 1065 patients used the 1-800-NOCLOTS pediatric stroke telephone consultation service. 60% of callers had not initiated antithrombotic therapy. For Acute Ischemic Stroke, questions concerned the selection and interpretation of etiological investigations [80]. Telemedicine has been used in the diagnosis of Duchenne's muscular dystrophy, profound mental retardation, peripheral neuropathy, spastic diplegia, autism, Tourette syndrome, Rett's syndrome, and myotonia [15].

10. Stroke

Stroke is a universal problem. Time is crucial for effective intervention in acute ischemic stroke. Today community hospitals are exploring methods to enhance and expedite acute stroke care. In addition to lack of stroke care coverage in rural areas, there is a shortage of neurologists and radiologists to care for approximately 700 000 new stroke and nearly 1 million new TIA patients every year in the United States alone [81].

Less than 1.5% of acute stroke victims are treated with thrombolytics and few benefit from the expertise and experience of stroke teams. "Telestroke" management using state-of-the-art video telecommunications increases the number of patients given effective acute stroke treatment [82].

Data were prospectively documented in the databank of the telestroke service, in the Bavarian Stroke Registry. The telemedicine service included, a 24 h/day 'strokologist' with access to high-speed videoconferencing and receiving CT/MRI images. With this, indicators for stroke management quality improved compared with other hospitals without stroke unit (12%). Eighty-six (2.1%) of the patients received systemic thrombolysis compared to 10 patients in the preceding year. The paper proves that a stroke network leads to a substantial improvement in stroke management and fills the gap of non-availability of specialized stroke expertise in neurologically underserved areas [83].

Wiborg analyzed the impact of telemedicine in routine stroke management. Teleconsultation using a videoconference system is a feasible method to improve stroke care in rural areas where management is hindered by long transportation distances. Relevant contributions could be made in > 75% of the cases concerning diagnostic workup, CT assessment, and therapeutic recommendations. A total of 153 stroke patients were examined by teleconsultation. 2 patients received "teleguided" thrombolysis [84]. Choi, has pointed out that telemedicine facilitates thrombolytic therapy for acute stroke patients. A time- and spatially related emergency need is addressed. In the 13 months preceding the telemedicine project (January 2003 – March 2004), 2 (0.8%) of 327 patients received rt-PA, compared with 14 (4.3%) of 328 patients during the telemedicine project (April 2004 – May 2005), p < .001) [85]. Seven rural hospitals in the southern part of Germany in Swabia were connected to the stroke unit of Günzburg with the use of a videoconference link (Telemedicine in Stroke in Swabia [TESS] Project). Teleconsultation in cases of acute stroke was found to be reliable and practicable [86].

Telestroke would enhance stroke education [87]. Health-care professionals would gain experience and expertise through the interaction with a remote expert – telementoring. In fact the NIH Stroke Scale, has been successfully administered remotely and its feasibility and reliability confirmed [88].

Prehospital use of telemedicine for stroke is already being piloted, linking patients in the ambulance to the emergency department. In ischemic stroke, recombinant tissue plasminogen activator (rtPA) is a major breakthrough and if administered within 3 hours of onset of stroke it results in improved survival and outcome [89]. Safe rt-PA administration for ischemic stroke during telemedicine consultation has been documented [90,91].

Many institutes lack the resources and specialized teams for providing fulltime response to acute stroke patients [92]. These institutes depend on the rapid transfer of patients to nearby regional stroke centers for therapy. The primary reason for patients not receiving this therapy is late arrival after the 3 hours of window period. Telemedicine is emerging as a time-saving efficient means. In the University of Maryland Medical center, employing a pair tilt and zoom camera with remote site control allowing 2-way real time audiovisual communication and CT image transfer, 50 stroke consultations between 1999 and 2001 were reviewed. Of these, 23 were managed through telemedicine linkage and 27 by traditional telephone conversation followed by transfer. Of the 23 telemedicine consultations, 2 were aborted because of technical difficulties. Of the patients evaluated by the traditional method 3.8% (1/27) received rtPA whereas

23.8% (5/21) in the telemedicine group received rtPA and there were no complications of this therapy. Telemedicine provided a treatment option not previously available at a remote hospital. For the administration of rtPA, telemedicine was safe, feasible and was well received [61]. Barber has reviewed the validity of the Telephone Interview for Cognitive Status (TICS) in post-stroke subjects [93].

11. Parkinson's Disease

Studies have confirmed that valid motor assessments of patients with Parkinsonism can be made via Inter active Video Conferencing (IVC) [94]. In one study involving nine patients Hubble independently examined and scored (UPDRS) by two movement disorder specialists. One examination was performed in-person and the other via IVC over a distance of 350 miles by a tele consultant. Individual patient scores did not differ [24].

12. Dementia

Using telecomputing to provide information and support to caregivers of persons with dementia has been reported [95]. Inherent features of telecomputing make computer-mediated information and support systems like the Alzheimer's Disease Support Center a viable complement [96,97]. Telephone and e-mail, has been used by specially trained nurse/counselors who record the caller's query, provide emotional support and practical advice for demented patients [98,99]. A telephone interview, although not a substitute for a face-to-face diagnostic evaluation, is a reliable procedure for evaluating cognitive, functional and behavioral functioning in an elderly population with normal aging and dementia Computer-mediated intervention for Alzheimer's caregivers has also been documented [100].

13. Telepsychiatry

Several reports in the last decade of the twentieth century reveal that telepsychiatry was coming of age [101–113]. Telemedicine for patients with obsessive-compulsive disorder was reported as early as 1996 [114]. In 1998 Brown reported on the use of telemedicine in "rural psychiatry" [115]. This was followed by reports on computer-based psychiatric assessment [116]. Use of videophones and low-cost standard telephone lines to provide a social presence in telepsychiatry was reported in 1998 by Cukor et al. [117]. Telemedicine has also been used for intensive support of psychiatric inpatients admitted to local hospitals [118]. Telepsychiatry in children and adolescents has proved to be effective [119–121]. Telepsychiatry has also been used in the very elderly [122].

14. Telerehabilitation

Virtual reality techniques through telemedicine has been used in the rehabilitation of patients afflicted with cognitive impairment [123]. Virtual Reality has been used in stroke rehabilitation. A platform for home rehabilitation controlled telemedically has been evaluated [124].

Telerehabilitation has also been achieved using web-based telecommunication [125]. Providing psychiatric backup to family physicians by telephone has been the subject matter of many communications [126–129].

15. Epileptology

It is well known that seizures may not always be simple tonic clonic grand mal seizures which can be recognized and managed by a family physician. The wide spectrum of clinical manifestations makes clinical observation by a specialist desirable. Ideally this should be accompanied by simultaneous video EEG analysis. These sophisticated tools are mostly available only in tertiary care centers not because the equipment cannot be deployed in smaller places but because experts are not available. Several studies [129] have now shown that current technology can be used to transmit EEG signals remotely. This will enable epileptologists to extend their reach considerably. Clinicians in Finland obtain a second opinion of digital (EEG) recordings, from a centre of excellence, using interactive data and video consultations [130]. Of the emergencies, status epilepticus and stroke have high potential for improving patient management.

16. Tele Neuropathology

Neuropathology consultation via digitized images was reported as early as 1992 [131]. Due to increase in sub specialization and demand for more precise diagnosis, tele-neuropathology will become increasingly available [132,133]. However some pathologists are afraid of sampling errors in remote diagnosis [134]. Viewing digitized images of histological slides on a video monitor rather than directly through a light microscope will become commonplace. For the transmission of the digitized images from a telemicroscope to the remote diagnostic video monitor, different technologies can be used. These include ordinary telephone lines, broadband telecommunications channels, and the Internet. The transmitted images may serve for primary neuropathological diagnosis, teleconsultation, quality assurance, proficiency testing, and distance learning. Static-imaging systems are insufficient for diagnostic neuropathology. High levels of diagnostic accuracy can be achieved using dynamic-imaging systems and the transmission of live video images in real time. A robotized telemicroscope enables the remote tele neuropathologist to manipulate and examine the entire histological specimen [135]. In some European countries, pathology laboratories are linked and telediagnosis of frozen section histology specimens are made by experts from hundreds of miles away [136,137]. Teleneuropathology has been described as "Telemedicine of the future." Online internet based robotic telepathology has been used in the diagnosis of neuro-oncology cases. Correlation of histology, cytogenetics and proliferation fraction in meningiomas through image analysis done remotely has been reported [138]. Frozen section diagnosis using Telepathology is now available [139]. In one study (52 neurosurgical frozen sections) there was a good degree of concordance (45/52) between the diagnosis based on transmitted video images and the diagnosis based on direct evaluation. Remote evaluation was associated with a more rapid consultation from the standpoint of the consultant, who spent approximately 2 minutes less per case when using remote microscopy; this was achieved at the expense of considerably greater effort on the part of the referring pathologist, who spent approximately 16minutes per case to select a slide for transmission [140].

A new concept of a microscope system for Telepathology, named the World Wide Microscope (WWM) has been thought of [141]. The prototype is being implemented. WWM is constructed by the following three units; (1) microscope unit, (2) control unit and (3) internet unit. The microscope unit is a conventional light microscope equipped with a motor drive and a CCD camera. The Internet unit is a World Wide Web homepage in which a Java applet and a communication server are installed. The control unit relays request commands generated from the applet to the microscope unit, and captures the microscopic images. The WWM may become the all round Telepathology tool of the next generation.

As in several fields in Telemedicine several legal issues have been raised. Some consider Telepathology "a breach of registrational barriers." The G 8 states in Europe have recommended that the location of the remote health care professional defines the site not only of licensure but also of liability. Jurisdiction uncertainties add to the complexities. Data protection and data security require attention. It has been suggested that, the principles of minimum data exchange, anonymity, pseudonymity and cryptography must be established as a basis for all Telepathology procedures [35].

17. Tele-Neurophysiology

Needs analysis for tele-neurophysiology has been reviewed by Ronan et al. [142]. Digitized neurophysiological waveforms, textual annotations and interpretive reports facilitating data interchange between neurophysiological instruments and computer systems within the neurophysiology laboratory, other information systems in the hospital, and outside healthcare facilities or research laboratories have been developed [143]. This has resulted in remote access to neurosurgical ICU physiological data using the World Wide Web (WWW) [144,145]. The UCLA Neurosurgery ICU has developed a distributed computer system that provides access over the WWW to current and previously acquired physiological data, such as intracranial pressure, cerebral perfusion pressure, and heart rate from critical care patients. Physicians and clinical researchers can access these data through personal computers from their offices, from their homes, or even while on the road. Physicians can now pose a limited, predefined set of clinically relevant questions to the system without having to be at the patient's bedside [146]. PC-based multimedia telemedicine systems have been designed to receive and transmit various neuro physiological parameters that aid in the detailed remote assessment of brain function [147,148]. Quality assurance in clinical neurophysiology has been ensured through telematics. The acquisition, storage, interpretation and telecommunication of EMG between different clinical centers remotely has been successfully carried out in Europe [149]. Technology has progressed so fast that there are intelligent systems with EMG-based joint angle estimation, for telemanipulation [150]. Even remote continuous physiological monitoring at home has been reported [151].

18. Tele-Radiosurgery

Telemedicine has been used to provide connectivity and access to specialized high performance computing and advanced software resources, as those used in radiosurgery. This requires volume visualization of projected treatment data and imaging anatomy via photo realistic rendering and virtual scenario simulation techniques – all manipulated remotely [152].

19. Mobile Telemedicine

Wireless telemedicine enabling a clinician to receive images, text and voice messages on a hand held palmtop is in the offing. Preliminary reports have successfully demonstrated instant pocket wireless CT teleradiology [153,154]. This will further facilitate neurosurgical consultations and has enormous implications for the future. A portable telemedicine unit comprising a PC linked to an Inmarsat B earth station through a modem allowed videoconferencing at 64 kbit/s. Three and a half years of clinical experience has shown this to be quite adequate for the majority of clinical telemedicine. Portable telemedicine units have been a major benefit to medical commanders in the field [155]. With rapid advances in mobile computing and cell phone technology the author is confident that it will soon be possible to do clinical examinations and review investigations through a cell phone.

20. Other Issues

N-ISDN (Narrowband Integrated Services/Digital Network), was compared to an emerging technology, ATM (Asynchronous Transfer Mode) while transferring images in neurosurgical emergencies, from a general hospital to a 100 km distant university hospital [156]. New communication systems using international digital networks including the Internet may allow re-distribution of medical resources between advanced countries and developing countries in Neurosurgery. Telemedicine in Neurosurgery between Japan & Malaysia using international digital telephone services has been carried out [157,158].

An inexpensive, easily available, easy to operate digital camera is a helpful alternative to expensive, labor-intensive teleradiology systems particularly in small community-based hospitals without DICOM based systems. Digital photographs of CT images can be transmitted as a jpeg file through e-mail. The digital camera contains the necessary software. An image can be compressed to less than 150 kilobytes. There is no visually demonstrable difference in image quality between digital and hard copy images. Large number of images can be transferred in a reasonable time. Several publications deal with the various technical aspects involved in image transfers [159,160]. In a study involving 100 emergency cranial CTs Ludwig discusses whether image selection is a useful strategy to decrease the transmission time in teleradiology [161].

The internet [162] and the World Wide Web play a major role in making available the services of the limited number of specialists in neurosciences to a global audience. Publications dealing with applications of the World Wide Web to neurosurgical practice [163,164] and the use of electronic forums [165,166] reiterate this. Electronic communities are rapidly growing The phenomenal increase in the capacity of image processing in computers and in the rate of transmission of data over the net, are resulting in remote medical visits, video conferences, surgical simulation and even remote virtual surgery [167]. Virtual reality is being increasingly used in neurosurgery [168,169]. Neurosurgical resources on the net are also steadily increasing [170].

21. Educational Video conferencing – Global and National

Video conferencing is an inexpensive way of interacting with neurosurgeons and neurologists world wide In August 2001 on behalf of the Dept of Neurosurgery Apollo Hospitals Chennai; the author organized a two-hour teleconference with Prof Tetsuo Kanno of the Dept of Neurosurgery Fujitha Health University, Nagoya Japan. This international grand round went of without a hitch. A similar meeting followed – with Prof. Michael Schulder of the Dept of Neurosurgery, UDMNJ New Jersey in December 2001. In 2002 a multipoint intercontinental neuro-surgery/trauma – emergency medicine & disaster management conference was simultaneously conducted with Tunisia – Chennai – Geneva and Paris Subsequently ten teleconferences have taken place periodically with Neurosurgery centers worldwide. This included the postgraduate course organized by the World Federation of Neurosurgical Societies at Riyadh and the 6th World Congress on Minimally Invasive Neurosurgery from Japan. Need-based neurology educational teleconferencing on a regular basis, is being conducted between Sanjay Gandhi Post Graduate Institute of Medical Sciences, Lucknow and SCB Medical College, Cuttack which are 1500 km apart using desktop video conferencing system with PTZ camera, and 126 KBPS ISD telephone lines More than 35 sessions have been conducted [171]. The pediatrics department of the Apollo hospitals has for the last 5 years been conducting weekly tele CME programmes (400) where specialist neurologists and neurosurgeons often participate.

22. The Future

Hospitals of the future will drain patients from all over the world without geographical limitations. In Cyberia, after all one is a netizen! High quality medical services can be brought to the patient, rather than transporting the patient to distant and expensive tertiary care centers. Telemedicine has not yet made a significant impact on mainstream neurosciences However it appears that this innovative technology is here to stay. Questions are often raised – and rightly so – whether Telemedicine is the result of technology push rather than clinical pull. Information Technology has changed, is changing, and will continue to change the delivery of health care, worldwide. Humankind is witnessing a growth in technology unprecedented in the annals of history. Previous generations of physicians will find the new concepts of telemedicine unfathomable. To many, it may sound blasphemous. What will happen to the individual doctor patient relationship considered sacrosanct for centuries? Is it not sacrilegious and bordering on heresy to treat a patient in another continent without knowing his family and cultural background? Yes, say the diehards. No, say the technology enthusiasts. The truth, as in all great truths, is probably somewhere in between.

Telemedicine enthusiasts should not forget that technology should be used as a support to treat patients, not viewed as a goal in itself. The challenge today is not confined to overcoming technological barriers, insurmountable though they may appear. It is true that available technology still has considerable scope for improvement. Rather the challenge is why, where and how, to implement which technology and at what cost. A needs assessment is critical. The take off problems, facing telemedicine is legion. Telemedicine today sounds hep and cool, but the reality may be quite different. The future however promises to be exciting. Telemedicine will be more than a roller coaster trip. The journey will well be worth the wait. Time alone will tell Cushing once remarked in another context, whether Telemedicine is a "forward step in a backward direction" or to paraphrase Neil Armstrong "one small step for man but one giant leap for mankind."

It is the author's dream and hope that within the next few years there will be telemedicine units in most parts of suburban and rural India. Feasibility and proof of concept validation studies have been completed and the first phase of execution is starting. ISRO hopes that eventually there would be almost a million teleconsultations a day in India. Eventually no Indian will be deprived of a specialist consultation wherever he/she is. This is not impossible. What is required is not implementing better technology and getting funds but changing the mindset of the people involved. Neurological consultation in suburban and rural India and many other regions will soon be only a mouse click away!!

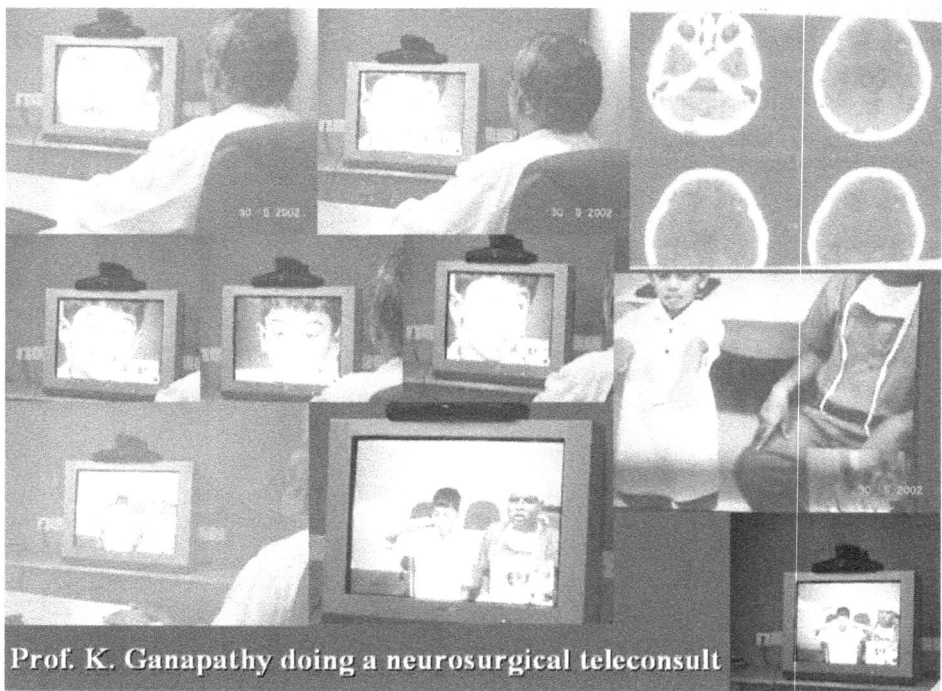

Prof. K. Ganapathy doing a neurosurgical teleconsult

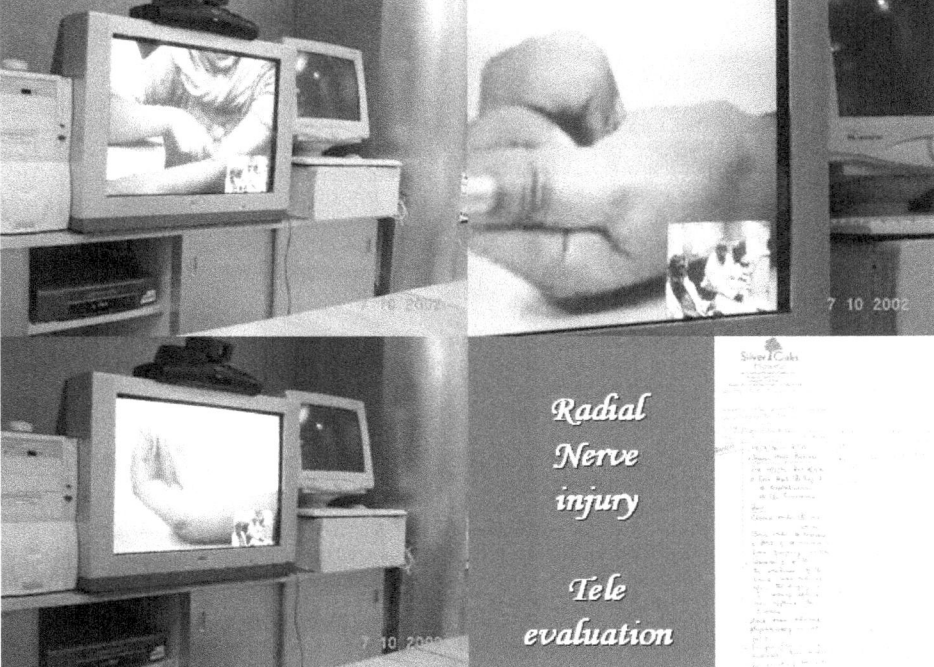

References

[1] Todd Dorman: Telemedicine in anesthesia Anesthesiology Clinics of North America: 2000;18:663.
[2] Ganapathy K: Role of Telemedicine in Neurosciences in Progress in Clinical Neurosciences 2002; 17:1-10.
[3] Ganapathy K: Telemedicine in action. The Apollo experience. 95-102. Proceedings of the International Conference on Medical Informatics. Editors ML Saikumar, Nirmala Sekhar Institute of Public Enterprise 2001.
[4] Moser PL, Hauffe H, Lorenz IH, Hager M, Tiefenthaler W, Lorenz HM, Mikuz G, Soegner P, Kolbitsch C: Publication output in telemedicine during the period January 1964 to July 2003. J Telemed Telecare 2004;10(2):72-7.
[5] Ganapathy K: Telemedicine in India in "Medical Informatics Around the World" editor Andrew Steele 2002. Universal Publishers. USA.
[6] Ganapathy K: Telemedicine in neurology: underutilized potential. Letters to the Editor Neurology India 2005. Accepted for publication.
[7] Ganapathy K: Telemedicine in the Indian context. An overview p. 178-181 in "Establishing telemedicine in developing countries: from inception to implementation". Editor Rifat Latifi. Studies in health technology and Informatics. vol. 104. IOS Press 2004.
[8] Ganapathy K: Relevance of telemedicine in caring for the less than abled. P. 137-139. Report of the Conference on Information Technology Enablers for persons with Disability. Institution of Electronics and Telecommunications Engineers 2001.
[9] Ganapathy K: Telemedicine and Neurosciences in developing countries. Surgical Neurology 2002; 58:388-395.
[10] Misra UK, Kalita J, Mishra SK, Yadav RK: Telemedicine in neurology: Underutilized potential. Neurol India 2005;53:27-31.
[11] Ganapathy K: Telemedicine in neurology. Neurol India 2005;53:242-242.
[12] Patterson V: Teleneurology. J Telemed Telecare 2005;11(2):55-9.
[13] Bremner F, Kennedy C, Rees A, Acheson J, Murdoch I: Usefulness of teleconsultations in neuro-ophthalmology. J Telemed Telecare 2002;8(5):305-6.

[14] Megan A. Letourneau, Daune L. MacGregor, Paul T. Dick, E.J. McCabe, Anita J. Allen, Valerie W, Chan, Lynn J. MacMillan, Meredith R. Golomb. Use of a Telephone Nursing Line in a Pediatric Neurology Clinic: One Approach to the Shortage of Subspecialists. PEDIATRICS Vol. 112 No. 5 November 2003, pp. 1083-1087.

[15] Warren B. Karp, R. Kevin Grigsby, Maureen McSwiggan-Hardin, Suzanne Pursley-Crotteau, Laura N. Adams, Wyndolyn Bell, Max E. Stachura, William P. Kanto. Use of Telemedicine for Children With Special Health Care Needs. PEDIATRICS Vol. 105 No. 4 April 2000, pp. 843-847.

[16] Garaizar C, Sobradillo I, Martinez-Gonzalez MJ, Prats JM: Telephone consultation in child neurology practice: quantification and contents. Rev Neurol 1999;29:999-1002.

[17] Paiva T, Coelho H, Araujo MT, Rodrigues R, Almeida A, Navarro T, Cruz M, Carneiro G, Belo C: Neurological teleconsultation for general practitioners. J Telemed Telecare 2001;7(3):149-54.

[18] Maulden SA: Information technology, the internet, and the future of neurology. Neurologist 2003 May;9(3):149-59.

[19] Paiva T, Coelho H, Almeida A, Navarro T, Araujo MT, Belo C: Teleconsulta en neurology in a health unit: preliminary approach. Acta Med Port 2000 Jul-Aug;13(4):149-58.

[20] Campanella N, Francioni O, Taus M, Giovagnoli M, Morosini P: Medicina Generale, Azienda Ospedaliera Umberto I, Ancona. When and how is medical teleconsultation to doctors practising in remote areas of developing countries convenient and reliable? About eight clinical cases. Recenti Prog Med 2004 Jan;95(1):5-10.

[21] Araujo MT, Paiva T, Jesuino JC, Magalhaes M: General practitioners and neurotelemedicine. Stud Health Technol Inform 2000;78:45-67.

[22] Steven MW: Telemedicine in developing countries. BMJ 2001;323:524-525.

[23] Schoffer KL, Patterson V, Read SJ, Henderson RD, Pandian JD, O'Sullivan JD: Guidelines for filming digital camera video clips for the assessment of gait and movement disorders by teleneurology. J Telemed Telecare 2005;11(7):368-71.

[24] Hubble JP, Pahwa R, Michalek DK, Thomas C, Koller WC: Interactive video conferencing: a means of providing interim care to Parkinson's disease patients Mov Disord 1993 Jul;8(3):380-2.

[25] Vassallo DJ, Hoque F, Farquharson Roberts M, Patterson V, Swinfen P, Swinfen R: An evaluation of the first year's experience with a low-cost telemedicine link in Bangladesh. J Telemed Telecare 2001; 7:125-38.

[26] Yellowless P: Successful development of telemedicine systems-seven core principles. J Telemed Telecare 1997;3:215-22.

[27] Rottger J, Irving AM, Broere J, Tranmer B: Use of telecommunications in a rural emergency. Brain surgery by fax. J Telemed Telecare 1997;3:59-60.

[28] Bailes JE, Poole CC, Hutchison W, Maroon JC, Fukushima T: Utilisation and cost savings of a wide area computer network for Neurosurgical consultation. Telemed J 1997;3:135-9.

[29] Chua R, Craig J, Wootton R, Patterson V: Cost implications of out-patient teleneurology. J Telemed Telecare 2001;1:62-64.

[30] Craig J, Chua R, Russell C, Patterson V, Wootton R: The Cost-effectiveness of teleneurology consultations for patients admitted to hospitals without neurologist on site. 1: A retrospective comparison of the case-mix and management at two rural hospitals. Int J Geriatr Psychiatry 1998;13:381-8.

[31] Craig J, Chua R, Russell C, Patterson V, Wootton R: The cost-effectiveness of teleneurology consultations for patients admitted to hospitals without neurologist on site. A retrospective comparison of the case-mix and management at two rural hospitals. J Telemed Telecare 2000;61(1):46-9.

[32] Maass M, Kosonen M, Kormano M: Transportation savings and medical benefits of a teleneuroradiological network. J Telemed Telecare 2000;6(4):225-8.

[33] Stoeger A, Stromayr W, Giacomuzzi SM, Dessl A, Buchberger W, Jaschke W: A cost analysis of an emergency computerized tomography teleradiology system. J Telemed Telecare 1997;3(1):35-9.

[34] Trott P, Blignault I: Cost evaluation of a telepsychiatry service in northern Queensland. J Telemad Telecare 1998;4:66-8.

[35] Dierks C: Legal aspects of Telepathology. Anal Cell Pathol 2000;21:97-99.

[36] Ganapathy K: Management and prevention of Head injuries in India using telemedicine in "ICRAN 2002 – International conference on Recent Advances in Neurotraumatology Bali Aug 2002". Monduzzi editore International Proceedings Division.

[37] Ganapathy K: Telemedicine in the Management of Head Trauma. The Indian Journal of Neurotraumatology 2004;1:1-7.

[38] Ganapathy K: Role of telemedicine in neurosciences. p. 116-124 in "Establishing telemedicine in developing countries: from inception to implementation". Editor Rifat Latifi. Studies in health technology and Informatics. Vol. 104. IOS Press 2004.

[39] Smith RS: Telemedicine and trauma care. South Med J 2001;8:825-9.

[40] Walters KA: Telephoned head injury referrals: the need to improve the quality of information provided. Arch Emerg Med 1993;10:29-34.

[41] Wang LM, Huang YT, Chern CH, Lo HC, Lee CH, Tang D, Ho LT: Tele-emergency medicine: the evaluation of Taipei Veterans General Hospital and Kinmen-Granite Hospital in Taiwan. Zhonghua Yi Xue Zhi 2001;64: 621-8.

[42] Hazebroucq V, Fery-Lemonnier E: The value of teleradiology in the management of neuroradiologic emergencies. J Neuroradiol 2004 Sep;31(4):334-9.

[43] Hersh WR, Helfand M, Wallace J, Kraemer D, Patterson P, Shapiro S, Greenlick M: Clinical outcomes resulting from telemedicine interventions: a systematic review. BMC Med Inform Decis Mak 2001;1:5. Epub 2001 Nov 26.

[44] Daucourt V, Petitjean ME, Chateil JF, Michel P: Evaluation of the benefits for the patient arising from an inter-hospital teleradiology network in a French administrative area. J Telemed Telecare 2005; 11(4):178-84.

[45] Aucar J, Granchi T, Liscum K, Wall M, Mattox K: Is regionalization of trauma care using telemedicine feasible and desirable? Am J Surg 2000;180:535-9.

[46] Beach M, Miller P, Goodall I: Evaluating telemedicine in an accident and emergency setting. Comput Methods Programs Biomed 2001;64:215-23.

[47] Tachakra S, Loane M, Uche CU: A follow up study of remote trauma teleconsultations. J Telemed Telecare 2000;6:330-4.

[48] Gray W, O'Brien D, Taleb F, Marks C, Buckley T: Benefits and pitfalls of Telemedicine in neurosurgery. J Telemed Telecare 1997;3:108-10.

[49] Gray WP, Somers J, Buckley TF: Report of a national neurosurgical emergency teleconsulting system. Neurosurgery 1998;42:103-108.

[50] Gray WP, Somers J, Buckley TF: Report of a national neurosurgical teleradiology system. J Telemed Telecare 1997;3:36-7.

[51] Gray WP: Report of a national neurosurgical teleradiology system based on optical scanning technology. Proceedings of the 9th European Congress of Radiology. Eur Radiol 1995;5:296.

[52] Gray WP, Somers Jack, Buckley Timothy F: Report of a National Neurosurgical Emergency Teleconsulting System. Spencer JA, Dobson D, Hoare M, Molyneux AJ, Anslow PL: The use of a computerized image transfer system linking a regional neuroradiology center to its district hospitals. Clin Radiol 1991;44:342-344.

[53] Goh KY, Lam CK, Poon WS: The impact of teleradiology on the inter-hospital transfer of Neurosurgical patients. British Journal of Neurosurgery 1997;11:52-56.

[54] Goh KY, Tsang KY, Poon WS: Does teleradiology improve inter-hospital management of head-injury? Can J Neurol Sci 1997;24:235-9.

[55] Poca MA, Sahuquillo J, Domenech P, Pedraza S, Maideu J, Vila X, Arikan F, Sanchez E, Garnacho A: Use of teleradiology in the evaluation and management of head-injured patients. Results of a pilot study of a link between a district general hospital and a neurosurgical referral center. Neurocirugia (Astur) 2004;15:17-35.

[56] Eljamel MS, Nixon T: The use of a computer-based image link system to assist inter-hospital referrals. Br J Neurosurg 1992;6:559-62.

[57] Moulin T, Retel O, Chavot D: Impact of new information and communication technologies (NTIC) on hospital administration and patient management. Care Network for Diagnosing and Treating Neurologic Emergencies. Sante Publique 2003 Apr;15 Spec No:191-200.

[58] Elger CE, Burr W: Advances in telecommunications concerning epilepsy. Epilepsia 2000; 41 Suppl 5:S9-12.

[59] Elger CE, Burr W: Advances in telecommunications concerning epilepsy. Technol Health Care 2000; 8:25-34.

[60] Nardi BA, Schwarz H, Kuchinsky A, Leichner R, Whittaker S, Sclabassi R: "Turning away from talking heads: the use of video-as-data in neurosurgery", Human Factors in Computing Systems INTER-CHI '93 pp. 327-334.

[61] Oizumi T, Ohira T, Kawase T: The use of computers and networking in the neurosurgical field. Rinsho Byori 1999;47:119-25.

[62] Meyer BC, Lyden PD, Al-Khoury L, Cheng Y, Raman R, Fellman R, Beer J, Rao R, Zivin JA: Prospective reliability of the STRokE DOC wireless/site independent telemedicine system. Neurology 2005 Mar 22;64(6):1058-60. Comment in: Neurology 2006 Feb 14;66(3):460.

[63] Chua R, Craig J, Wooton R, Patterson V: Randomised controlled trial of telemedicine for new neurological outpatient referrals. J Neurol Neurosurg Psychiat 2001;71:63-6.

[64] Craig J, Chua R, Russell C, Wootton R, Chant D, Patterson V: A cohort study of early neurological consultation by telemedicine on the care of neurological inpatients J Neurol Neurosurg Psychiatry 2004;75:1031-5.

[65] Craig J, Chua R, Wootton R, Patterson V: A pilot study of telemedicine for new neurological outpatient referrals. J Telemed Telecare 2000;6:225-8.
[66] Craig JJ, McConville JP, Patterson VH, Wootton R: Neurological examination is possible using telemedicine. Journal of Telemedicine and Telecare 1999;5:177-81.
[67] Chaves-Carballo E: Diagnosis of childhood migraine by compressed interactive video. Kans Med 1992;93(12):351-2.
[68] Patterson VH, Craig JJ, Wootton R: Effective diagnosis of spinal cord compression using telemedicine Br J Neurosurg 2000 Dec;14(6):552-4.
[69] Patterson VH, Craig JJ, Wootton R: Effective diagnosis of spinal cord compression using telemedicine Int J Med Inf 2001 May;61(2-3):217-27.
[70] Shiomi T: Telemedicine and lifestyle modifications in obstructive sleep apnea patients. Nippon Rinsho 2000;58:1689-92.
[71] Hurlen P, Osthye T: Electronic House call. Tulsskr Nor Laegeforen 1998;118:2984-7.
[72] Zamzam N, Luther F: Comparison of lip incompetence by remote video surveillance and clinical observation in children with and without cerebral palsy. Eur J Orthod 2001 Feb;23(1):75-84.
[73] Wheeler T: Telemedicine and special needs children. Telemed Today 1998;6:16-20.
[74] Davis MC: MR Teleradiology network serving remote imaging centers. J Digit Imaging 1998; 11(3 Suppl 1):88-92.
[75] Heautot JF, Gibaud B, Catroux B, Thoreux PH, Cordonnier E, Scarabin JM, Carsin M, Gandon Y: Influence of the teleradiology technology (N-ISDN and ATM) on the inter-hospital management of neurosurgical patients. Br J Neurosurg 2000;14:552-4.
[76] Kroeker KI, Diamond R, Jennet PA, Johnston RV: Video-capture teleradiology for the after-hours reading of computerized tomography scans. J Telemed Telecare 2000;6(4):229-32.
[77] Lee T, Latham J, Kerr RS, et al.: Effect of a new computed tomographic image transfer system on management of referrals to a regional neurosurgical service. Lancet 1990;336:101-3.
[78] Sherry L Apple, John H Schmidt: Technique for Neurosurgically Relevant CT Image Transfers Using Inexpensive Video Digital Technology. Surg Neurol 2000;53:411-16.
[79] Spencer JA, Dobson D, Hoare M, Molyneux AJ, Anslow PL: The use of a computerized image transfer system linking a regional neuroradiology center to its district hospitals. Clin Radiol 1991; 44:342-344.
[80] Kuhle S, Mitchell L, Andrew M, Chan AK, Massicotte P, Adams M, deVeber G: Urgent clinical challenges in children with ischemic stroke: analysis of 1065 patients from the 1-800-NOCLOTS pediatric stroke telephone consultation service. Stroke 2006 Jan;37(1):116-22. Epub 2005 Dec 1. Comment in: Stroke 2006 Jan;37(1):3.
[81] David Z, Wang DO: Editorial Comment—Telemedicine: The Solution to Provide Rural Stroke Coverage and the Answer to the Shortage of Stroke Neurologists and Radiologists. Stroke 2003;34:2957.
[82] LaMonte MP, Bahouth MN, Hu P, Pathan MY, Yarbrough KL, Gunawardane R, et al.: Telemedicine for acute stroke Triumphs and Pitfalls. Stoke 2003;34:725-8.
[83] Audebert HJ, Wimmer ML, Hahn R, Schenkel J, Bogdahn U, Horn M, Haberl RL: Can telemedicine contribute to fulfill WHO Helsingborg Declaration of specialized stroke care? Cerebrovasc Dis 2005;20(5):362-9. Epub 2005 Sep 2.
[84] Andreas Wiborg, MD Bernhard Widder. Teleneurology to Improve Stroke Care in Rural Areas- The Telemedicine in Stroke in Swabia (TESS) Project. Stroke 2003;34:2951.
[85] Choi JY, Porche NA, Albright KC, Khaja AM, Ho VS, Grotta JC: Using telemedicine to facilitate thrombolytic therapy for patients with acute stroke. Jt Comm J Qual Patient Saf 2006 Apr;32(4): 199-205.
[86] Wiborg A, Widder B, Riepe MW, Krauss M, Huber R, Schmitz B: Contribution by telemedicine on comprehensive care for stroke patients in rural areas. Akt Neurol 2000;27:119-124.
[87] Levine SR, Gorman M: "Telestroke": the application of telemedicine for stroke. Stroke 1999;30: 464-9.
[88] Shafqat S, Kvedar JC, Guanci MM, Chang Y, Schwamm LH: Role for telemedicine in acute stroke: feasibility and reliability of remote administration of the NIH Stroke Scale. Stroke 1999;30: 2141-2145.
[89] Tissue plasminogen activator for acute ischemic stroke. National Institute of Neurological Disorders and stroke rt-PA stroke study group. N Eng J Med 1995;333:1581-7.
[90] LaMonte MP, Bates V, Bahouth MN, Gunawardane RD, Yarbrough KL, Pathan MY, Page CW, Mehlman I, Crarey PE: Safe rt-PA administration for ischemic stroke during telemedicine consultation: poster presentation. Stroke 2000;32:374-a.
[91] Wang DZ, Rose JA, Honings DS, Garwacki DJ, Milbrandt JC: Treating acute stroke patients with intravenous tPA: the OSF Stroke Network expertise. Stroke 2000;31:77-81.

[92]   Wilborg A, Widder B: Teleneurology to improve stroke care in rural areas: The Telemedicine in Stroke in Swabia (TESS) Project. Stroke 2003;34:2951-6.

[93]   Barber M, Stott DJ: Validity of the Telephone Interview for Cognitive Status (TICS) in post-stroke subjects. Int J Geriatr Psychiatry 2004;19:75-9.

[94]   Hubble JP: Interactive vide conferencing and Parkinson's disease. Dept. of Neurology, Kans Med 1992;93:351-2.

[95]   Monteiro IM, Boksay I, Auer SR, Torossian C, Sinaiko E, Reisberg B: Reliability of routine clinical instruments for the assessment of Alzheimer's disease administered by telephone. J Geriatr Psychiatry Neurol 1998;11:18-24.

[96]   Smyth KA, Harris PB - TI: Using telecomputing to provide information and support to caregivers of persons with dementia. Gerontologist 1993 Feb;33(1):123-7.

[97]   Smyth KA, Harris PB: Using telecomputing to provide information and support to caregivers of persons with dementia. Kans Med 1992;93:351-2.

[98]   Harvey R, Roques PK, Fox NC, Rossor MN: CANDID – Counseling and diagnosis in dementia: a national telemedicine service supporting the care of younger patients with dementia. Int J Geriatr Psychiatry 1998;13:381-8.

[99]   Harvey R, Roques PK, Fox NC, Rossor MN: CANDID – Counselling and Diagnosis in Dementia: a national telemedicine service supporting the care of younger patients with dementia. Med Inform Internet Med 1999;24(2):121-34.

[100]   Mahoney DF, Tarlow B, Sandaire J: A computer-mediated intervention for Alzheimer's caregivers. Comput Nurs 1998;16:208-16.

[101]   Dreyer NC, Dreyer KA, Shaw DK, Wittman PP: Efficacy of telemedicine in occupational therapy: a pilot study. J Allied Health 2001;30:39-42.

[102]   Gammon D, Bergvik S, Bergmo T, Pedersen S: Videoconferencing in psychiatry: a survey of use in northern Norway. J Telemed Telecare 1996;2:192-8.

[103]   Mannion L, Fahy TJ, Duffy C, Borderick M, Gethins E: Telepsychiatry: an island pilot project. J Telemad Telecare 1998;4:62-3.

[104]   May C, Gask L, Ellis N, Alkinson T, Mair F, Smith C, Pidd S, Esmail A: Telepsychiatry evaluation in the north-west of England: preliminary results of a qualitative study. J Telemed Telecare 2000;6:820-2.

[105]   McLaren PM, Ball CJ: Interpersonal communications and telemedicine: hypotheses and methods. J Telemed Telecare 1997;3:5-7.

[106]   Miclonen ML, Ohinmaa A, Moring J, Isohanni M: The use of videoconferencing for telepsychiatry in Finland. J Telemed Telecare 1998;4:125-31.

[107]   Paul NL: Telepsychiatry, the satellite system and family consultation. J Telemad Telcare 1997;3:52-3.

[108]   Rappaport N: Emerging models. Chil Adolesc Psychiatr Clin N Am 2001;10:13-24.

[109]   Ruskin PE, Reed S, Kumar R, Kling MA, Siegel E, Rosen M, Hauser P: Reliability and acceptability of psychiatric diagnosis via telecommunication and audiovisual technology. Psychiatr Serv 1998; 49:1086-8.

[110]   Seemann O, Soyka M: Psychiatry and psychotherapy on the internet. Current overview. Nervenarzt 199;70:76-80.

[111]   Souza D: Telemedicine for intensive support of psychiatric inpatients admitted to local hospitals. J Telemed Telecare 2000;6:826-8.

[112]   Stevens A, Doidge N, Goldbloom D, Voore P, Farewell J: Pilot study of televideo psychiatric assessments in an underserviced community. Am J Psychiatry 1999;156:783-5.

[113]   Yellowless P, Kennedy C: Telemedicine applications in an integrated mental health service based at a teaching hospital. J Telemed Telecare 1996;2:205-9.

[114]   Baer L, Cukor P, Jenike MA, Leah L, Laughlen J, Coyle JT: Pilot studies of telemedicine for patients with obsessive-compulsive disorder. Am J Psychiatry 1996;153:968.

[115]   Brown FW: Rural telepsychiatry. Psychiatr Serv 1998;49:963-4.

[116]   Cawthorpe D: An evaluation of a computer-based psychiatric assessment: evidence for expanded use. Cyberpsychol Behav 2001;4:503-10.

[117]   Cukor P, Baer L, Willis BS, Leahy L, OLaughlen J, Murphy M, Withers M, Martin E: Use of video-phones and low-cost standard telephone lines to provide a social presence in telepsychiatry. Telemed J 1998;4:313-21.

[118]   Souza D: Telemedicine for intensive support of psychiatric inpatients admitted to local hospitals. J Telemed Telecare 2000;6:826-8.

[119]   Gelber H: The experience in Victoria with telepsychiatry for the child and adolescent Mental Health Services. J Telemed Telecare 2001;7:32-4.

[120]   Gelber H: The experience of the Royal Childrens Hospital Mental Health Service videoconferencing project. J Telemed Telecare 1998;4:71-3.

[121] Kopel H, Nunn K, Dossetor D: Evaluating satisfaction with a child and adolescent psychological telemedicine outreach service. J Telemed Telecare 2001;7:35-40.
[122] Tang WK, Chiu H, Woo J, Hjelm M, Hui E: Telepsychiatry in psychogeriatric services: a pilot study. Int J Geriatr Psychiatry 2001;16:88-93.
[123] Gourlay D, Lun KC, Liya J: Telemedicinal virtual reality for cognitive rehabilitation. Stud Health Technol Inform 2000;77:1181-6.
[124] Rydmark M, Broeren J, Pascher R. Mednet: Stroke rehabilitation at home using virtual reality, haptics and telemedicine. Stud Health Technol Inform 2002;85:434-7.
[125] Grimes GJ, Dubois H, Grimes SJ, Greenleaf WJ, Rothernberg F, Cunnigham D: Telerehabilitation services using web-based telecommunication. Stud Health Technol Inform 2000;70:113-8.
[126] Kates N, Curstolo AM, Nikolaou L, Craven MA, Farrar S: Providing psychiatric backup to family physicians by telephone. Can J Psychiatry 1997;42:955-9.
[127] Kavanagh SJ, Yellowlees PM: Telemedicine clinical applications in mental health. Aust Fam Physician 1995;24:1242-7.
[128] Kavangh S, Hawker F: The fall and rise of the South Australian telepsychiatry network. J Telemed Telecare 2001;7:41-3.
[129] Vaz, Francisco, Pacheco, Osvaldo, Martins da Silva, Antonio: A telemedicine application of EEG signal transmission. Proceedings of the Annual Conference on Engineering in Medicine and Biology NJ, USA. 1991;466-467.
[130] Loula P, Rauhala E, Erkinjuntti M, Tary E, Hirvonen K, Hakkinen V: Distributed clinical neurophysiology. J Telemed Telecare 1997;3(2):89-95.
[131] Cronenberger JH, Hsiao H, Falk RJ, Jennette JC: Neuropathology consultation via digitized images. Ann N Y Acad Sci 1992;670:281-92.
[132] Walter GF, Malthies HK, Brandis A, von Jan U: Telemedicine of the future: Teleneuropathology. Technol Health Care 2000;8:25-34.
[133] Walter GF, Matthies HK, Brandis A, von Jan U: Telemedicine of the future: tele Neuropathology. J Telemed Telecare 2000;8(3):142-6.
[134] Mairinger T, Netzer TT, Schoner W, Gschwendtner A: Pathologists' attitudes to implementing Telepathology. J Telemed Telecare 1998;4(1):41-6.
[135] Szymas J, Wolf G, Papierz W, Jarosz B, Weinstein RS: Online internet based robotic telepathology in the diagnosis of neuro-oncology cases: a teleneuropathology feasibility study. Hum Pathol 2001; 32:1304-8.
[136] Becker RL Jr, Specht CS, Jones R, Rueda-Pedraza ME, O'Leary TJ: Use of remote video microscopy (Telepathology) as an adjunct to neurosurgical frozen section consultation. Hum Pathol 1993;24: 909-11.
[137] Eide TJ, Nordrum I, Stalsberg H: The validity of frozen section diagnosis based on video microscopy. Zentralbl Pathol 1992;138:405-7.
[138] Striepecke E, Handt S, Weis J, Koch A, Cremerius U, Reineke T, Bull U, Schroder JM, Zang KD, Bocking A: Image analysis in meningiomas. Correlation of histology, cytogenetics and proliferation fraction. Pathol Reo Pxact 1996;192:816-24.
[139] Steffen B, Gianom D, Winkler C, Hosch HJ, Oberholzer M, Famos M: Frozen section diagnosis using Telepathology. Swiss Surg 1997;3:25-9.
[140] Becker RL Jr, Specht CS, Jones R, Rueda-Pedraza ME, O'Leary TJ: Use of remote video microscopy (Telepathology) as an adjunct to neurosurgical frozen section consultation. Hum Pathol 1993 Aug; 24(8):909-11.
[141] Nagata H, Mizushima H: World wide microscope: new concept of Internet Telepathology microscope and implementation of the prototype. Medinfo 1998;9:286-9.
[142] Ronan L, Murphy K, Browne G, Connolly S, McMenamin J, Lynch B, Delanty N, Fitzsimons M: Needs analysis for tele-neurophysiology in the Irish North-Western Health Board. Ir Med J 2004; 97(2):46-9.
[143] Jacobs EC, Lagerlund TD, Collura TF, Burgess RC: A data interchange standard for clinical neurophysiology Proc Annu Symp Comput Appl Med Care 1993;813-7.
[144] Monteiro IM, Boksay I, Auer SR, Torossian C, Sinaiko E, Reisberg B, Nenov V, Kiopp J: Remote access to neurosurgical ICU physiological data using World Wide Web. Stud Health Technol Inform 1996;29:242-9.
[145] Nenov V, Kiopp J: Remote access to Neurosurgical ICU physiological data using World Wide Web. Stud Health Technol Inform 1996;29:242-9.
[146] Nenov V, Klopp J: Remote analysis of physiological data from Neurosurgical ICU patients. J Am Med Inform Assoc 1996;3:318-27.
[147] Yoo SK, Kim SH, Kim NH, Kang YT, Kim KM, Bae SH, Vannier MW: Design of a PC-based multimedia telemedicine system for brain function teleconsultation. Int J Med Inf 2001;61:217-27.

[148] Yoo SK, Kim SH, Kim NH, Kang YT, Kim KM, Bae SH, Vannier MW: Design of a PC-based multi-media telemedicine system for brain function Teleconsultation. Eur J Orthod 2001;23(1):75-84.
[149] Vingtoft S, Johnsen B, Fuglsang-Frederiksen A, Veloso M, Barahona P, Vila A, Fawcett P, Scofield I, Ladegaard J, Otte G, et al.: ESTEEM: a European telematic project for quality assurance within clinical neurophysiology. Medinfo 1995;2:1047-51.
[150] Suryanarayanan S, Reddy NP, Gupta V: An intelligent system with EMG-based joint angle estimation for telemanipulation. Stud Health Technol Inform 1996;29:546-52.
[151] Johnson P, Andrews DC: Remote continuous physiological monitoring in the home. J Telemed Telecare 1996;2;107-13.
[152] Von Hanwehr R, Popescy GF, Taylor HE, Winkler KH, Swenberg CE: Interventional telemedicine for noninvasive neuroradiosurgery: remote-site high-performance computing, mathematical optimization, and virtual scenario simulation. Journal of Medical Systems 1995;19:219-62.
[153] Yamamoto LG, Williams DR: A demonstration of instant pocket wireless CT teleradiology to facilitate neurosurgical consultation and future telemedicine implications. Am J Emerg Med 2000;18:423-6.
[154] Yamamoto LG: Wireless teleradiology and fax using cellular phones and notebook PCs for instant access to consultants. Am J Emerg Med 1995;13:184-187.
[155] Navein J, Fisher A, Geiling J, Richards D, Roller J, Hagmann J: Portable satellite telemedicine in practice. J Telemed Telecare 1998;4 Suppl 1:25-8.
[156] Heautot JF, Gibaud B, Catroux B, Thoreux PH, Cordonnier E, Scarabin JM, Carsin M, Gandon Y: Influence of teleradiology technology (N-ISDN and ATM) on the inter-hospital management of neurosurgical patients. Med Inform Internet Med 1999;24:121-34.
[157] Houkin K, Fukuhara S, Selladurai BM, Zurin AA, Ishak M, Kuroda S, Abe H: Telemedicine in Neurosurgery using international digital telephone services between Japan and Malaysia – technical note. Neurologia Medico-Chirurgica 39(11):773-7; discussion 777-8, 1999 Epilepsia 2000;41 Suppl 5: S9-12.
[158] Houkin K, Fukuhara S, Selladurai BM, Zurin AA, Ishak M, Kuroda S, Abe H: Telemedicine in Neurosurgery using international digital telephone services between Japan & Malaysia – technical note. Neurologia Medico—Chirugrgica 1999;39(11):773-7.
[159] Yamamoto LG: Using JPEG image compression to facilitate telemedicine. Am J Emerg Med 1995; 13:55-57.
[160] Urban V, Busart C, Huwel N, Perneezky A: Teleconsultation: A new neurosurgical image transfer system for daily routine and emergency cases—a four year study. Eur J Emerg Med 1996;3:5-8.
[161] Ludwig K, Bick U, Oelerich M, Schuierer G, Puskas Z, Nicolas K, Koch A, Lenzen H: Is image selection a useful strategy to decrease the transmission time in teleradiology? A study using 100 emergency cranial CTs – Eur Radiol 1998;8:1719-21.
[162] Yamamoto LG, Herman MI, Elliott P, et al: Telemedicine using the internet. Am J Emerg Med 1996; 14:416-420.
[163] Fujimaki T: Applications of the World Wide Web to neurosurgical practice. Neurosurgery 1997; 41:995-6.
[164] Yamamoto LG, Suh PJ: Accessing and using the internet's world wide web for emergency physicians. Am J Emerg Med 1996;14:302-308.
[165] Botia E: The Internet application to neurology: electronic forums of Revista de Neurologia. How the Internet, Medicine and Neurology Forum has been developed. Rev Neurol 1998;26:578-80.
[166] Mola S, Botia E, Belmonte MA, Bravo R, Casado A, Moreno P, Osorno M, Vega-Gama JG: Electronic forum of revista de neurologia: 'Internet, Medicine and Neurologia'. Rev Neurol 1998;26: 625-32.
[167] Pareras LG, Martin-Rodriguez JG: Neurosurgery and the Internet: a critical analysis and a review of available resources. Neurosurgery 1996 Jul;39(1):216-32; discussion 232-3.
[168] Tronnier VM, Staubert A, Bonsanto MM, Wirtz CR, Kunze S: Virutal reality in Neurosurgery. Radiologe 2000;40:211-7.
[169] Viirre E: Vestibular telemedicine and rehabilitation. Application for virtual reality. Stud Health Technol Inform 1996;29:299-305.
[170] Sakovich VP, Kolotvinov VS: The current neurosurgical resources on the Internet. Zh Vopr Neirokhir Im N N Burdenko 1999;2:3-7.
[171] Misra UK, Kalita J, Mishra SK, Yadav RK: Telemedicine for distance education in neurology: Preliminary experience in India. J Telemed Telecare 2004 (in the press).

Current Principles and Practices of Telemedicine and e-Health
R. Latifi (Ed.)
IOS Press, 2008

Telemedicine in Primary Health Care

Anastasia KASTANIA
Department of Informatics, Athens University of Economics and Business, Greece

Abstract. Here, the possibilities to build integrated primary health care telemedicine services are presented accompanied with available epistemic criteria for quality evaluation purposes. Given that the cost of sanitary care is increasing continuously the telemedicine approach is a challenge for providing quality care and at low cost to the rural citizens.

Keywords. Telemedicine infrastructures, integrated information systems, quality

Introduction

The concepts for telemedical services design and development are the same, independent of whether they have to be provided within a clinic (local setting), between clinics and general practitioners (regional or metropolitan area), or on the wide area scale [1]. The goals for applying telemedicine in primary health care should include:

- the immediate and complete participation of the specialist in the treatment of a medical incident that cannot be treated completely by the general practitioner
- the overall estimation not only in diagnosis and therapy but also in the transfer of the patient to secondary care services
- the reduction of the socio-economic consequences of a disease to the patient, his family and in the society
- the systematic training of general practitioners in the use of real-time communication systems.

1. Basic Requirements to Practice Telemedicine in Primary Care

Primary health establishments can be grouped in Health Centers (HCs) or Health Posts (HPs) [2]. The set of various HPs depending on one HC configures what is called a 'health micronet', which is the basic unit in primary health-care systems [2]. Every Health Post and Health Center should have:

- physician (general practitioner trained in pre-hospital emergencies handling)
- basic diagnostic medical technology (digital electrocardiograph, medical scanner, spirometer, otoscope, ophthalmoscope, electronic stethoscope, vital signs monitor, holter, pharyngoscope, dermascope, colposcope, fetal monitor)
- necessary equipment and materials to handle the emergencies
- telephone devices (with ISDN connection if possible) to communicate, transfer data and connect with the Internet

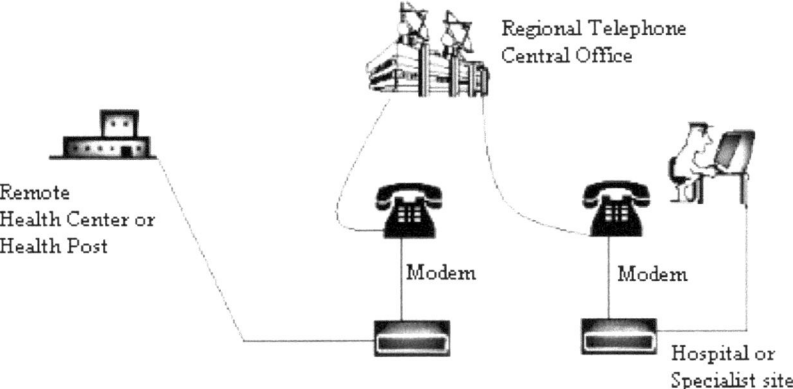

Figure 1. Telephone in primary healthcare telemedicine.

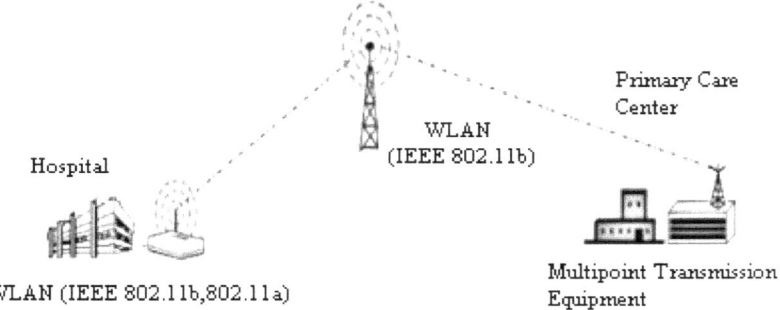

Figure 2. Wireless and terrestrial communications.

- a computer capable to send and receive high quality medical images and biosignals, connected with a printer and a document scanner.

2. Primary Care Telemedicine Infrastructures

Telemedicine systems should be as easy to use as the telephone [3]. The wired networking architectures used in primary care telemedicine are the plain old telephone services (POTS) and the integrated services digital network (ISDN) (Fig. 1).

Rural telemedicine networks have also been designed using the IEEE 802 (Fig. 2).

Also air/wireless communications, radio frequency, microwaves, satellite, the global mobile system (GSM) and the cellular digital packet data (CDPD) have been used. To be successful, telemedicine technologies must adapt to the needs of practitioners and patients [3]. Fortunately, the Internet is able to support the data transmission needs projected for telemedicine [4].

Satellites are extremely important for the communication between the primary care centers and the hospitals [5]. Multimedia technology plays a critical role in developing telemedicine applications. New broadband technology of networking (DVB-RCS: Digital Video Broadcasting-Return Channel by Satellite, DVB-S: Digital Video Broad-

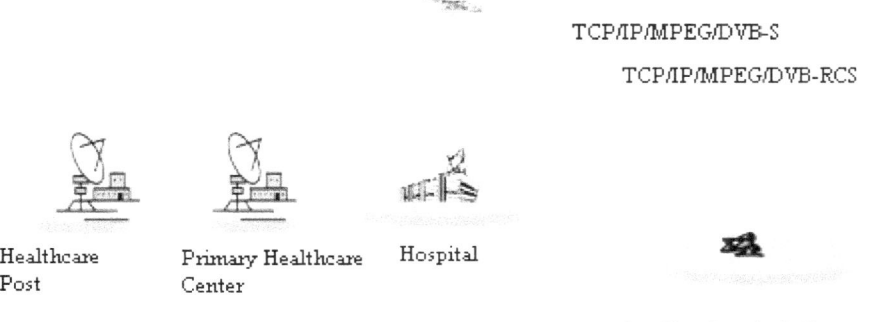

TCP/IP/MPEG/DVB-S

TCP/IP/MPEG/DVB-RCS

Healthcare
Post

Primary Healthcare   Hospital
Center

Satellite Terminals Access   Satellite Terminals/Gateway

Figure 3. Broadband satellite multimedia network.

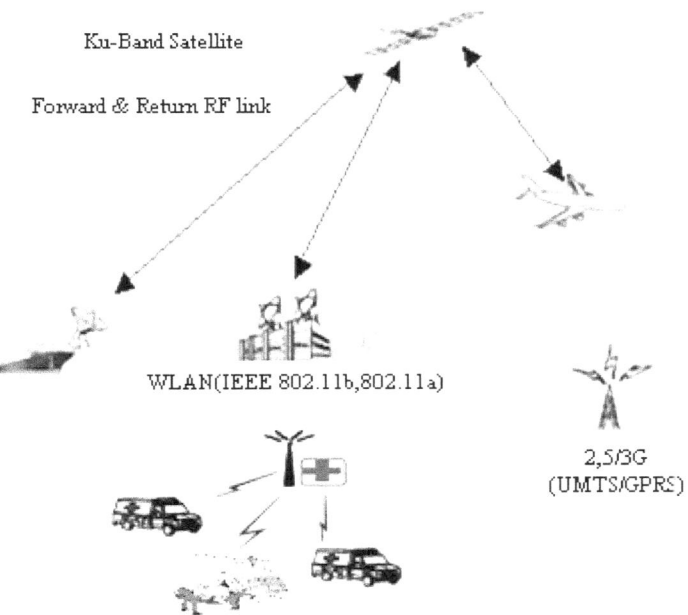

Ku-Band Satellite

Forward & Return RF link

WLAN(IEEE 802.11b,802.11a)

2,5/3G
(UMTS/GPRS)

Figure 4. Pre-hospital health emergency care.

casting by Satellite) is the current challenge in transferring medical multimedia data (Fig. 3).

Also integrated systems need to be developed and be operational providing telematics tools and services for the best planning, and response management of pre-hospital health emergencies (Fig. 4).

3. Primary Care Integrated Information Systems

The design of telemedicine information systems for primary health care is a non-trivial task (Fig. 5).

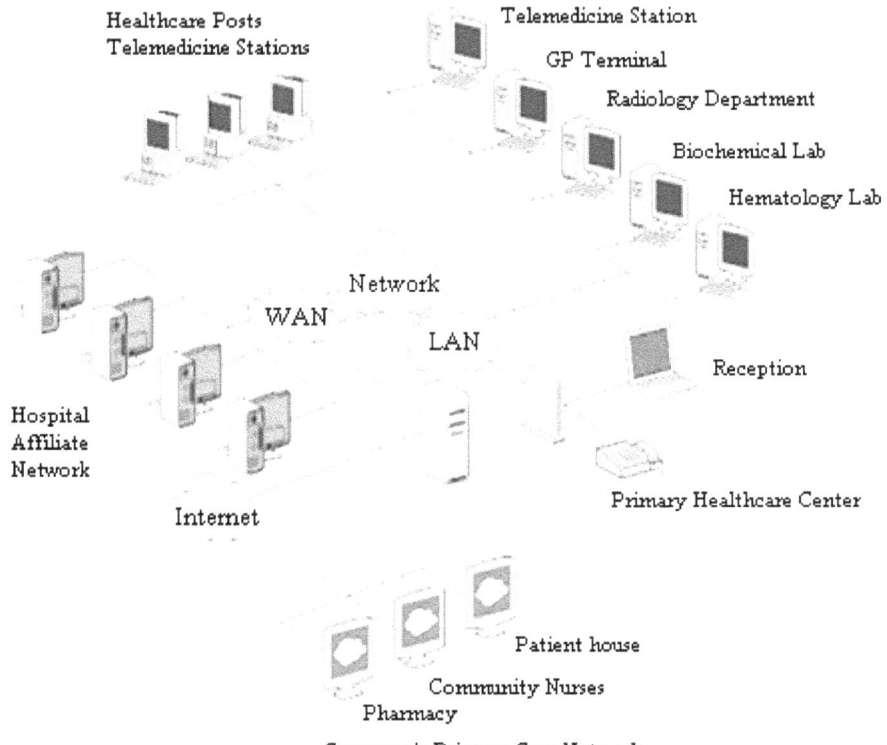

Figure 5. Communities of communication in regional or national networks.

The primary care has a main role in the delivery of preventive health care and in the triaging of patients needing a specialist or hospital services [6]. In the primary care center or in the health post a database server is needed to act as a central repository for patient information, which can be made available on request from the physician's personal computer. The physician should have access to software modules integrated into his or her patient management system [6]. Use of the longitudinal clinical record for clinical management of at risk patients is an important tool for optimizing outcomes and minimizing costs in general practice [6]. The areas of clinical decision support, computerized clinical measurement and patient education are given particular attention as they represent novel and emerging activities in the computerization of general practice. Smart cards, which use computer chips embedded in a plastic card, are used for healthcare purposes in primary care in some European countries [7]. Such smart cards could potentially enable individual patients to access their electronic medical records or control access of others to those records [7].

An obstacle to carry out the standardized electronic medical record is the lack of a full-standardized medical vocabulary [8]. Physicians urged that SNOMED III vocabulary could be used because it includes symptoms, findings and modifiers [8]. There are also electronic medical records implementations that use ICPC-2 (International Classification of Primary Care) in combination with the more granular classification ICD10 (International Classification of Diseases), to describe every clinical situation in general practice in proper detail [9].

Primary care integrated information systems should support the provision of telemedicine services. The importance of network communications to practice telemedicine is obvious. Basic asynchronous health care communication can be carried out using general-purpose computer-mediated-communication software that allows for improved communication channels (including Internet delivered interactive video for telemedicine consultations), e-mail and Web-based chat and discussion forums [10]. Various encryption and authentication methods have emerged for e-mail, including secure multi-purpose Internet mail extensions (S/MIME) and Internet applications including secure sockets layer (SSL), secure HTTP (S-HTTP) and secure electronic transactions (SET). Effective asynchronous health care communication will give telemedicine a greater reach and support the connectivity and clinical care goals of e-health. Physicians need to be experienced in medical records processing, scheduling and intrafaculty communication [10]. Furthermore they need to be trained to practice telemedicine effectively.

4. Quality Assurance Models for Primary Care Telemedicine Networks

According to Grigsby and Barton [11] usefulness and usability must have a central role in the assessment of telemedicine technology. Although health services have the appropriate technology, high quality data transmission is also necessary.

Ribière et al. [12] propose a loss-function as a quality tool to measure how customer dissatisfaction can affect cost and healthcare quality. Bailey et al. [13] proposed a technique to measure and analyze computer user satisfaction, using a weighted sum of a set of thirty-nine factors. These approaches can be used as a basis for the assessment of both patient and physician satisfaction since in telemedicine applications they are both users of computers and other medical equipment.

There are many dimensions to exploit quality in primary care teleapplications. These include the following quality evaluation issues: telehealth network [14–16], information standards [15], medical services provision [17,18], communications [19], interaction [18], data transmission [18], teleconsultations [20], software [21], health care [22–28], life [29,30], multimedia [31], equipment [32,33] and patient satisfaction [12,13].

The planned level in the construction of a National Standard for primary care telemedicine services provision based on improvement of quality should take into account the "Good Enough Quality Framework" [34] and the "Success model of an Information System" proposed by DeLone and McLean [35]. Good enough quality is assured via assessment of the benefits, the problems and the overall quality of the product. The "Success model of an Information System" supports a socio-technical analysis of the systems and recognizes quality as a demand for success. The components in DeLone and McLean model are [35]: quality of service, quality of the system, quality of information, use, user satisfaction, individual impact and organizational impact. Furthermore, questionnaires can be designed to assess user, provider and organization satisfaction [14,36–41].

Conclusions

The computer and communication technologies to practice primary care telemedicine have been sufficiently developed. Technology allows physicians to "visit" using computer networks the primary care patients and are capable to consult each other for complex medical cases using teleconferencing in real-time.

Proper application of information technology in primary health care and use of telemedicine will extend traditional diagnosis and patient management beyond the physician's office. On going technical aid and support is critical to continue a telemedicine service. Special attention should be given to the fact that it is not so much the technology that makes the difference but that the rural patients respond positively to consistent access, care, monitoring and attention provided by telemedicine.

References

[1] A.N. Kastania, Telemedicine models for primary care, Chapter in the Book *Establishing Telemedicine in Developing Countries: from inception to implementation* (ed. R. Latifi), IOS Press, Amsterdam (2004) 89-98.

[2] A. Martínez, V. Villarroel, J. Seoane, and F. del Pozo, Analysis of Information and Communication Needs in Rural Primary Health Care in Developing Countries, *IEEE Transactions On Information Technology In Biomedicine* 9(1) (2005) 66-72.

[3] D.S. Puskin and J.H. Sanders, Telemedicine Infrastructure Development, *Journal of Medical Systems* 19(2) (1995) 125-129.

[4] B.A. Houtchens, A. Allen, T.P. Clemmer, D.A. Lindberg and S. Pedersen, Telemedicine Protocols and Standards: Development and Implementation, *Journal of Medical Systems* 19(2) (1995) 93-119.

[5] H.W. Tyrer, P.D. Wiedemeier, R.W. Cattlet, Rural Telemedicine: Satellites and Fiber Optics, *Biomed Sci Instrum* 37 (2001) 417-422.

[6] N.H. Lovell and B.G. Celler, Information technology in primary health care, in the Proceedings of APAMI- HIC 97, 55(1) (1999) 9-22.

[7] L.L. Dickey and J.D. Piette, Promoting the Delivery of Preventive Medicine in Primary Care, Chapter in the Book *Public Health Informatics and Information Systems* (eds. P.W. O'Carroll, W.A. Yasnoff, M.E. Ward, L.H. Ripp and E.L. Martin), Springer, London (2003) 513-531.

[8] G.J. Arvary, The Limited Use of Digital Ink in the Private-sector Primary Care Physician's Office, *Journal of the American Medical Informatics Association* 6 (2) (1999) 134-142.

[9] D.K. Kounalakis, C. Lionis, I. Okkes and H. Lamberts, Developing an Appropriate EPR System for the Greek Primary Care Setting, *Journal of Medical Systems* 27(3) (2003) 239-246.

[10] V. Wilson, Asynchronous Health Care Communication, Communications of the ACM 46(6) (2003) 79-84.

[11] J. Grigsby and P.L. Barton, Telecommunications Technology, Health Services & Technology Assessment, in the Proceedings of Medical Technology Symposium (1998) 12-15.

[12] V. Ribière, A.J. LaSalle, R. Khorramshahgol, Y. Gousty, Hospital Information Systems Quality: A Customer Satisfaction Assessment Tool, in the Proceedings of the 32nd Hawaii International Conference on System Sciences (1999).

[13] J.E. Bailey and S.W. Pearson, Development of a tool for measuring and analyzing user satisfaction, *Management Science* 29(5) (1983) 530-545.

[14] M. Hebert, Telehealth success: evaluation framework development, in the Proceedings of Medinfo 10(Pt 2) (2001) 1145-9.

[15] J.C. Hogenbirk, KO Telehealth Evaluation Framework, Centre for Rural and Northern Health Research, Laurentian University, Canada (2005).

[16] C. LeRouge, A. Hevner, R. Collins, Telemedicine Encounter Quality: Comparing Patient and Provider Perspectives of a Socio-Technical System, in the Proceedings of the 37th Hawaii International Conference on System Sciences (2004).

[17] S.E. Cross, S.M. Stevens and J.E. Bailes, A Digital Video Library Application in Health Care, in the Proceedings of the IEEE International Joint Symposia on Intelligence and Systems (1996) 254-260.

[18] A. Tiwana and B. Ramesh, From Intuition to Institution: Supporting Collaborative Diagnoses in Telemedicine Teams, in the Proceedings of the 33rd Annual Hawaii International Conference on System Sciences (2000).

[19] V. Bharadwaj, R. Raman, R. Reddy and S. Reddy, Empowering Mobile Healthcare Providers via a Patient Benefits Authorization Service, in the Proceedings of the Tenth IEEE International Workshop in Enabling Technologies: Infrastructure for Collaborative Enterprises (2001) 73-78.

[20] A.W. Powell, Reengineering Health Care Delivery using Telemedicine, in the Proceedings of the Medical Technology Symposium (1998) 371-374.
[21] G. Harris, India: Telemedicine's Great New Frontier, *IEEE Spectrum* (2002) 16-17.
[22] S. Dembeyiotis, N. Katevas, G. Konnis, D. Koutsouris and S. Pavlopoulos, An Image Processing and Management System for Radiology, in the Proceedings of the Fourth International Conference in Image Management and Communications (1995) 250-255.
[23] R. Sacile, Telemedicine Systems for Collaborative Diagnosis over the Internet. Towards Virtual "Collaboratories", in the Proceedings of Academia/Industry Working Conference on Research Challenges (2000) 191-196.
[24] D.L. Paul, Wicked Decision Problems in Remote Health Care: Telemedicine as a Tool for Sensemaking, in the Proceedings of the 32nd Annual Hawaii International Conference on System Sciences (1999).
[25] M. Gurstein Chair, Panelists: Peter Day, Gert-Jan de Vreede, Michael Miller, Celia T. Romm, Vanessa Whitehead, Community Informatics: International Experiences and Case Studies, in the Proceedings of the 20th international conference on Information Systems (1999) 578-581.
[26] D.G. Kilman and D.W. Forslund, An International Collaboratory Based on Virtual Patient Records, *Communications of the ACM* 40(8) (1997) 111-117.
[27] J.C. Lowery, Getting started in Simulation in Healthcare, in the Proceedings of the 1998 Winter Simulation Conference, Vol. 1 (1998) 31-35.
[28] M.A. Smith, Some Social Implications of Ubiquitous Wireless Networks, *ACM SIGMOBILE Mobile Computing and Communications Review* 4(2) (2000) 25-36.
[29] J.F. Winchester, W.G. Tohme, B. Levine, J. Collmann, K.A. Schulman, J.W. Turner, S. Rathore, N. Khanafer, A. Alaoui, N. Pania, A. Al-Aama, L. Hoffman, M. Hofilena and S.K. Mun, Telemedicine and Dialysis, in the Proceedings of Medical Technology Symposium (1998) 116-118.
[30] K.A. Stroetmann, M. Pieper and V.N. Stroetmann, Understanding Patients: Participatory Approaches for the User Evaluation of Vital Data Presentation, in the Proceedings of the 2003 ACM conference on Universal usability (2002) 93-97.
[31] D. Won-Kyu Hong and C. Seon Hong, A QoS management framework for distributed multimedia systems, *International Journal of Network Management*, John Wiley & Sons Ltd 13(2) (2003) 115-127.
[32] V.W.A. Mbarika, Is Telemedicine the Panacea for Sub-Saharan Africa's Medical Nightmare, *Communications of the ACM* 47(7) (2004) 21-24.
[33] W.G. Tohme and S. Olsson, Developments and Directions of Technology Assessment in Telemedicine, in the Proceedings of the Fourth International Conference on Image Management and Communications (1995) 79-85.
[34] J. Bach, Good Enough Quality: Beyond the Buzzword, *IEEE Computer* 30(8) (1997) 96-98.
[35] W.H. DeLone and E.R. McLean, Information Systems Success Revisited, in the Proceedings of the 35th Annual Hawaii International Conference on System Sciences (2002) 2966-2976.
[36] G.L. Knatterud, F.W. Rockhold, S.L. George, F.B. Barton, C.E. Davis, W.R. Fairweather, T. Honohan, R. Mowery and R. O'Neill, Guideliness for Quality Assurance in Multicenter Trials: A Position Paper, *Controlled Clinical Trials* 19 (1998) 477-493.
[37] Office of Health and the Information Highway Health Canada, Evaluating Telehealth 'Solutions' A Review and Synthesis of the Telehealth Evaluation Literature (2000) 1-71.
[38] A. Ohinmaa, D. Hailey and Risto Roine, The Assessment of Telemedicine General principles and a systematic review, INAHTA Project on Telemedicine (1999).
[39] J. Grigsby, R.E. Schlenker, M.M. Kaehny, P.W. Shaughnessy, EJ. Sandberg Perspective: Analytic framework for evaluation of Telemedicine, Telemed J. 1(1) (1995) 31-39.
[40] M.J. Field (Ed.), A Guide to Assessing Telecommunications for Health Care, Committee on Evaluating Clinical Applications of Telemedicine, Institute of Medicine, The National Academies Press (1996) 1-288.
[41] S.M. Capalbo and C.N. Heggem, Evaluating Telemedicine Technologies in Rural Settings, Montana State University, Policy Issues Paper 10 (1999) 1-19.

Current Principles and Practices of Telemedicine and e-Health
R. Latifi (Ed.)
IOS Press, 2008

Telemedicine for Home Health and the New Patient: When Do We Really Need to Go to the Hospital?

Elizabeth A. KRUPINSKI, PhD
University of Arizona, Tucson, AZ 85724

Abstract. This chapter will review the current state-of-the-art of home health services in the telemedicine environment. Two aspects in particular will be discussed that reflect where most of the efforts in home telehealth care are being directed. The first aspect is the more traditional implementation in which the healthcare practitioner "visits" the patient (typically chronically ill or at home recovering from a hospital visit) virtually at a distance using telemedicine technologies to assess their health status, obtain a select set of vital signs (e.g., blood pressure), and converse with them about how they feel and so on. The second application is the growing field of distance monitoring, especially as it pertains to prevention and health maintenance. In this application, the users may be patients with chronic conditions such as asthma or diabetes that require regular monitoring to achieve or maintain healthy functioning, but they are typically not in an acute phase. More and more often, however, the users of distance monitoring technologies are relatively healthy people looking to enhance their health awareness and healthy status by monitoring various vital signs to alert them of any potential changes in their health status that would require actual medical attention.

Keywords. Telehealth, home care, monitoring

Introduction

Telemedicine is a rapidly evolving field that is continually branching out to encompass more and more clinical specialties and applications. Home telehealth care is not one of the newer applications, but it is one that has seen an incredible amount of growth and expansion into new environments over the past few years. In part due to the growing aging population in the United States and around the world, it is expected that telehealth technologies and applications will continue to have an increasing role in the home healthcare industry [1]. At the 2006 American Telemedicine Association (ATA) Annual Meeting, the Kenneth Bird Annual Distinguished Lecture was given by Bill Crounse, MD the Healthcare Industry Director for the Microsoft Corporation, who noted certain trends in the healthcare arena that are likely to impact positively the spread of telehealth services, especially those related to home health. The first trend relevant to the spread of home telehealth care is the probable end of employer-paid health insurance as we know it. Additionally, changes in the Medicare payment system in October of 2000 mandated that home health agencies must find ways to improve the quality of care and outcomes, while at the same time effectively managing costs [2]. The burden of financing healthcare is falling increasingly on the patient, requiring major innovations and change in the way that healthcare systems need to address the growing needs of patient populations. The shift to the patient also requires that patients begin thinking about new ways of protecting and maintaining their health, getting them much more involved in their own healthcare than in the past.

Another trend Crounse noted is the commoditization of healthcare services outside the traditional hospital or clinic-based provider setting. For many people, "home" is not simply the house we return to every day after work, but "home" extends to wherever we conduct our daily business – the office, the mall, the grocery store, the sports arena. We have already seen in the past few years the proliferation of devices such as blood pressure monitors in drug stores, but increasingly we are seeing more health monitoring devices appearing in shopping malls and other public gathering places. These non-traditional healthcare settings may seem odd or even inappropriate to many people, but clearly the "one-stop-shopping" idea has great appeal to people living in an increasingly busy world. Additionally, patients with diabetes and other chronic conditions require monitoring 24 hours a day not just when they are at home, and many companies are developing telemonitoring devices to facilitate and improve monitoring in diverse environments.

The focus on "lifestyle monitoring" was echoed by the ATA's 2006 Opening Keynote speaker Astro Teller, CEO of Body Media, Inc. One of his main messages was that telemedicine may need to focus more on consumer attitudes about healthcare and technology and try to understand what he called the "sequencing of the human lifestyle." His contention was that by promoting the use of personal monitoring devices for not only those with immediate healthcare needs, but also the general public, we may be able to collect a large quantity of data that could reveal much about subtle changes that take place in person's health status on a day to day basis, and thereby understand longitudinal disease and aging processes in a more refined manner. In traditional healthcare and even with many of the remote monitoring devices we have now, data is only collected on a periodic basis. How many people have been put on high blood pressure medicine because of a single high reading in the doctor's office and the "white coat" reaction? By moving towards near continuous monitoring, we may be able to identify trigger events for certain health conditions and understand the probable cyclical nature of many health conditions over the day. Pharmaceutical companies could improve the way medications are delivered, clinicians could improve the way therapy is provided, and people could adjust their lifestyles based on the feedback they receive about their health status.

Finally, the explosion of health information availability is a trend that nearly everyone has experienced. For many people, cruising the Internet from home or work in search of health and medical information has become a standard practice. It is becoming more common for people to turn to their computer for healthcare advice, often as a complement or even an alternative to seeking out direct advice from healthcare professionals [3–6]. The resources on the Internet for patients with chronic diseases are numerous [7–9]. In general it seems that most searches by the average patient yield adequate results, although having some guidance from a physician regarding what keywords to use during a search may improve results [10]. There is evidence that Internet use for seeking health information varies as a function of age [11], race and cultural factors [8], but as computer use and training [11] spreads these differences may diminish. Whether or not the patients actually use the information they find on the Internet to alter their behavior or care may also vary with these factors. Campbell and Nolfi [11] found that although elderly patients were willing to learn how to surf the Internet for health care information, when it came to making decisions about the health care they were more likely to adhere to a physician-centered model of care and rely on their physician to make recommendations and give advice.

This chapter will explore some of the current trends in home telehealth care. Two aspects in particular will be discussed that reflect where most of the efforts in home telehealth care are being directed. The first aspect is the more traditional implementation in which the healthcare practitioner "visits" the patient (typically chronically ill or at home recovering from a hospital visit) virtually at a distance using telemedicine technologies to assess their health status, obtain a select set of vital signs (e.g., blood pressure), and converse with them about how they feel and so on. The second application is the growing field of distance monitoring, especially as it pertains to prevention and health maintenance. In this application, the users may be patients with chronic conditions such as asthma or diabetes that require regular monitoring to achieve or maintain healthy functioning, but they are typically not in an acute phase. More and more often, however, the users of distance monitoring technologies are relatively healthy people looking to enhance their health awareness and healthy status by monitoring various vital signs to alert them of any potential changes in their health status that would require actual medical attention.

1. Home Telehealth & Virtual Visits to the Home

Home telehealth is defined as "remote care delivery or monitoring between a health care provider and a patient outside of a health facility, in his or her place of residence, whether a patient's home, assisted living facility or nursing home" [12]. For those not yet involved in home telehealth care but are interesting in finding out where to start and what procedures to follow, the Home Telehealth Special Interest Group of the American Telemedicine Association has published the "ATA Home Telehealth Toolkit" that provides everything from how to carry out a needs assessment to choosing the proper technology and how to market your program [13]. Pellegrino and Kobb [14] have even developed a "recipe for success" in identifying the skill sets required for a successful home health telepractitioner that center around abilities, work style and attitudes.

In this more traditional version of home telehealth care, the practitioner is intimately involved in the monitoring and care of the patient at home. In many cases the telehealth visits either replace some of the in-person visits by the practitioner or are additional visits, but it most cases the traditional in-person visit is not completely eliminated [15,16]. This combination of traditional and telecare has been shown repeatedly to be an extremely useful and valuable mechanism for delivering care. For example, Pare et al. [17] compared chronic obstructive pulmonary disease (COPD) patients receiving home telecare versus those receiving traditional home care. Those in the telecare group received fewer home visits by nurses (4.2 vs 7.5), although the visits were longer (57.5 vs 46.6 minutes). They also had fewer hospitalizations (5% vs 40%), although the stays were longer than the traditional group (13.5 vs 7.3 days). The telecare patients also made more (2.5 vs 1.4) and longer (22.2 vs 19.9 minutes) telephone calls to the on-call telephone service than the traditional patients. IN terms of costs savings however, they were significant. The nurses saved on traveling time (96.0 vs 168.0 minutes) and distance (55.6 vs 99.0 km) per patient with the telecare group. When all expenses were accounted for, the telecare group was also shown to be more cost-efficient than the traditional group ($2,424 vs $2,779 per patient for a 6-month period). Patient attitudes in the telecare group were also quite high with respect to ease of use of the system, quality of technical support and perceived usefulness of the care (gave them a sense of security and helped them adopt new practices that stabilized their health). Mair et al. [18] also found similar positive attitudes in COPD patients towards telecare.

Diabetes is another chronic disease where home telehealth care is being used successfully. The Veterans Health Administration has a rather extensive care coordination/home-telehealth (CC/HT) program for diabetes management and have shown success on a variety of important outcome variables. Comparing records of patients before and after enrolling in the CC/HT program, they had significantly fewer hospitalizations (50% reduction), lower emergency room use (11% reduction), fewer bed days of care (decreased by 3.0 on average) and overall improvement in quality of life, pain reduction and social functioning [19]. They also found that although clinical outcomes did not differ between two groups receiving different intensities of telecare (daily vs weekly), those receiving daily monitoring had fewer hospital admissions with fewer bed days of care, and fewer unscheduled clinic visits [20,21]. Clemensen et al. [22] have found that it is also possible to treat diabetic foot ulcers using a combination of videophones and Internet-based patient records.

Home telehealth has also been used successfully for treating acute infections [23], chronic respiratory failure [24], lung transplant recipients [25], stroke recovery [26], asthma self-management [27], patients with cystic fibrosis [28], chronic heart failure [29,30], and even follow-up care of patients with spinal cord injuries [31] and children with brain and other injuries [32,33]. The evidence is even mounting for effective use of home telecare for patients with various mental disabilities, including schizophrenia [34], and Alzheimer's disease [35]. One very interesting application in this area was the delivery of Dignity Psychotherapy for patients with advanced cancers [36]. Patients reported a high level of satisfaction with the intervention and felt that they had benefited greatly from it. Those delivering the therapy felt that the interventions were timely, with minimal length between sessions and transcript delivery and few technical difficulties.

1.1. Challenges & Solutions

Although delivery of care to the patient at home via telehealth technologies has been shown to be effective, cost efficient and satisfactory to both patients and providers in a wide variety of situations, there are still some challenges to be met. Proper training of the people installing the telecare units in the patients' homes is essential. Starren et al. [37] found that for a group of nurses responsible for installing units, technology-related problems (especially those related to telecommunications) were the primary cause of difficulties. They stressed the importance of the installers having not only the clinical skills to teach patients how to use the various unit attachments (e.g., blood pressure cuffs), but also the need for them to be trained sufficiently themselves to have the technical knowledge to complete the equipment installation successfully. Once home telehealth systems are installed in the patient's home, there is also evidence that the home health staff needs to assess the manner in which care is delivered because they may need to alter their work routines. Those who are better prepared and go into the home telehealth care arena with a more open attitude about technology and innovation are more likely to be successful [38]. In a related vein, Nesbitt et al. [38] also found that it is necessary to have the required core staff to dedicate someone with the proper skill set and interest. Those sites with limited staff, heavy caseloads and multiple staff responsibilities found it a significant challenge to incorporate home telehealth care into their routine. These types of challenges can be met with careful planning, use of existing tools such as the ATA Telehealth Toolkit [13], and proper training. It may also help to have existing protocols in place that staff can follow to safely and effectively monitor patients [39]. Demiris et al. also note that have a clear understanding of the ethical considerations involved in home telehealth care is essential for efficient delivery of services to the home [40]. These considerations include privacy, confidentiality, informed consent, equity of access, promoting dependency vs independence, lack of human touch and the impact of technology on the patient-nurse relationship, and the medicalization of the home environment.

Another challenge, not unique to home telecare, is cost, reimbursement and sustainability. The issue for home telecare, however, is compounded by the variety of environments considered home (e.g., the patient's house, a nursing home, assisted living facilities, hospice) and the variety of health care professionals providing services in these environments [41–43]. There is little doubt that a solid business case can be made for home telecare. Models for analyzing the factors that contribute to the financial effectiveness of a home health organization have shown that home telehealth can have a positive impact on an organization's financial status [44,45], and numerous studies have demonstrated clear savings [15–17,46]. The challenge here, aside from revising legislation to approve more reimbursement codes, is to get home health agencies past the break-even point. As Rumberger and Dansky [45] note, there may not be an immediate return on investment (ROI) after initial adoption. It may take at least a year before sustainability starts to look feasible and up top five before it can be achieved. The key is to keep in mind the various challenges already noted regarding appropriately skilled providers, taking the effort to integrate telecare into the existing workflow, having set protocols and so on, so the infrastructure is in place that will facilitate a more rapid ROI.

The final challenge relates to some extent to some of the hesitation in getting more codes approved for reimbursement. Although some studies of home telehealth have adequate sample size to carry out valid and reliable statistical analyses [19–21], a large number of studies do not, making it difficult to generalize the results. The focus on patient and provider satisfaction and technical aspects rather than clinical outcomes is also a challenge. Cost effectiveness studies and models have had a significant impact on acceptance and growth in this area, but many of these are based on relatively small samples as well. According to a recent paper "Research Recommendations for the American Telemedicine Association," designing studies with adequate sample sizes, proper comparison (i.e., control) groups, and a focus on clinical outcomes is crucial to advancing telehealth applications and the acceptance of telehealth at all levels, from users to payers [47].

2. Home Telehealth & Electronic Monitoring

As noted by both Dr. Crounse and Mr. Teller at the ATA 2006 meeting as well as many others [48], there is a very strong trend now towards the commoditization of healthcare, patient-centric healthcare, and personalized healthcare. In other words, even healthy people are starting to monitor their own health much more intensely than at any time in the past and are spending more money and time doing so. Although home telehealth as described in the previous section relies heavily on monitoring devices to obtain patient information, many of these same devices are being used in healthier populations simply to maintain health status and prevent health problems. One population in particular that seems to be focus point for these monitoring technologies is the elderly [49]. Rather than relying on long-term care facilities, more and more people prefer to age in place or grow old at home. In order to facilitate the aging in place desire, many researchers are developing tools for the "smart" home that will hopefully extend the time people can live at home. Although the home health practitioner has a role in this type of environment should some health event arise or if someone needs regular attention if they are ill, there is less of a role for the health practitioner in this type of scenario than the one discussed previously for patients who are chronically ill. In this scenario the "patients" are generally healthy individuals who are at risk for potential ill health events (e.g., the elderly) and would like to be monitored so that such an event might be predicted and prevented or if an event occurs immediate intervention can take place. It is quite likely that this type of monitoring and care scenario, especially for the elderly, will be cost efficient [50]. Most of the studies to date in this area, however, have been proof-of-concept or feasibility studies so eventual outcomes and true cost effectiveness are unknown at this point.

In this area of the "smart" home and newer electronic monitoring devices there is quite a bit of interesting research and development occurring. In some cases the goal is to transform existing home health monitoring devices that typically sit on a table for use and make them smaller and more transportable. Instead of always having to go to a certain room at a certain time to obtain a sensor reading, a compact device can be used anywhere at anytime. For example, Yoon et al. developed a compact device (palm-sized) that obtained photoplethysmography signals that could be analyzed to measure simultaneously hematocrit, pulse, respiration rate, and saturated oxygen in arterial blood [51]. Blood pressure could also be measured with an additional finger cuff. When tested on over 500 people, error rates were within clinically acceptable ranges.

Beyond simple sensors, large or compact, to measure specific physiological parameters, is the idea of a more ubiquitous context-aware infrastructure that not only measures discrete functions, but expends electronic monitoring to detect and interpret patient movements, patterns within these movements, aberrations in these movements and so on [52]. The concept is to monitor patients in their practically on a 24-hour basis. The URSafe project is developing a portable device with three sensors to detect electrocardiogram (ECG) signals, oxygen rate (SpO2) and a fall detection signal. Through regular monitoring of the signals, abnormalities can be detected and a medical center notified. If there are no abnormalities detected, the device simply continues to passively monitor the patient [53]. Sum et al. are also developing a wearable vital sign monitor for pulse rate, motion, and skin temperature. This device is only $2 \times 2.5 \times 4$ cm^3 and uses a wireless transceiver to communicate with the data terminal [54]. The size and weight are key factors when developing a portable device for the elderly. Suzuki et al. developed a completely passive motion monitoring system using a single infrared sensor [55]. Although they only did a pilot test with three subjects, the trial recorded a 7-day baseline then tested over 28 days. Using the sensor they were able to characterize the subjects' sleeping, waking activities, indoor activities around the house, dinner activities and going to bed. Given the baseline patterns they then established a set criterion during the 28-day period that was used to detect aberrations from "normal" activity patterns. Again, the idea is to passively monitor patients as much as possible, but only call for intervention if something out of the ordinary occurs. Early evidence suggests that these types of position and motion sensors may also make a feasible to build a home-based telerehabilitation system for sensing and tracking the motion of stroke patients [56]. Combined with a whole-house type monitoring system, this could prove very useful not only for therapy but for more continuous monitoring of adherence to exercises and movement around the house in general.

The electronic sensors being developed today for distance monitoring are not just focused on vital signs and movement. Istrate et al. are working on sound surveillance sensors [57]. The system they are working on has two stages. The first stage is sound detection using a discrete wavelet based transform algorithm that specifically detects non-stationary sound signals (e.g., impulsive or "crash" sounds). The second stage uses another set of statistically based operations to classify the detected sounds. The goal is to monitor the sound environment in the home, filtering out general background noise, and detecting sounds of distress. Early results indicate that they can achieve 97% alarm detection rate. Although presently geared towards in-home hemodialysis patients, researchers are also developing sensors for beds that might find other uses in the future for home telecare and monitoring. These bed sensors are designed to detect liquids released during the night from infusion leaks, bleeding due to infusion-tube pullout and urine due to incontinence [58,59]. Early results are promising, although false positives occur for example when one's dog jumps on the bed and drools! [59]

Wearable devices are also being developed for daily continuous monitoring, avoiding the problem that even portable systems face – the devices are less likely to be forgotten, recording is automatic, and there is very little for the patient to do but put it on. One such system is simply a wristband that has sensors for blood pressure, pulse oximetry, ECG, respiration rate, heart rate, body surface temperature and fall detection sensors [60]. This group is also developing an add-on blood glucometer, a device to measure ECG while the patient is in bed or on a chair, another one to measure ECG, body temperature, bodyfat ratio and weight while on the toilet seat, and a motion sensing/analysis device to monitor activity. Other systems being developed incorporate many of the same monitoring sensors, but in "smart" clothes. The main idea here is that other devices such as portable ones or even something like the wristband have only a single contact point or area, while a vest or shirt covers a much wider area and is in contact with about 90% of the covered skin surface [61,62]. The potential here is to integrate these types of sensors not only into specialized pieces of clothing, but to integrate them into everyday where that anyone could purchase. The goal with these everyday continuous monitoring devices would be illness prevention in otherwise fairly healthy people, as well as monitoring of those needed healthcare attention.

2.1. Challenges & Solutions

One challenge to overcome in this area of continual monitoring to detect aberrations in both healthy and ill populations is finding ways to keep the false positive rate low. Systems that rely on finding deviations from regular movement patterns must be flexible enough to incorporate the fact that even the elderly are not always regular in their habits around the home. Just because they stay in bed 15 minutes longer one day than usual does not mean there is an emergency. The criteria for intervention may have to be something that is individualized for each person, using the patient's input for when they would consider something an emergency. The balance between true and false positives must be carefully weighed. Just as with home alarm systems, the homeowner, the alarm company and the police department will tolerate only so many false alarms before they all stop responding. Companies developing these sensors and alarm systems for healthcare monitoring should look to other monitoring areas for methods they have adopted to avoid too many false alarms while still maintaining high true positive detection rates.

Another challenge that will have to be faced once these monitoring technologies really take off and a multitude of healthy and ill people start using and wearing them, is what to do with all the data coming in and how and when are health professionals notified when there is an emerging healthcare event? Clearly we will need computer-based analysis systems that monitor the incoming data from multiple sources and analyze them with sophisticated algorithms using established, validated and accepted standards for points of intervention. Additionally, all of this analysis needs to be done in real time with mechanisms in place to react to an event should it occur. There are groups working on solutions to this challenge, developing multi-agent systems to monitor and interpret these huge volumes of data [63]. Another fruitful area for investigation in data analysis is the integrative interpretation of the data from the various sensors. If we are going to continuously collect data from all these vital signs, motion activities and so on, it seems inefficient to simply record and interpret each individual signal as if it was the only one being recorded. Changes in one parameter may trigger or be the results of changes in another, and it is only by looking at the complete integrated signal pattern that subtle changes in health status may be evident. This is not simply and informatics or engineering problem but is one that physiologists, clinicians, psychologists and other researchers must start to consider.

3. The Future

It is impossible to predict exactly what the future of home health care will look like, but it is more than certain that home telehealth care will play an increasing large role in the way that patients are cared for. More sophisticated monitoring sensors that are less intrusive, more accurate and more reliable are going to be developed and more people are going to be using them in their everyday lives. Electronic monitoring will not just be for the chronically ill or the elderly, but will be something that the majority of people rely on for feedback about their health status. When this occurs, the impact on the healthcare system in general should be significant. Patients should be able to return home more quickly from hospital to stay with their family, yet still receive the same high quality of care and follow-up they would have received if they had stayed in the hospital. Ideally of course, we would like to see improved and expanded care compared to what we have now, not only through continuous monitoring but also through expansion of services. Patients would not just be monitored, but rehabilitative therapy sessions could be conducted at a distance, and interactive education sessions across multiple households could be presented. People with chronic conditions such as asthma or diabetes as well as generally healthy people could prevent visits to the hospital for acute problems because they and their healthcare providers are more aware of the subtle signs that predict health events that require attention. Cost effectiveness studies for these daily-monitoring scenarios have not yet been conducted, but it is clear that measures to prevent acute healthcare events should reduce healthcare costs in the long run.

4. Conclusions

Home telehealth care is on the verge of an explosion of widespread use and acceptance. Commonly used and widely available technologies such as cell phones and miniature sensors are going to revolutionize health for everyone. The chronically ill are already benefiting from these technologies, although more studies with larger sample sizes and clear assessment of clinical are required. The expansion to daily wear continuous monitoring devices for both ill and healthy populations is happening. What we need to consider is what will we do with all this data, and what constitutes a medical event that requires attention (and at what point do we intervene). Very soon we will also have to consider more societal and ethical issues such as who gets monitored, how much do we "invade" the home with monitoring technologies, who will pay for these monitoring technologies and emergency response services, and at what point is there too much monitoring? These are questions that are going arise in the very near future and we would be wise to consider them now rather than later because home telehealth care and personalized monitoring are clearly in the future of healthcare for everyone.

References

[1] Office for the Advancement of Telehealth 2001 Report to Congress on Telehomecare. Washington DC: Office for the Advancement of Telehealth, 2002.
[2] P.B. Dray, When it comes to prospective payment, home health agencies can learn from the experiences of acute care hospitals with DRGs. Health Manage Technol **23** (2002), 44-50.
[3] J. Alexander, S. Zeibland, The Web – bringing support and health information into the home: the communicative power of qualitative research. Intl J Nursing Studies **43** (2006), 389-391.
[4] R. Lowes, Models of online success. Medical Economics **83** (2006), 8-10.
[5] ADA Division of Communications, ADA Council on Scientific Affairs, For the dental patient – surfing for substance: evaluating oral health information on the Internet. J Am Dental Assoc **137** (2006), 692.
[6] J. Kivits, Informed patients and the internet: a mediated context for consultations with health professionals. J Health Psych **11** (2006), 269-282.
[7] G.E. Deitrick, R.C. Polomano, Findingt a balanced diet on the World Wide Web: nutrition at the end-of-life. J Pain & Palliative Care Pharmacotherapy **19** (2005), 53-59.
[8] D. Schatell, K. Klicko, B.N. Becker, In-center hemodialysis patients' use of the Internet in the United States: a national survey. Am J Kidney Disease **48** (2006), 285-291.
[9] W. Himmel, J. Meyer, M.M. Kochen, H.W. Michelmann, Information needs and visitors' experience of an Internet expert forum on infertility. J Medical Internet Research **7** (2005), e20.
[10] H.A. Liszka, T.E. Steyer, W.J. Hueston, How to guide patients for online information: Focus on chronic disease. J South Carolina Med Assoc **101** (2005), 378-380.
[11] R.J. Campbell, D.A. Nolfi, Teaching elderly adults to use the Internet to access health care information: before-after study. J Medical Internet Research **7** (2005), e19.
[12] American Telemedicine Association Home Telehealth Special Interest Group, Frequently asked questions for home telehealth-providers. http://atmeda.org/ICOT/sighomehealth.htm (Last accessed August 23, 2006).
[13] American Telemedicine Association Home Telehealth Special Interest Group, ATA Home Telehealth Toolkit. http://atmeda.org/ICOT/sighomehealth.htm (Last accessed August 23, 2006).
[14] L. Pellegrino, R. Kobb, Skill sets for the home telehealth practitioner: a recipe for success. Telemed J & e-Health **11** (2005), 151-156.
[15] E.A. Krupinski, Home health and telemedicine: where are we today? In E. Latifi (ed) Establishing telemedicine in developing countries: from inception to implementation. IOS Press, Washington, DC, 2004.
[16] S.K. Bohnenkamp, P. MacDonald, A.M. Lopez, E. Krupinski, A. Blackett, Traditional versus telenursing outpatient management of patients with cancer with new ostomies. Oncology Nursing Forum **31** (2004), 1005-1010.
[17] G. Pare, C. Sicotte, D.St. Jules, R. Gauthier, Cost-minimization analysis of a telehomecare program for patients with chronic obstructive pulmonary disease. Telemed & e-Health **12** (2006), 114-121.
[18] F.S. Mair, P. Goldstein, C. May, R. Angus, C. Shiels, D. Hibbert, J. O'Connor, A. Boland, C. Roberts, A. Haycox, S. Capewell, Patient and provider perspectives on home telecare: preliminary results from a randomized control trial. J Telemed & Telecare **11** (2005), 95-97.

[19] N.R. Chumbler, B. Neugaard, R. Kobb, P. Ryan, H. Qin, Y. Joo, Evaluation of a care coordination/home-telehealth program for veterans with diabetes: health services utilization and health-related quality of life. Evaluation & Health Professions **28** (2005), 464-478.

[20] N.R. Chumbler, B. Neugaard, P. Ryan, H. Qin, Y. Joo, An observational study of veterans with diabetes receiving weekly or daily home telehealth monitoring. J Telemed & Telecare **11** (2005), 150-156.

[21] N.R. Chumbler, W.B. Vogel, M. Garel, H. Qin, R. Kobb, P. Ryan, Health services utilization of a care coordination/home-telehealth program for veterans with diabetes: a matched-cohort study. J Ambulatory Care Management **28** (2005), 230-240.

[22] J. Clemensen, S.B. Larsen, N. Ejskjaer, Telemedical treatment at home of diabetic foot ulcers. J Telemed & Telecare **11** (2005), S14-16.

[23] L. Eron, P. King, M. Marineau, C. Yonehara, Treating acute infections by telemedicine in the home. Clin Infectious Diseases **39** (2004), 1175-1181.

[24] T. Koizumi, M. Takizawa, K. Nakai, Y. Yamamoto, S. Murase, T. Fujii, T. Kobayashi, O. Hatayama, K. Fujimoto, K. Kubo, Trial of remote telemedicine support for patients with chronic respiratory failure at home through a multistation communication system. Telemed J & e-Health **11** (2005), 481-486.

[25] B.C. Karl, S.M. Finkelstein, W.N. Robiner, The design of an Internet-based system to maintain home monitoring adherence by lung transplant recipients. IEEE Trans Inform Tech in Biomed **10** (2006), 66-76.

[26] K.M. Buckley, B.Q. Tran, C.M. Prandoni, Receptiveness, use and acceptance of telehealth by caregivers of stroke patients in the home. Online J Issues Nurs **9** (2004), 9.

[27] J.A. Fonesca, A. Costa-Pereira, L. Delgado, L. Fernandes, M.G. Castel-Branco, Asthma patients are willing to use mobile and web technologies to support self-management. Allergy **61** (2006), 389-390.

[28] F. Magrabi, N.H. Lovell, R.L. Henry, B.G. Celler, Designing home telecare: a case study in monitoring cystic fibrosis. Telemed J & e-Health **11** (2005), 707-719.

[29] N. Smart, B. Haluska, L. Jeffriess, T.H. Marwick, Predictors of a sustained response to exercise training in patients with chronic heart failure: a telemonitoring study. Am Heart J **150** (2005), 1240-1247.

[30] J.G. Cleland, A.A. Louis, A.S. Rigby, U. Janssens, A.H. Balk, TEN-HMS Investigators, Noninvasive home telemonitoring for patients with heart failure at high risk of recurrent admission and death: the Trans-European Network-Home-Care Management System (TEN-HMS) study. J Am Coll Cardiol **45** (2005), 1654-64.

[31] J.H. Bloeman-Vrencken, L.P. de Witte, M.W. Post, Follow-up care for persons with spinal cord injury living in the community: a systematic review of interventions and their evaluation. Spinal Cord **43** (2005), 462-475.

[32] A. Tura, L. Quareni, D. Longo, C. Condoluci, A. van Rijn, G. Albertini, Wireless home monitoring and health care activity management through the Internet in patients with chronic diseases. Medical Informatics & Internet Med **30** (2005), 241-253.

[33] N.L. Young, W. Barden, P. McKeever, P.T. Dick, Tele-HomeCare Team, Taking the call-bell home: a qualitative evaluation of Tele-HomeCare for children. Health & Social Care Commun **14** (2006), 231-241.

[34] S. Frangou, I. Sachpazidis, A. Stassinakis, G. Sakas, Telemonitoring of medication adherence in patients with schizophrenia. Telemed J & e-Health **11** (2005), 675-683.

[35] J.M. Alisky. Integrated electronic monitoring systems could revolutionize care for patients with cognitive impairment. Med Hypotheses **66** (2006), 1161-1164.

[36] S.D. Passik, K.L. Kirsh, S. Leibee, L.S. Kaplan, C. Love, E. Napier, D. Burton, R. Sprang, A feasibility study of dignity psychotherapy delivered via telemedicine. Palliative & Supportive Care **2** (2004), 149-155.

[37] J. Starren, C. Tsai, S. Bakken, A. Aidala, P.C. Morin, C. Hillman, R.S. Weinstock, R. Goland, J. Teresi, IDEATel Consortium. The role of nurses in installing telehealth technology in the home. Comp, Inform, Nursing **23** (2005), 181-189.

[38] T.S. Nesbitt, S.L. Cole, L. Pellegrino, P. Keast, Rural outreach in home telehealth: assessing challenges and reviewing successes. Telemed & e-Health **12** (2006), 107-113.

[39] E.M. Martin, M.K. Coyle, Nursing protocol for telephonic supervision of clients. Rehab Nursing **31** (2006), 54-57.

[40] G. Demiris, D.P. Oliver, K.L. Courtney, Ethical considerations for the utilization of tele-health technologies in home and hospice care by the nursing profession. Nursing Admin Quart **30** (2006), 56-66.

[41] J.M. Daly, G. Jogerst, J.Y. Park, Y.D. Kang, T. Bae, A nursing home telehealth system: keeping residents connected. J Gerontol Nursing **31** (2005), 46-51.

[42] G.C. Doolittle, P. Whitten, M. McCartney, D. Cook, N. Nazir, An empirical chart analysis of the sustainability of telemedicine for hospice visits. Telemed J & e-Health **11** (2005), 90-97.

[43] M. Walsh, J.R. Coleman, Trials and tribulations: a small pilot telehealth home care program for medicare patients. Geriatric Nursing **26** (2005), 343-346.

[44] J. Frey, C.M. Harmonosky, K.H. Dansky, Performance model for telehealth use in home health agencies. Telemed J & e-Health **11** (2005), 542-550.

[45] J.S. Rumberger, K. Dansky, Is there a business case for telehealth in home health agencies? Telemed J & e-Health 12 (2006), 122-127.

[46] S.M. Finkelstein, S.M. Speedie, S. Potthoff, Home telehealth improves clinical outcomes at lower cost for home healthcare. Telemed J & e-Health **12** (2006), 128-136.

[47] E. Krupinski, S. Dimmick, J. Grigsby, G. Mogel, D. Puskin, S. Speedie, B. Stamm, B. Wakefield, J. Whited, P. Whitten, P. Yellowlees, Research recommendations for the American Telemedicine Association. Telemed J & e-Health, In Press.

[48] P.J. Heinzelmann, N.E. Lugn, J.C. Kvedar, Telemedicine in the future. J Telemec & Telecare **11** (2005), 384-390.

[49] P. Cheek, L. Nikpour, H.D. Nowlin, Aging well with smart technology. Nurs Admin Quart **29** (2005), 329-338.

[50] L. Magnusson, E. Hanson, Supporting frail older people and their family carers at home using informatics and communication technology: cost analysis. J Advanced Nurs **51** (2005), 645-657.

[51] G. Yoon, J.Y. Lee, K.J. Jeon, K.K. Park, H.S. Kim, Development of a compact home health monitor for telemedicine. Telemed J & e-Health **11** (2005), 660-667.

[52] D. Zhang, Z. Yu, C.Y. Chin, Context-aware infrastructure for personalized healthcare. Studies Health Tech & Informatics **117** (2005), 154-163.

[53] F. Castanie, C. Mailhes, S. Henrion, End-t0-end signal processing from the embedded body sensor to the medical end user through QoS-less public commincation channels: the U-R-SAFE experience. Studies Health Tech & Informatics **117** (2005), 172-179.

[54] K.W. Sum, Y.P. Zheng, A.F. Mak, Vital sign monitoring for elderly at home: development of a compound sensor for pulse rate and motion. Studies Health Tech & Informatics **117** (2005), 43-50.

[55] R. Suzuki, S. Otake, T. Izutsu, M. Yoshida, T. Iwaya, Monitoring daily living activities of elderly people in a nursing home using an infrared motion-detection system. Telemed J & e-Health **12** (2006), 146-155.

[56] H. Zheng, N.D. Black, N.D. Harris, Position-sensing technologies for movement analysis in stroke rehabilitation. Med & Biol Engineer & Comput **43** (2005), 413-420.

[57] D. Istrate, E. Castelli, M. Vacher, L. Besacier, J.F. Serignat, Information extraction from sound for medical telemonitoring. IEEE Trans Inform Tech Biomed **10** (2006), 264-274.

[58] Y. Yonezawa, Y. Miyamoto, H. Ogawa, I. Ninomiya, K. Sada, S. Hamada, W.M. Caldwell, A new intelligent bed care system for hospital and home patients. Biomed Intrum & Tech **39** (2005), 313-319.

[59] J.A. Cafazzo, A.C. Easty, P.G. Rossos, K. Leonard, C.T. Chan, Complex tele-monitiring: facilitating hospital-at-home. Telemed J & e-Health **12** (2006), 202.

[60] H. Chun, J. Kang, K.J. Kim, K.S. Park, H.C. Kim, IT-based diagnostic instrumentation systems for personalized healthcare services. Studies Health Tech & Informatics **117** (2005), 180-190.

[61] F. Axisa, P.M. Schmitt, C. Gehin, G. Delhomme, E. McAdams, A. Dittmar, Flexible technologies and smart clothing for citizen medicine, home healthcare, and disease prevention. IEEE Trans Inform Tech Biomed **9** (2005), 325-336.

[62] J. Yao, R. Schmitz, S. Warren, A wearable point-of-care system for home use that incorporates plug-and-play and wireless standards. IEEE Trans Inform Tech Biomed **9** (2005), 363-371.

[63] V.G. Koutkias, I. Chouvarda, N. Maglaveras, A multiagent system enhancing home-care health services for chronic disease management. IEEE Trans Inform Tech Biomed **9** (2005), 528-537.

.

Current Principles and Practices of Telemedicine and e-Health
R. Latifi (Ed.)
IOS Press, 2008

Telerehabilitation: Current Perspectives

Deborah THEODOROS[a] and Trevor RUSSELL[b]

[a]Division of Speech Pathology, School of Health and Rehabilitation Sciences,
The University of Queensland, Brisbane, Australia
[b]Division of Physiotherapy, School of Health and Rehabilitation Sciences,
The University of Queensland, Brisbane, Australia

Abstract. Telerehabilitation in which rehabilitation services are provided at a distance using communication technologies is a new and developing field of telehealth. Primarily developed to provide equitable access to individuals who are geographically remote and to those who are physically and economically disadvantaged, telerehabilitation also has the capacity to improve the quality of rehabilitation health care. Online delivery of rehabilitation enables the rehabilitation therapist to optimize the timing, intensity and duration of therapy that is often not possible within the constraints of face-to-face treatment protocols in current health systems. This chapter outlines the advances made to date in telerehabilitation applications in the fields of physiotherapy, speech-language pathology, occupational therapy, and biomedical engineering and provides evidence for the success of these applications. Applications to date encompass systems ranging from low-bandwidth low-cost videophones, to highly expensive, fully immersive virtual reality systems with haptic interfaces. A number of barriers to the establishment and advancement of telerehabilitation within health care systems have been outlined and include professional issues relating to the inherent hands-on approach of some treatments, licensure laws, professional skill development, patient disability, reimbursement, and the paucity of online assessment and treatment tools and outcomes data. In response, possible solutions to these barriers such as the development and validation of alternative assessment and treatment procedures, involvement in the international policy debate, as well as the resolution of national professional policies which hinder the wider uptake of telerehabilitation technologies, have been outlined. The future of telerehabilitation is promising as a new, yet complex form of telehealth with the capacity to provide a wide range of services specifically designed to suit the needs of the individual.

Keywords. Telerehabilitation, advances, technology

Introduction

Telerehabilitation provides a range of rehabilitation services at a distance via communication technologies. Such services may include therapeutic intervention, remote monitoring of progress, education and training to families and rehabilitation professionals, and a means for networking for people with disability [1]. Primarily, the development of telerehabilitation has been driven by the need to provide equitable access to rehabilitation services for individuals who are geographically remote from rehabilitation specialists. The ongoing, long-term rehabilitation requirements of many people as a result of stroke, traumatic brain injury, progressive neurological disorder, and developmental disorder are frequently unmet in the individual's local community. The difficulty in the recruitment and retention of rehabilitation professionals in non-metropolitan centers and rural and remote areas is well recognized [2,3] and contributes significantly to this dilemma. In addition, many individuals with disability, and their families, have significant mobility issues associated with physical impairment, access to transport, and socioeconomic factors which preclude them from accessing any service regardless of distance. The establishment of an alternate model to face-to-face treatment that is accessible, flexible, and equally therapeutic and economic has the potential to enhance the rehabilitation process for these individuals.

While equitable access to rehabilitation services has been the primary impetus for the development of telerehabilitation, it has been suggested that the quality of care may also be enhanced by this service delivery model. Telerehabilitation has the potential to optimize the timing, intensity, and sequencing of intervention that is likely to produce the greatest functional outcome for the patient [4]. With health-care systems worldwide experiencing the need to operate with ever-increasing restrictions in relation to inpatient, outpatient, and community service models, optimal face-to-face treatment regimens are unsustainable. Indeed, they are unable to support intensive therapy regimens recommended for neurorehabilitation based on increasing evidence of neural plasticity and brain reorganization following brain damage [5]. Telerehabilitation provides the opportunity for flexible implementation of a range of treatment protocols that can enhance optimal outcomes [4]. Continuity of care by rehabilitation specialists, and the capacity to readily monitor progress and intervene in a timely manner are other advantages of this service delivery platform [6]. Furthermore, the opportunity for the individual to continue rehabilitation within their own social and vocational environment via telerehabilitation should lead to greater functional outcomes and enhanced integration [7].

Over the last decade, telerehabilitation applications for physical and communication rehabilitation, and home environment evaluation have been steadily developing and have provided assessment and intervention services to children and adults with a wide variety of physical and communication disabilities. The technology involved in these applications has included the simple telephone [8,9], Internet-based videoconferencing systems with dedicated software tools [10–16], physical sensors [17] and expensive, fully immersive virtual reality systems with haptic feedback [18,19]. This chapter will review the current developments in telerehabilitation applications, identify barriers to the implementation of telerehabilitation into mainstream health care, discuss possible solutions to these barriers, and propose future directions for telerehabilitation.

1. Current Developments: Evidence-Based Practice

1.1. Physical Rehabilitation

The term 'physical rehabilitation' can be applied to any rehabilitation process that involves an interaction between a patient and a practitioner resulting in the diagnosis or treatment of any physical dysfunction. Within the context of telerehabilitation, physical rehabilitation refers to assessment and treatment services that are delivered remotely through the use of telecommunications technologies. Many disciplines are involved in physical rehabilitation, the primary contributors being physical therapists, biomedical engineers and occupational therapists. To date, there are very few research teams with programs of research in this field, with the majority of telerehabilitation research being driven by small, creative research groups seeking to address specific clinical needs. The literature is primarily composed of case reports or small pilot studies and while much of the research is encouraging, there is an obvious lack of highly controlled and large scale research studies to demonstrate improved patient outcomes or cost-effectiveness [20].

Compared to other areas in telemedicine, telerehabilitation for physical disorders has had a short history. This undoubtedly stems from the nature of rehabilitation consultations and the conceptual difficulty experienced by many practitioners when imagining how to perform what is traditionally 'hands-on' therapy via a virtual medium. The mantra from the uninitiated clinician is invariably the same: "I cannot possibly treat my patients if I cannot touch them." In addition to perceptual barriers, the rehabilitation practitioner relies heavily on *measuring* their patients to both inform the diagnostic process and to monitor the outcomes of their interventions. Early telerehabilitation technologies, such as conventional videoconferencing, did not offer the clinician with any means of obtaining these measurements. This presented as an insurmountable barrier to many practitioners and stifled the use of telemedicine systems for rehabilitation consultations. However, recent years have seen a dramatic increase in the number and complexity of technology solutions available, many of which include the capacity to actively measure the performance of their remote patients in real-time (see below). In response, an almost palpable shift has begun in the attitudes of rehabilitation practitioners towards the use of telerehabilitation technology in clinical practice This is evidenced in the growing murmur of support for these technologies emanating from professional associations both in America and throughout the world [21,22], and the number of telerehabilitation research papers being presented at conferences traditionally dominated by medical fields.

The state of the art technologies that are paving the way for telerehabilitation applications for physical disorders can be broadly classified as 1) image-based telerehabilitation systems, 2) sensor based telerehabilitation and 3) virtual environments and virtual reality technologies.

1.2. Image Based Telerehabilitation

Unquestionably, throughout the history of telemedicine, videoconferencing has been a staple technology and it has been used consistently since the 1960's. Within the field of telerehabilitation, the first description of the use of videoconferencing appears in the early 90's where Delaplain et al. (1993) [23] describes a service (including physical therapy) provided via a satellite-based videoconferencing system. Soon after this, and concurrent with a reduction in the cost of videoconferencing systems, a flurry of telerehabilitation research ensued which utilized videoconferencing technology, making this the most widely used technology for telerehabilitation consultations. Projects were conducted in the fields of general physiotherapy [24–26], for ankle-foot orthotics [27], neurological physiotherapy [28,29] seating and wheelchair evaluations [30], and the rehabilitation of patients with spinal cord injuries [31]. In addition, telerehabilitation interventions have been evaluated in the areas of wheelchair prescription, foot care, gait problems, orthotics, prosthetics, arm weakness/joint degradation and communication disorders [32]. A recent study by Lai et al. (2004) [33], examined the feasibility of using videoconferencing to conduct a community-based stroke rehabilitation program. Nineteen subjects completed an eight week program during which they received education, exercises and psychosocial support via a videoconferencing system installed in a community centre for seniors. They found significant improvements in the Berg Balance Scale (BBS), State Self-Esteem Scale (SSES), Medical Outcomes Study 36-item Short Form (SF-36) and a stroke knowledge outcome measure.

While many projects utilizing videoconferencing technology have demonstrated encouraging outcomes, the inability to measure patient performance remotely has been a major limitation. To address this, a team of researchers from the University of Queensland, Australia developed a PC based telerehabilitation system which is based on videoconferencing technology, but also includes measurement tools that are able to objectively quantify the participant's physical performance (such as range of motion, muscle strength and gait) across a low-bandwidth Internet link. These tools were designed to perform the measurements optically, from the videoconferencing image, therefore eliminating the need for expensive sensors or equipment at the patient end of the consultation. To date the metrological properties of the system and it's validity for the measurement of knee range of motion [14], muscle strength [34], swelling [34] and assessment of gait [12] in the orthopaedic population has been evaluated. In yet unpublished work, the diagnostic accuracy of the telerehabilitation system for evaluating balance in the elderly and the functional ability of patients with Parkinson's Disease as also been tested and found to be accurate and reliable when compared to traditional face-to-face means of assessing these patients.

Using the same telerehabilitation system, Russell and colleagues have conducted the first Randomized Controlled Trial (RCT) in telerehabilitation to evaluate the efficacy of the system when used to provide outpatient rehabilitation to patients who have received total knee replacement surgery [35,13,15]. A total of sixty-five patients were randomized to receive rehabilitation either face-to-face with a physiotherapist or by interacting with a physiotherapist via the telerehabilitation system. Following a six-week intervention program, equivalent statistical improvements were seen across twelve physical and functional outcome measures across the two groups. At the conclusion of the RCT the authors concluded that: 1) rehabilitation via the telerehabilitation application produced physical and functional results that were comparable with those achieved through traditional face-to-face therapy, 2) patients were satisfied with receiving treatment via telerehabilitation, and 3) the telerehabilitation intervention was successful despite participants having limited computer skills.

1.3. Virtual Environments

A virtual environment (VE) is a three-dimensional, computer-generated environment which enables the user to interact with a simulated real-world environment in real time. VE systems, often called virtual reality (VR), vary in complexity and range from a simple PC running VE software, to costly systems that use various human-machine interfaces. Interfaces such as head-mounted visual displays can be used to 'immerse' the user in a three-dimensional virtual environment. The sensory information (e.g. vision, hearing, touch) gained from the VE can be manipulated such that certain desirable motor responses are elicited from the user. These motor responses are, in turn, integrated back into the VE thus completing the feedback loop and enabling the user to manipulate and interact with the VE. Using these systems, rehabilitation specialists can construct environments and tasks that incorporate key rehabilitation concepts such as task repetition, feedback and motivation that are able to produce motor skills which translate to the real world [36,37].

Several research teams have been working to adapt and develop virtual reality based systems that can specifically be used to monitor and provide treatment to patients in their own homes. To date much of the research surrounding the use of VR in telerehabilitation has utilized single case study or very small sample study designs. Holden and colleagues, a research team based at the Massachusetts Institute of Technology, Cambridge, Massachusetts have adapted a previous VE system to include telerehabilitation functionality [38,39]. Their system provides real-time videoconferencing together with a synchronised VR session between a patient who is located in their own home and a remote therapist. Both the patient and the therapist are able to visualise the VR session synchronously and the therapist may view the patient via the videoconference. In a preliminary study, seven patients with chronic stroke underwent 30 one-hour VR sessions over a six-week period via a high-speed Internet connection. Participants demonstrated significant improvements (range 16–67%, $P = 0.003$–0.05) on the main outcome measures of the Fugal-Meyer Test of Motor Recovery, the Wolf Motor Function Test and strength tests of the shoulder and hand [39,40].

Another low-cost system developed by Reinkensmeyer and colleagues [41] for hand and arm therapy uses a web interface and a force feedback joystick that is capable of assisting or resisting movements. The patient uses the system autonomously by logging into a web site and a therapist can periodically review their performance statistics and modify their treatment program if necessary. Results of a single case study of a patient following a stroke have demonstrated encouraging results. A similar system, called the 'Jerusalem Telerehabilitation System' combines the concept of this system with videoconferencing technologies. This enables the system to be used in either a stand-alone mode where the patient practices the exercises independently, or in a cooperative mode where therapist and patient are online simultaneously and interact during the session [42].

Using a similar concept, but a much more sophisticated system, Burdea and colleagues from Rutgers University, New Jersey have developed a home based VR telerehabilitation system that makes use of a hardware videoconferencing system, a VR system equipped with and a three-dimentional Polhemus tracking sensor and a multipurpose haptic grove called the Rutgers Master II (RMII). The RMII is an exoskeleton structure which is able to deliver accurate resistive forces to the users fingertips. This novel arrangement of human-machine interface can be used not only to sample the patients hand position in space, but also to provide resistive exercises for the patient. Preliminary testing of the system for both upper and lower limb applications in orthopaedic patients has produced promising results [18,19]. A more recent system, the 'Rutgers Arm' has also been reported by this research group. The Rutgers Arm system does not include a haptic glove however the addition of a low friction table enables exercises of the shoulder and elbow to be incorporated [43].

While VR technologies undoubtedly have a significant place in the future development of telerehabilitation, large scale studies are needed to examine the validity and cost-benefit of the employment of such systems in a remote context.

1.4. Sensor Based Rehabilitation

The use of sensor technologies in telerehabilitation applications has long been heralded by experts in the field as an essential ingredient for the development of evidence based diagnostic and treatment programs. Whether it is using a sophisticated SmartShirt™ (Sensatex, Maryland USA) to retrieve real-time biometric parameters or a simple electronic pedometer to asynchronously relay statistics to a remote therapists, the accurate quantification of physical parameters of the remote patient is an appealing concept to rehabilitation therapists. As is so often seen in the field of telemedicine, the challenge in the production of clinically useful sensor-based telerehabilitation systems has not primarily been in the development of the technologies. Rather, the difficulty is in managing, sorting, analysing and producing clinically relevant outputs from the inexorable quantity of data retrieved from the sensors [44]. The process has come to be known as 'information reduction' or 'data mining' and considerable resources and effort are being invested in optimizing algorithms to produce meaningful outputs from large amounts of data, which are congruent with the types of outcomes and functional assessment tools that clinicians are accustomed to interpreting [45].

Zheng and colleagues (2005) [46] provide an extensive overview of current sensor technologies that are commercially available and appropriate for incorporation into telerehabilitation systems. Sensors can be largely grouped into two categories, position-sensing technologies and motion-sensing technologies. Position-sensing technologies include sensors such as pedometers, goniometers, electromechanical switches or pressure sensors, inertial sensors, accelerometers and gyroscopes and are used to measure motion and orientation change in limbs and body positions. Motion-sensing technologies can be classified according to motion-tracking techniques which include: electromagnetic, acoustic, mechanical, and electrostatic position and orientation trackers, and video and electro-optical tracking systems. Motion-sensing trackers are used to generate real-time data that represents human movement through space [46].

Despite the great promise of sensor based telerehabilitation, and the emergence of start-up companies to exploit the technologies, there has been limited recent research activity in the research arena evaluating the clinical applications and efficacy of the technology. Mathie et al. (2004) [17] conducted a pilot study using a wireless triaxial accelerometer to monitor human movement in a group of six elderly subjects. The sensor was used to monitor for falls, metabolic energy expenditure and to detect changes in functional status over a period of two to three months. The researchers concluded that the device was practical for long term unsupervised home monitoring. This team has proceeded to use the technology as a means for producing real-time human movement classification [47], a topic that others have also addressed [48,49].

Telerehabilitation for physical disorders is a rapidly expanding area that is being driven by a proliferation of new technologies. As with any new research area, there is a need for well controlled and large scale research, utilising patients with a wide range of conditions, to fortify the preliminary findings reported in the literature to date. Such research should consider the cost-benefit factors of the interventions, a critically important factor in establishing a positive business case for the future expansion and uptake of telerehabilitation services into health care systems.

1.5. Communication and Swallowing

The clinical services provided by speech-language pathologists involve the assessment and treatment of a range of communication and swallowing disorders in children and adults. The communication disorders may involve speech, voice and/or language impairment. Speech-language pathology intervention is based largely on an auditory and visual interaction between the client and the clinician, and therefore readily lends itself to an online environment. Indeed, the Mayo Clinic [50] has incorporated teleconsultations in speech-language pathology since 1987 with the general consensus being that the telehealth approach represented a viable alternative to face-to-face consultation where distance precluded a timely and cost-effective service, or where specialized expertise was unavailable. To date, applications have been developed to assess and/or treat acquired adult neurological speech and language disorders, stuttering, voice disorders, speech and language disorders in children, head and neck oncology cases, and swallowing dysfunction. While some of these applications have utilized simple communication technologies, others have involved the use of sophisticated Internet-based videoconferencing systems with dedicated software tools enabling assessment and treatment procedures that mirror the face-to-face environment.

The assessment and treatment of acquired adult speech and language disorders has been one of the major areas of development in telerehabilitation for communication disorders. Researchers at the National Rehabilitation Hospital in Washington DC and the Rehabilitation Engineering Research Center (RERC) on Telerehabilitation have developed a custom software package called RESPECT (Remote SPEech-language Cognitive-communication Treatment) which combines real-time videoconferencing with the capacity to deliver assessment and treatment materials to the patient's computer. Using this system, researchers have established the validity of measuring the performance of adults with acquired brain injury on the standardized Story Retelling Procedure via an Internet-based videoconferencing system [10,51]. Results indicated that no significant differences in performance were identified between the face-to-face and telehabilitation settings, and that participants were highly accepting of the online assessment. Intervention studies using this system are ongoing.

Research currently being conducted in Australia, in the Telerehabilitation Research Unit at the University of Queensland has involved the development and validation of telerehabilitation applications for the assessment and treatment of acquired neurological speech and language disorders. In particular, this research has focused on the assessment and treatment of the speech disorder in Parkinson's Disease and on the assessment of aphasia and apraxia of speech. A specifically designed PC based videoconferencing system connected to the Internet at a relatively low bandwidth has been developed for this purpose. Specifically developed software tools enable the administration of informal and standardized speech and language assessments. Researchers have validated the assessment of dysarthria, a motor speech disorder, in 19 participants using informal and standardized assessments of speech production and intelligibility via an Internet-based videoconferencing system [16]. Results indicated that measurements of severity of dysarthria, percentage intelligibility in sentences, and perceptual ratings made in the telerehabilitation environment fell within a predetermined clinical accuracy level and were, therefore, comparable to those made in the face-to-face environment. A more extensive study of the assessment of 40 persons with hypokinetic dysarthria associated with Parkinson's Disease has revealed high levels of agreement between assessments conducted online and face-to-face for ratings of speech intelligibility, articulatory precision, vocal qualities, and oromotor function, and for objective measurement of sound pressure level and pitch range [52].

Similarly, preliminary data by these researchers has shown that language disorders following brain impairment can be validly assessed via the Internet using a standardized aphasia test [11]. Eighteen participants with aphasia following stroke and traumatic brain injury were simultaneously assessed face-to-face and online on the short form of the Boston Diagnostic Aphasia Examination, 3rd edition [53]. Across the 25 subtests, weighted kappa values revealed high levels of agreement for 23 of the subtests while the remaining three subtests demonstrated moderate levels of agreement between face-to face and online assessments. Ratings of melodic pattern sentence repetition, articulatory agility, grammatical form, presence of paraphasias, phrase length, word-finding, auditory comprehension and level of severity demonstrated high levels of agreement (83–100%).

At present, there is a paucity of research involving telerehabilitation applications for the treatment of acquired neurological speech and language disorders. However, a recent pilot study by researchers at the University of Queensland has shown that significant improvements in the speech of 10 people with Parkinson's Disease could be achieved using the Lee Silverman Voice Treatment (LSVT®) via the Internet [54]. Participants attained significant improvements in vocal pitch range and sound pressure levels of speech on various tasks, and were perceived to have significant improvements in the degree of breathiness in their voices, and in loudness level and variation. Further research designed to validate this treatment in comparison to face-to-face treatment is currently ongoing.

Telerehabilitation has also been shown to be an effective vehicle for the assessment and treatment of voice disorders. Mashima et al. (2003) [55], at the Tripler Army Medical Center in Hawaii conducted a study in which 23 participants with a voice disorder were treated online using an Internet-based videoconferencing system connected to the Internet with speech analysis software. The performance of these participants was compared to a similar group of 28 participants treated face-to-face. Positive treatment effects were obtained in both groups with no significant difference in the measures obtained for the traditional and telerehabilitation environments. This mode of service delivery was considered to be cost and time effective allowing active defense personnel to be treated at their assigned location rather than returning to a central base.

Treatment programs for stuttering have been successfully adapted to a telerehabilitation environment using both simple and more complex communication technology. In Australia, researchers have adapted the Lidcombe program for childhood stuttering to a distance format [56]. The technology used in these studies involved the Plain Old Telephone System (POTS) for regular consultations together with offline video recordings. In all, 6 children were successfully treated in this manner. Overall, the parents and children responded positively to the program delivered at a distant. In a recent Canadian study, a high speed videoconferencing intranet link was used by Sicotte, Lehoux, Fortier-Blanc and Leblanc (2003) [57] to assess and treat six children and adolescents who stuttered. A reduction in the frequency of dysfluency was achieved in these children and this was maintained six months later. Kully (2000) [58] reported on the successful follow-up treatment of an adult male with a severe stutter who had previously completed an intensive three-week program. A videoconferencing link via the Internet was established between a metropolitan and a rural site through which the participant practiced specific speech skills under the direction of the clinician and discussed problem-solving strategies. Both the clinician and the participant reported satisfaction with treatment sessions.

To date, there has been limited research published in the area of pediatric speech and language disorders despite educational and health agencies in several countries being regularly involved in teleconsultations via videoconferencing with children in rural and remote areas. Researchers in Western Australia where the population is distributed to many remote areas of the state saw the need to develop an alternate means of delivering speech pathology services to children living in these areas. Fairweather, Parkin, and Rozsa (2004) [59] conducted a study involving the assessment of the speech, oral muscular function, and language of 13 school-aged children (6–14 years) via interactive videoconferencing over an ISDN connection. Each child was assessed by two speech pathologists on standardized articulation and language assessments, an informal oromotor examination, and via a language sample analysis. All assessments were conducted by the remote clinician, while the on-site clinician manipulated stimulus materials. Both clinicians simultaneously rated each assessment. Results indicated 69% and 92% total agreement between the clinicians for the level of severity of the articulation and language disorder, respectively. Several discrepancies between the raters were found to occur for certain speech sounds in children with severe articulatory disorders. Despite the inflexibility of the camera views and lighting, the researchers concluded that this mode of service delivery had potential for the assessment of the speech and language disorders in children of this age group.

A recent pilot study conducted by researchers at the University of Queensland has further developed this concept and investigated the feasibility of an Internet-based assessment of speech disorder in children aged four to six years [60]. The system used in this study is similar to that used in all speech-language pathology research at the University of Queensland with dedicated software supporting the specific requirements of the assessment tasks. In this research all test materials were transmitted to the remote site computer thus negating the need for onsite assistance. This study involved the administration of a simple articulation test and an oromotor assessment with the child's performance being simultaneously assessed face-to-face and online. High levels of agreement between the online and face-to-face clinicians for single-word articulation (92%), speech intelligibility (100%), and oro-motor tasks (91%) were obtained suggesting that the Internet-based protocol had the potential to be a reliable method for assessing paediatric speech disorders. Further research is ongoing to validate the assessment of speech, language and literacy disorders online as well as the treatment of literacy disorder across the Internet.

Despite the obvious limitations, attempts have been made to perform assessments of swallowing function within an online environment. A clinical swallowing assessment involves an evaluation of oromotor function and trial swallows of small samples of food and liquid of varying consistencies. During the trial swallows, the speech-language pathologist observes and feels for rate and height of laryngeal elevation. While the oromotor function assessment can be adequately achieved online and food and liquid administered by a third party, the physical assessment of laryngeal elevation is not possible in this environment. However, this limitation may be partially overcome through strategic positioning of web cameras to view laryngeal elevation more closely. There have not been any studies reported in the literature that have investigated the validity of online clinical assessment of swallowing function. To date, only a single case study has indicated that an initial assessment of the nature and extent of swallowing dysfunction in an adult via videoconferencing was achieved, although a more complete evaluation was restricted due to the inability to physically determine the degree of laryngeal movement [61]. In contrast, in order to achieve an objective, remote assessment of oral/pharyngeal swallowing function, Perlman and Witthawaskul (2002) [62] reported on a procedure for the real-time videofluoroscopic examination of swallowing via the Internet. A computer at the patient end was connected to a fluoroscope to capture video signals and transmit these across the network to the controller's computer. This system enabled the successful capture and display of images in real-time with only a three to five second delay. This application to assess swallowing function has yet to be validated in persons with a range of swallowing disorders.

A very recent topic of research interest in telerehabilitation has been the speech pathology management of head and neck cancer patients. Myers (2005) [63] reported on the successful use of videoconferencing to provide speech rehabilitation and psychosocial support to one patient post laryngectomy and to another patient following radical chemoradiotherapy living in rural areas. In addition, the videoconferencing link provided education to families and clinicians inexperienced in the care of head and neck cancer patients. In the case of a third patient, the system was used to remove and reinsert a new tracheoesophageal puncture (TEP) voice prosthesis with the assistance of a relative and local nurse. This procedure was effectively accomplished and highlighted the potential for telehealth technology to facilitate the rehabilitation and ongoing management of persons with head and neck cancer. Research currently being conducted at the University of Queensland has focused on establishing the validity of using a telehealth application to conduct post discharge review assessments of the communication and swallowing function for individuals following total laryngectomy compared to face-to-face assessment. The PC-based videoconferencing system currently being used at the University of Queensland provided the platform for this study. Preliminary results from this research have indicated that the majority of parameters relating to evaluating current alaryngeal communication and swallowing status could be reliably measured online. Overall, both patient and clinician satisfaction with the online interaction were found to be high.

Although telerehabilitation applications in speech-language pathology have been steadily increasing, there is an ongoing need for research to develop and validate the use of these applications in a greater range of adult and pediatric communication and swallowing disorders. In particular, there is an urgent need for online treatment efficacy studies to determine the comparability of this form of service delivery with face-to face treatment.

2. Barriers and Issues at Hand

In comparison to many other areas of telemedicine, telerehabilitation is in its infancy. While there is enormous potential for future development in this field, there are a number of barriers and issues that need to be addressed to ensure that telerehabilitation becomes an integral part of rehabilitation health care. Some of these obstacles such as professional portability and training are generic to the field of telehealth. Other issues such as the degree of physical contact required in rehabilitation therapy, patient characteristics, reimbursement, the paucity of outcomes data, and the availability of assessment and treatment tools that can replicate face-to-face practice are more specific barriers to the advancement of telerehabilitation.

2.1. Professional Issues

The nature of the work of a rehabilitation therapist involves a *hands on* approach with significant physical contact between the therapist and the patient. For the physiotherapist and occupational therapist, and to a lesser extent, the speech-language pathologist, this interaction can make it difficult for some treatment techniques to be applied online. For example, performing spinal manipulation is not a possible treatment technique via telerehabilitaiton. In these situations, adaptations to the assessment or treatment procedure may be required to accommodate these changes. For example, the consultation may need to be conducted with an assistant at the patient end who will assist in the performance of tasks as directed by the online therapist. The need for a hands on approach in some areas of rehabilitation is one of the main reasons for professional skepticism towards telerehabiltation as an alternate service delivery model.

Professional portability between states within a country is also seen as a possible barrier to the establishment of telerehabilitation. In most countries, rehabilitation therapists must be licensed to practice in the state in which the patient receives treatment as well as in the state from which they are providing services. Licensing requirements in many states in the US and other countries can be financially onerous due to the cost of initial application fees, annual renewal fees, and the need to satisfy the state's educational requirements [64]. As a result, licensure laws and limited reimbursement impede the use of telerehabilitation services.

The current lack of comprehensive *training for professionals* in telerehabiltation applications constitutes an additional barrier to the inclusion of this service delivery model in health care. The future of telerehabilitation will depend on prior training in the use of the technology and specific practice issues for rehabilitation therapists at both the clinician and student levels.

2.2. Patient Characteristics

Many of the patients accessing rehabilitation services demonstrate significant levels of disability, particularly those requiring neurorehabilitation. The greater the level of disability (physical, cognitive, and communication), the more difficult it becomes to conduct a rehabilitation consult online. In some cases, the individual requires considerable assistance to execute various physical tasks while others with significant cognitive dysfunction (e.g., distractability, impulsiveness, short term memory etc.) are precluded from participating online. Selection of patients for telerehabilitation is a critical factor in successful outcomes and requires careful consideration by the health care professional to achieve this.

2.3. Reimbursement

Reimbursement for telerehabilitation services is limited in health care systems throughout the world and remains one of the most significant barriers to the expansion of telerehabilitation. A recent survey of Medicaid programs in the US by Palsbo (2004) [65] revealed that only ten states (Hawaii, Minnesota, and Nebraska, Arizona, Colorado, Georgia, Iowa, Montana, South Dakota and Utah) reimbursed for telerehabilitation or telemedicine. At the discipline level, it has been reported that 71% of telepractice services in speech-language pathology were not being reimbursed in 2002. The major barrier to reimbursement was the lack of strong outcome data supporting telerehabiltation applications and the need to develop specific telerehabilitation procedure codes for payment. The challenge to the rehabilitation specialists, therefore, is to provide the clinical evidence base for telerehabilitation, and to advocate for the use of telerehabilitation applications with health insurance providers.

2.4. Assessment and Treatment Tools

One of the major barriers to the progression of telerehabilitation lies in the fact that there is no single protocol for this type of health care. Inevitably, any one patient requires a different treatment protocol to another, as well as the services of various rehabilitation specialists. As a result, a range of technologies designed to enable assessment and treatment may be required in the rehabilitation program for that individual. The complexity of these requirements can be problematic for the establishment of telerehabilitation as a core component of health care. The development of assessment and treatment procedures that can be conducted online, as effectively and reliably as face-to-face procedures, are critical to the advancement of telerehabilitation.

2.5. Outcomes Data

The uptake of telerehabilitation into mainstream health care is also impeded by the paucity of outcomes research for this method of service delivery. Until this data is available, telerehabilitation is unlikely to be fully accepted by professional, government, and health funding bodies. Clinical research is needed to develop appropriate applications in telerehabilitation, set minimal technical specifications and standards, validate clinical protocols, and investigate the effectiveness of clinical outcomes, client and clinician satisfaction, quality of care, and cost-effectiveness of telerehabilitation [66]. Research in telerehabilitation has increased steadily over the last few years and is likely to continue to do so as rapid advances in communication technologies occur. In recognition of the growth in telepractice, several rehabilitation professions such as speech-language pathology, physiotherapy and occupational therapy, have recently drafted position statements for their members citing issues such as clinical standards, ethics, professional licensing, liability and malpractice, privacy and confidentiality, and reimbursement as important considerations in maintaining standards in this area [66,67].

3. Suggested Solutions to Overcome Barriers

Like many areas in telemedicine, the barriers restricting the widespread uptake of telerehabilitation technologies do not have simple solutions. Many political, professional and institutional changes, at the local, national and international level, are required before the clinician can truly utilize the technologies in a coordinated and endorsed way. In addition, clinicians must also be willing to approach the technologies with an open mind and adopt alternative practices to enable them to perform complex assessments and treatments within the confines of a virtual world. Strategies to overcome the various barriers that hinder the wider uptake of telerehabilitation applications into clinical practice may be considered from political and clinical perspectives.

3.1. Political Considerations

The emerging evidence in the literature regarding the efficacy of telerehabilitation interventions, coupled with the ever advancing telecommunication technologies makes it possible, at least in theory, to deliver effective rehabilitation services around the world. The concept of Global e-Health, a convergence of health care throughout the world, offers great benefit, especially to the heath and wellbeing of the developing world. However, the absence of inter-jurisdictional policy, or even guidelines to regulate and support global e-Health initiatives [68] threatens to undermine the possibilities offered by telerehabilitation technologies. There are many key policy issues that must be addressed. These include issues of licensure and certification across state and national boarders, equivalence of international clinical standards, regulation on privacy issues and the access and protection of patient health information, issues on costs and remuneration of services, the complexities of accountability and liability and the unification of international rules effecting clinical consultations, among others. Many of these issues are complex and culturally sensitive and can only be effectively addressed at the global level [68]. A number of International organizations such as the World Summit of the Information Society (WSIS), the World Health Organisation (WHO), the Pan American Health Organisation (PAHO), the World Trade Organisation (WTO) and the Universitas 21 Organisation (U21) are entering debate around many of the issues surrounding global health, however there yet remains a lack of leadership and focus on e-health policy [68]. The significant challenge for the subspecialty of telerehabilitation is to ensure that as the debate on e-health policy intensifies, there is adequate representation from the rehabilitation sciences and that policy is determined for all areas of e-health not just medicine per se. To ensure this, rehabilitation specialists need to take an active role in the debate and must be represented in these global organizations.

To facilitate the ultimate goal of internationally accepted policies for the practice of telerehabilitation, a great deal needs to be achieved at a local and national level. Professional association and registration bodies must play a fundamental role in the development of policies and guidelines which are applicable country-wide. While these guidelines should cover issues such as best practice and the minimum training requirements for telehealth practice, a paramount issue that must be addressed in the short term is that of professional portability. Professional portability has been defined as "the ease with which any health-care professional, recognized as an appropriately skilled practitioner, expert or trainee, is able to move in person or virtually across barriers (including political, cultural, social and temporal barriers), and among and between jurisdictions, to transfer knowledge, skills and care" [69]. To date, many of the rehabilitation professions require registration in the individual state in which they practice. This presents as a significant problem for telepractice across state boarders. While there are concerted efforts being made by a number of professional associations throughout the USA and Canada to address this issue and move towards a national registration [66,70,71] the issues remains largely unaddressed in the wider international community. Hailey et al. (2005) [70] highlights some of the challenges in achieving this, including the fact that licensing bodies for some professions are absent in some jurisdictions. This makes it difficult to establish minimum educational requirements and core competencies for a nationally recognized registration. However, regardless of these difficulties, rehabilitation professions in each country must address the issue of professional portability before significant progress can be made on a global scale.

With the issues of professional portability aside within jurisdictions, the issue of reimbursement for services is a primary factor limiting the use of telerehabilitation technologies. The fact that only five states in the USA alone [64] currently reimburse for telerehabilitation services, reflects the early developmental stage of telerehabilitation and the limited evidence for the clinical and cost effectiveness of telerehabilitation practices. Driving the debate from the perspective of the policy makers is the fear that if telerehabilitation practices were to be reimbursed, there would be a massive utilization of services by individuals who currently are unable to access care, precipitously increasing the system-wide expenditure on health care [1]. Ironically, from the perspective of the rehabilitation practitioners, an increase in the utilization of services from those currently unable to access services is the primary motivation for adopting telerehabilitation practices. In order to convince the policy makers to pay for services, there is a desperate need for high quality research in the field of telerehabilitation. This research should be directed at not only at demonstrating the diagnostic accuracy of the assessments and the efficacy of treatment interventions, but also at firmly establishing the cost effectiveness of the services. Once the elusive factor of cost-effectiveness begins to emerge in the literature, it must be followed up with a strong lobbying by both clinicians and professional associations for the right for reimbursement of services. Furthermore, the rehabilitation professions need to ensure that all drafted legislation is sufficiently broad to cover all aspects of the rehabilitation process, not just core medical service [1].

3.2. Clinical Considerations

At the grass roots level, the most significant challenge to the integration of telerehabilitation services may lie in changing the attitude of rehabilitation therapists towards telerehabilitation technologies. Many therapists remain skeptical of the ability to perform remote patient assessments and have reservations about the diagnostic accuracy of these assessments. This is primarily due to a lack of exposure to telerehabilitation technologies and the scant number of published diagnostic equivalence studies. Similarly, many practitioners have great difficulty in conceptualizing how to apply what a traditionally 'hands on' therapy through a virtual medium. This is a considerable problem especially for the physiotherapy and occupational therapy professions where 'hands on' treatment forms a significant component of their daily practice. However, there is emerging evidence which demonstrates that equivalent patient outcomes can be achieved without the use of 'hands-on' techniques. For example, Russell and colleagues (2003) [13] conducted a RCT investigating the efficacy of providing outpatient telerehabilitation to patients who had received a total knee replacement surgery. In this study, equivalent patient outcomes were achieved through telerehabilitation when compared to traditional face-to-face treatment even though 'hand-on' techniques were not able to be applied. Rather, outcomes were achieved by instructing the patient how to self-apply manual techniques and perform relevant exercises via the videoconference. The self-management strategies adopted in this study are not a new concept and have been demonstrated to be effective in many other areas of practice [72]. Embracing these concepts and adapting traditional treatments so that they can be delivered without the use of hands is paramount for the wider adoption of telerehabilitation technologies.

A factor that has been shown to be important for the adoption of telemedicine technologies [73–76] and is particularly important for telerehabilitation consultation is the design of the telemedicine system. Due to the nature of the telerehabilitation consultation, the therapist must interact with the telemedicine system to quantify the performance of the patient. This is particularly true with sensor based systems and virtual reality systems where the therapist must deal with a complex array of data. Telerehabilitation systems must be designed with this in mind and utilize leading concepts in interface design such as the human factors development approach suggested by Salvemini (1999) [77].

Finally, exposure to the possibilities and the emerging evidences for telerehabilitation technologies is a critical requirement for a greater uptake of telerehabilitation technology in everyday practice. Education covering e-health concepts and principles should be introduced into the curricular of professional rehabilitation courses such that using telerehabilitation technologies is not a new concept to the next generation of practitioners. For those practicing already, continuing education courses and workshops sponsored by professional associations should introduce rehabilitation practitioners to the possibilities of telerehabilitation technologies.

4. Future

The future of telerehabilitation is indeed a bright one. In the few years since its inception, progress has been made on many fronts including the development of innovative technologies and an earnest start towards the validation of assessment and treatment outcomes through clinical research. Due to the unique requirements of measurement and the various nuances of telerehabilitation practice, much of the emphasis to date has been on the development of new technologies. These technologies, which exceed the complexity of systems in other areas of practice (e.g. telepsychiatry), have been progressing rapidly. However much of the research has utilized single case cr small study samples designs to evaluate the potential of the new devices. Additionally, many studies have opted to test the device in controlled laboratory environments rather than in target communities. As a staple array of technologies slowly emerges, the challenge from here is to implement and evaluate the technologies on a large scale in real world environments. Such studies must employ controlled research methodologies and large populations to firmly explore the advantages and disadvantages of telerehabilitation practice. The broader issues of cost-benefit and cost-effectiveness must be considered, especially in the area of telerehabilitation where many of the complex technologies come at a high cost. Additionally, the feasibility of deploying highly complex systems, that require large communication bandwidths, into the areas where telerehabilitation application are needed most, such as rural and remote areas, must be evaluated.

Further work is also required to refine and develop new technologies to enable care to be delivered to a larger array of patients. With the development of complex evaluation systems, such as the use of sensor based rehabilitation, partnership opportunities arise with research teams in other areas such as those developing tele-homecare solutions. Many tele-homecare technologies which are designed to monitor patient status remotely in the home could be adapted to provide the objective data required for successful telerehabilitation consultations. Collaboration between these researchers may result in the generation of systems that not only offers continuous patient monitoring, but also enables the delivery of therapeutic intervention when altered physiological parameters are detected. For example, imagine a cell phone developed for people with Parkinson's Disease that not only continuously monitors their movement and speech parameters, but that schedules and facilitates real-time telerehabilitation consultations when these parameters reach critical levels.

Looking further into the future, technologies are likely to be developed which offer even more possibility for remote rehabilitation. For example robot assisted therapy, a concept which is already being explored in the literature, may be combined with haptics to give therapists the vital sense of touch and the ability to guide and facilitate movement remotely. The exciting area of nanotechnology, new concepts in neurorehabilitaiton, increasing telecommunication speeds and accessibility, and the miniaturization and mobilization of devices all open the door to endless possibilities for telerehabilitation researchers, and a greater potential of providing global access to timely and high quality rehabilitation services.

5. Conclusion

Telerehabilitation has the potential to have a significant impact on the outcomes of many persons requiring rehabilitation of physical and communication disorders. Equitable access to rehabilitation services and improvements in quality of care are expected to occur. While the evidence for the efficacy of telerehabilitation in physical rehabilitation and speech-language pathology is steadily increasing, the development of further innovative applications in these areas and others remains critical to the success and sustainability of this method of service delivery. Political and clinical barriers, however, continue to impede the integration of telerehabilitation into mainstream health care. Solutions to these barriers encompass global, international, national, and local levels of interaction amongst rehabilitation professionals and governments to facilitate this process. The future of telerehabilitation, however, is an exciting one with the possibility of the development and use of new, innovative technologies that will transform current practice and make telerehabilitation an integral part of health care.

References

[1] Rosen MJ. Telerehabilitation. *Neurorehabilitation* 1999; *3*: 3-18.
[2] Pickering M, McAllister L, Hagler P, et al. External factors influencing the profession in six societies. *American Journal of Speech-Language Pathology* 1998; *7*: 5-17.
[3] Yarrow S. (1999). Members' 1998 survey of the Parkinson's Disease Society of the United Kingdom. In R. Percival & P. Hobson (Eds.), *Parkinson's disease: Studies in psychological and social care* (pp. 79-92). Leicester: BPS Books.
[4] Winters JM, & Winters JM. A telehomecare model for optimizing rehabilitation outcomes. *Telemedicine Journal and e-Health* 2004; *10*: 200-212.
[5] Bach-y-Rita P. (2000). Conceptual issues relevant to present and future neurologic rehabilitation. In H. Levin & J. Grafman (Eds.), *Neuroplasticity and reorganization of function after brain injury* (pp. 357-379). New York: Oxford University Press.
[6] Bashshur R. Telemedicine effects: Cost, quality and access. *Journal of Medical Systems* 1995; *19*: 81-91.
[7] Temkin AJ, Ulieny GR, & Vesmarovich SH. Telerehabilitation: a perspective of the way technology is going to change the future of patient treatment. *Rehab Management* 1996; *9*: 28-30.
[8] Vaughan GR. Tel-communicology: Health care delivery system for persons with communication disorders. *ASHA Supplement* 1976; *18*: 13-17.
[9] Wertz RT, Dronkers NF, Bernstein-Ellis E, et al. (1987). Appraisal and diagnosis of neurogenic communication disorders in remote settings. In R. H. Brookshire (Ed.), *Clinical Aphasiology* (Vol. 17, pp. 117-123). Minneapolis: BRK Publishers.
[10] Georgeadis AC, Brennan DM, Barker LN, & Baron CR. Telerehabilitation and its effect on story retelling by adults with neurogenic communication disorders. *Aphasiology* 2004; *18*: 639-652.
[11] Hill A, Theodoros D, Russell T, Ward E, & Wootton R. (2006). *Assessing acquired neurogenic communication disorders via the Internet.* Paper presented at the American Telemedicine Association 11th Annual Meeting, San Diego.
[12] Russell T, Wootton R, & Jull G. The diagnostic reliability of Internet based observational kinematic gait analysis. *Journal of Telemedicine and Telecare* 2003; *9*: 48-51.
[13] Russell T, Buttrum P, Wootton R, & Jull GA. Low bandwidth physical rehabilitation for total knee replacement patients: Preliminary results. *Journal of Telemedicine and Telecare* 2003; *9*: 44-47.
[14] Russell T, Jull G, & Wootton R. Can the Internet be used as a medium to evaluate knee angle? *Manual Therapy* 2003; *8*: 242-246.
[15] Russell TG, Buttrum P, Wootton R, & Jull GA. Total knee replacement rehabilitation via low-bandwidth telemedicine. The patient and therapist experience. *Journal of Telemedicine and Telecare* 2004; *10*: 85-87.
[16] Hill AJ, Theodoros DG, Russell TG, et al. An Internet-based telerehabilitation system for the assessment of motor speech disorders: A pilot study. *American Journal of Speech Language Pathology* 2006; *15*: 1-12.
[17] Mathie MJ, Coster ACF, Lovell NH, et al. A pilot study of long-term monitoring of human movements in the home using accelerometry. *Journal of Telemedicine and Telecare* 2004; *10*: 144-151.
[18] Burdea G, Popescu V, Hentz V, & Colbert K. Virtual reality-based orthopaedic telerehabilitation. *IEEE Transactions on Rehabilitation Engineering* 2000; *8*: 430-432.

[19] Girone M, Burdea G, Bouzit M, Popescu V, & Deutsch JE. Orthopedic rehabilitation using the "Rutgers ankle" interface. *Studies in Health Technology and Informatics* 2000; *70*: 89-95.
[20] Winters JM. Telerehabilitation research: Emerging opportunities. *Annual Review of Biomedical Engineering* 2002; *4*: 287-320.
[21] Wakeford L, Wittman PP, White MW, & Schmeler MR. Telerehabilitation position paper. *American Journal of Occupational Therapy* 2005; *59*: 656-660.
[22] Australian Physiotherapy Association. (2005). *APA Vision for physiotherapy 2020*. Retrieved 13/10/2006, from http://apa.advsol.com.au/physio_and_health/public/download/APA_vision.pdf?CFID= 1921554&CFTOKEN=45679703.
[23] Delaplain CB, Lindborg CE, Norton SA, & Hastings JE. Tripler pioneers telemedicine across the Pacific. *Hawaii Medical Journal* 1993; *52*: 338-339.
[24] Chae YM, Heon Lee J, Hee Ho S, et al. Patient satisfaction with telemedicine in home health services for the elderly. *International Journal of Medical Informatics* 2001; *61*: 167-173.
[25] Clark P, Dawson S, Scheideman-Miller C, & Post M. Telerehab: Stroke teletherapy and management using two-way interactive video. *Neurology Report* 2002; *26*: 87-93.
[26] Nitzkin JL, Zhu N, & Marier RL. Reliability of telemedicine examination. *Telemedicine Journal* 1997; *3*: 141-157.
[27] Lemaire ED, & Jeffreys Y. Low-bandwidth telemedicine for remote orthotic assessment. *Prosthetics and Orthotics International* 1998; *22*: 155-167.
[28] Savard L, Borstad A, Tkachuck J, Lauderdale D, & Conroy B. Telerehabilitation consultations for clients with neurologic diagnoses: Cases from rural Minnesota and American Samoa. *Neurorehabilitation* 2003; *18*: 93-102.
[29] Forducey PG, Ruwe WD, Dawson SJ, et al. Using telerehabilitation to promote TBI recovery and transfer of knowledge. *Neurorehabilitation* 2003; *18*: 103-111.
[30] Malagodi M, Schmeler MR, Shapcott NG, & Pelleschi T. The use of telemedicine in assistive technology service delivery: results of a pilot study. *Technology: Special Interest Section Quarterly* 1998; *8*: 1-4.
[31] Phillips V, Vesmarovich R, Hauber E, Wiggers E, & Egner A. Telehealth: Reaching out to newly injured spinal cord patients. *Public Health Reports* 2001; *116*: 94-102.
[32] Lemaire ED, Boudrias Y, & Greene G. Low-bandwidth, internet-based videoconferencing for physical rehabilitation consultations. *Journal of Telemedicine and Telecare* 2001; *7*: 82-90.
[33] Lai JC, Woo J, Hui E, & Chan WM. Telerehabilitation – a new model for community-based stroke rehabilitation. *Journal of Telemedicine and Telecare* 2004; *10*: 199-205.
[34] Russell T, Wootton R, & Jull G. Physical outcome measurements via the Internet: reliability at two Internet speeds. *Journal of Telemedicine and Telecare* 2002; *8*: 50-52.
[35] Russell T. (2004). Establishing the efficacy of telemedicine as a clinical tool for physiotherapists: From systems design to randomised controlled trial., PhD thesis, University of Queensland, Brisbane.
[36] Bliss JP, Tidwell PD, & Guest MA. The effectiveness of virtual reality for administering spatial navigation training to firefighters. *Presence: Teleoperators and Virtual Environments* 1997; *6*: 73-86.
[37] Lintern G, Roscoe JM, Koonce JM, & Segal LD. Transfer of landing skills in begining flight simulation. *Human Factors* 1990; *32*: 319-327.
[38] Holden MK, Dyar T, Schwamm L, & Bizzi E. Virtual environment-based telerehabilitation in patients with stroke. *Presence: Teleoperators and Virtual Environments* 2005; *14*: 214-233.
[39] Holden MK. Virtual environments for motor rehabilitation: Review. *CyberPsychology and Behavior* 2005; *8*: 187-211.
[40] Holden MK, Dyar T, Dayan-Cimadoro L, Schwamm L, & Bizzi E. Virtual environment training in the home via telerehabilitation. *Archives of Physical Medicine and Rehabilitation* 2004; *85*: E12.
[41] Reinkensmeyer DJ, Pang CT, Nessler JA, & Painter CC. Web-based telerehabilitation for the upper extremity after stroke. *IEEE Transactions on Neural Systems and Rehabilitation Engineering* 2002; *10*: 102-108.
[42] Sugarman H, Dayan E, Weisel-Eichler A, & Tiran J. The Jerusalem TeleRehabilitation System, a new low-cost, haptic rehabilitation approach. *CyberPsychology and Behavior* 2006; *9*: 178-182.
[43] Kuttuva M, Boian R, Merians A, et al. The Rutgers Arm, a rehabilitation system in virtual reality: a pilot study. *CyberPsychology and Behavior* 2006; *9*: 148-151.
[44] Winters JM, & Wang Y. Wearable sensors and telerehabilitation. *IEEE Engineering in Medicine and Biology Magazine* 2003; *22*: 56-65.
[45] Bonato P, Mork PJ, Sherrill DM, & Westgaard RH. Data moining of motor patterns recorded with wearable technology. *IEEE Engineering in Medicine and Biology Magazine* 2003; *22*: 110-119.
[46] Zheng H, Black ND, & Harris ND. Position-sensing technologies for movement analysis in stroke rehabilitation. *Medical and Biological Engineering and Computing* 2005; *43*: 413-420.

[47] Karantonis DM, Narayanan MR, Mathie M, Lovell NH, & Celler BG. Implementation of a real-time human movement classifier using a triaxial accelerometer for ambulatory monitoring. *IEEE Transactions on Information Technology in Biomedicine* 2006; *10*: 156-167.

[48] Bouten CV, Koekkoek KT, Verduin M, Kodde R, & Janssen JD. Atriaxial accelerometer and portable data processing unit for the assessment of daily physical activity. *IEEE Trans Biomed Eng* 1997; *44*: 136-147.

[49] Uiterwaal M, Glerum EB, Busser HJ, & Van Lummel RC. Ambulatory monitoring of physical activity in working situations, a validation study. *Journal of Medical Engineering and Technology* 1998; *22*: 168-172.

[50] Duffy JR, Werven GW, & Aronson AE. Telemedicine and diagnosis of speech and language disorders. *Mayo Clinic Proceedings* 1997; *72*: 1116-1122.

[51] Brennan DM, Georgeadis AC, Baron CR, & Barker LM. The effect of videoconference-based telerehabilitation on story retelling performance by brain-injured subjects and its implications for remote speech-language therapy. *Telemedicine Journal and e-Health* 2004; *10*: 147-154.

[52] Constantinescu G, Theodoros D, Russell T, Ward E, & Wootton R. (2006). *A telerehabilitation application for assessing the speech and voice difficulties in Parkinson's Disease.* Paper presented at the American Telemedicine Association 11th Annual Meeting, San Diego.

[53] Goodglass H, Kaplan E, & Barresi B. *Boston Diagnostic Aphasia Examination.* 3rd edn. Baltimore: Lippincott Williams & Wilkins, 2001.

[54] Theodoros DG, Constantinescu G, Russell TG, et al. Treating the speech disorder in Parkinson's Disease online. *Journal of Telemedicine and Telecare* In press.

[55] Mashima P, Birkmire-Peters D, Syms M, et al. Telehealth: Voice therapy using telecommunications technology. *American Journal of Speech-Language Pathology* 2003; *12*: 432-439.

[56] Harrison E, Wilson L, & Onslow M. Distance intervention for early stuttering with the Lidcombe programme. *Advances in Speech Language Pathology* 1999; *1*: 31-36.

[57] Sicotte C, Lehoux P, Fortier-Blanc J, & Leblanc Y. Feasibility and outcome evaluation of a telemedicine application in speech: language pathology. *Journal of Telemedicine and Telecare* 2003; *9*: 253-258.

[58] Kully D. Telehealth in speech pathology: Applications in the treatment of stuttering. *Journal of Telemedicine and Telecare* 2000; *6*: S39-41.

[59] Fairweather C, Parkin M, & Rozsa M. (2004). *Speech and language assessment in school-aged children via videoconferencing.* Paper presented at the 26the World Congress of the International Association of Logopedics and Phoniatrics, Brisbane.

[60] Waite MC, Cahill LM, Theoodros DG, Russell TG, & Busuttin S. Online assessment of childhood speech disorders: A pilot study. *Journal of Telemedicine and Telecare.* In press.

[61] Lalor E, Brown M, & Cranfield E. Telemedicine: Its role in speech and language management for rural and remote patients. *Australian Communication Quarterly: Issues in Language, Speech and Hearing* 2000; *2*: 54-55.

[62] Perlman AL, & Witthawaskul W. Real-time remote telefluoroscopic assessment of patients with dysphagia. *Dysphagia* 2003; *17*: 162-167.

[63] Myers C. Telehealth applications in Head and Neck Oncology. *Journal of Speech-Language Pathology and Audiology* 2005; *29*: 125-129.

[64] Denton DR. Ethical and legal issues related to telepractice. *Seminars in Speech and Language* 2003; *24*: 313-322.

[65] Palsbo SE. Medicaid Payment for Telerehabilitation. *Archives of Physical Medicine and Rehabilitation* 2004; *85*: 1188-1191.

[66] American Speech-Language-Hearing Association. Speech-language pathologists providing clinical services via telepractice: Position statement. *ASHA Supplement.* In Press; *25*.

[67] National Initiative for Telehealth Guidelines. (2003). *National Initiative for Telehealth (NIFTE) Framework of Guidelines.* Retrieved 20/10/2006, from http://cst-sct.org/resources/FrameworkofGuidelines2003eng.pdf.

[68] Scott RE, & Lee A. E-health and the Universitas 21 organization: 3. Global policy. *Journal of Telemedicine and Telecare* 2005; *11*: 225-229

[69] Goldberg MA, Sharman Z, Bell B, Ho K, & Patil N. E-health and the Universital 21 organization: 4. Professional portability. *Journal of Telemedicine and Telecare* 2005; *11*: 230-233.

[70] Hailey D, Foerster V, Nakagawa B, et al. Achievements and challenges on policies for allied health professionals who use telehealth in the Canadian Arctic. *Journal of Telemedicine and Telecare 2005; 11 (Suppl. 2): S2:39-41* 2005; *11*: S2:39-41.

[71] Wakeford L, Wittman PP, White MW, & Schmeler MR. Telerehabilitation position paper. *The American Journal Of Occupational Therapy* 2005; *59*: 656-660.

[72] Guevara JP, Wolf FM, Grum CM, & Clark NM. Effects of educational interventions for self management of asthma in children and adolescents: systematic review and meta-analysis. *British Medical Journal* 2003; *326*: 1308-1309.

[73] Chimiak WJ, Rainer RO, Chimiak JM, & Martinez R. An architecture for naval telemedicine. *IEEE Transactions on Information Technology in Biomedicine* 1997; *1*: 73-79.

[74] Lathan CE, Kinsella A, Rosen MJ, Winters J, & Trepagnier C. Aspects of human factors engineering in home telemedicine and telerehabilitation systems. *Telemedicine Journal* 1999; *5*: 169-175.

[75] Salvemini AV. Improving the human-computer interface: A human factors engineering approach. *MD Computing* 1998; *15*: 1-6.

[76] Sengupta S, & Clayton PD. (1996). Clinical workstations: an architectural perspective. In J. Van Bemmel & A. T. McCray (Eds.), *IMIA Yearbook of Medical Informatics* (pp. 59-64). Stuttgart: Schattauer Vaerlag.

[77] Salvemini AV. Challenges for user-interface designers of telemedicine systems. *Telemedicine Journal* 1999; *5*: 163-168.

.

Current Principles and Practices of Telemedicine and e-Health
R. Latifi (Ed.)
IOS Press, 2008

Telemedicine and Wound Care

Cheri A. ONG, MD

Department of Plastic Surgery, Vanderbilt University, Nashville, Tennessee

Abstract. Although wound care has been practiced for centuries, telewound care is a relatively new concept. Currently, only a few pilot programs are in existence. Telewound care has yet to achieve the popularity and recognition of its other tele-medicine predecessors amongst members of the health care industry and public alike. The tremendous potential of incorporating the technology of telemedicine into wound care needs to be realized. Wound care is a representation of the care of chronic and debilitating conditions that require long-term specialized care. We have seen the positive effects of improved living conditions and advances in health care globally. The result: people are now living longer. Every day a small piece is added to the pie: the percentage of worlds' elderly and those with chronic medical conditions that would require medical attention is rising. With the escalating costs of health care, and the push of the industry towards outpatient care, this is a part of the health care crisis that is demanding our immediate attention. We have seen positive outcomes in the care of other chronic medial conditions using telemedi-cine such as home telecare programs. In addition, the effectiveness of several pro-grams using available advances in technology such as the field of radiology has been established. Wound care can build on success created in these fields to create an effective and useful method of care.

The aim of this chapter is to recognize the impact of this problem, to intro-duce several pilot programs in several different aspects of wound care and to build on current resources in order to achieve a novel method of wound care. The goal would be to create a technologically advanced, cost-effective and user-friendly program, and be able to bridge the gap between the sick and available specialized care. Both store-and-forward technology and televideo have a role to play in tele-wound care, the latter greater in the role of home telecare and teleconsultation, and the former in post-operative patients and the follow-up of chronic wounds. Either way, both have been underutilized and underdeveloped. With the advances in the field of telecommunications in connecting people across distances at a fraction of the time and costs, improved outcomes reported in other fields of telemedicine and positive legislative changes, there is an enormous potential in this field. We now have the ability, knowledge and resources to develop telewound care programs, which can provide high quality patient care in a more concise and cost-effective way. It is certainly a welcoming relief to a field that has traditionally been known to pose an emotional, physical and financial drain to all those involved.

Keywords. Telewound care, telemedicine, wound care

Introduction

In essence, the use of telemedicine in wound care is a subset of a bigger topic at hand: the management of chronic conditions associated with the aging population requiring long-term care. Chronic wound care can be a long process often requiring months and years of dedicated and specialized care. They include, but are not limited to post-surgical and medical patients with wound complications, vascular patients with ulcers; pressure sores in spinal cord injured and debilitated patients, and burn victims. Wound care is a field where timing and specialized appropriate care is of utmost importance. It is difficult to substitute the expertise of the "trained eye" of a wound care provider in terms of triage and wound care management decisions. Often times, poor patient outcomes can result from patient ignorance, the lack of specialized care and the delay in seeking timely and appropriate care due to barriers in time and distance. Months and years of suffering endured by a patient and their care providers, millions of health care dollars and resources utilized to manage the problem can be alleviated if patients can present to specialized providers in a timely fashion, or wound care programs which allow for interaction between the patient and specialized care providers across time and distances can be implemented for decision making purposes, and long-term preventive measures. Telewound care is a relatively new concept and medium to care for these patients. The goal is to provide the highest level of care to these patients in the safest and fastest method using the most user-friendly and cost-effective technologies that would be parallel in-person specialized care. In addition, unnecessary travel can be eliminated through proper patient triage.

1. Health Care Patterns: The Problems in Hand

With improvements in health care and technology, the global population of the elderly and those with chronic medical problems is increasing. Furthermore, the large majority of this population lives in rural parts of countries where accessibility to health care is limited. In the United States for example, greater than 60 million people live in rural areas. In addition, nearly fifteen percent (15%) of this rural population is over sixty-five (65) years of age. This is the population of greatest need of medical care due to the chronic nature of their diseases, disabilities and geographical isolation. As the push towards provision of medical care to the outpatient setting increases, many of these patients will be cared for in rehabilitation hospitals, nursing homes or in their own homes using home health care services. It is estimated that more than 1.5 million home health visits are being made each day in the United States [1]. Since most medical expertise is available in the urban setting, these patients are at a disadvantage in terms of obtaining the optimal specialized care for their problems. The care of chronic wounds is a field where experience counts. Trained personnel can make decisions quickly and correctly to prevent significant costs in morbidity and mortality. However the availability of trained personnel for example wound care nurses are currently too few to meet the demand. This problem will only escalate with time if the current trend continues.

The introduction of home telehealth programs is an example of a natural development in response to the demand of care at home. Management of several chronic medical problems including diabetes, congestive heart failure, chronic obstructive pulmonary disease (COPD), dementia, asthma and cerebrovascular accidents (CVA) has been managed successfully under this program.

Yet, in wound care management, telewound care is still in its infancy. Many pilot projects have been conducted in single-site institutions with small numbers of enrolled patients. The goal of this chapter is to introduce these programs, and to use them as a stepping-stone towards greater utilization of our current resources and towards the implementation of successful wound care programs. As the prevalence of chronic diseases and chronic wounds increases and the trend towards outpatient care rises, we must adapt to new technologies, and create new standards of care for the better interest of all involved.

"You see things; and you say, 'Why?' But I dream things that never were; and I say, 'Why not?' " George Bernard Shaw, (1856–1950).

2. Current Developments: Evidence Based Practice

Currently, most telewound care programs are based on store and forward, web-based technology. Live or interactive televideo is becoming increasingly popular, especially following the recent success of its use in the management of chronic medical illnesses via home telecare. The third type of interaction, which involves the review of taped televideo sessions of patients and their wounds have also been reported [2].

The use of store-and-forward in wound care is appealing because of the improved image resolution available in modern digital photography, the ability to compress large data files to be transferred at an acceptable time frame, the ease and wide availability of the internet in providing access to web based systems and the lower costs in terms of equipment and technological support. In addition, the information and images stored in these programs can be viewed at any time. Most of the work in store-and-forward programs is based on the success achieved in the fields of teledermatology and teleradiology. It is easy to see why these specialties have adopted telemedicine and created successful programs. They both rely on accurate and consistent projection of clear digital images and the timely transmission of their compressed versions for diagnosis and management.

In wound care however, there is still a lack of supported evidence for its widespread clinical use. The goals of current pilot projects have been to prove the reliability of digital images or televideo sessions to be comparable to onsite or face-to-face consultations. Once this initial point can be established, then the expansion of its use towards direct patient consultations, and wound monitoring can begin.

2.1. Digital Imaging

Digital images of wounds, technical aspects of surgeries, and postoperative pictures have been used in clinical practice for a long time, both for educational and clinical purposes. Presentations at a clinical conference or meeting would be quite difficult to follow and comprehend if they consist only of plain text, without images of clinical conditions, or operative techniques. The significant change made over the last few years has been the replacement of conventional slides by digital imaging as a medium to display these images.

Although not widely documented or spoken of, digital imaging has been incorporated in current patient care techniques across specialties. Hard copies of images from biopsy sites often accompany patients sent for evaluation by dermatologists to plastic surgeons and ENT surgeons for surgical excisions of cutaneous malignancies, which may be healed in the interim between the shave biopsy and consultation. Orthopedic trauma surgeons dealing with large soft tissue defects from traumatic injuries to the extremities often obtain intra-operative images which are sent to reconstructive surgeons for additional planning in tissue coverage.

Decision-making in wound care is based on sound clinical judgment made by specialists in the field. Because of this fact, the ability to see the actual wound and be able to make the right clinical decision in each situation is vital to patient care and outcomes. Across all surgical specialties, consultations are constantly being made by small hospitals, urgent care and emergency room personnel to surgeons and wound care specialists to "look at a wound," may it be acute or chronic in nature. It would be difficult for someone who is not well-versed in wound care to accurately describe the wound or to provide for these patients. In these patient consultations, clinical decisions can be made using transmitted images of the area of concern, in conjunction with patient information in the form of clinical notes or telephone conversations which will be less time consuming, decrease unnecessary patient and physician travel, allow for a better physician-physician relationship and provide better overall patient care.

One of the most important aspects of allowing one to do that is to ensure that the projection of digital images are a clear representation of the actual image of the wound in a face-to face situation. However, the clearest image may result in slow transfer times across communication lines, or long computer downloading times. This would not be time and cost effective. In addition, certain aspects of photography such as light projection, filtering, background color etc. can impact the appearance of images produced by the camera. Therefore, it is important that the clearest images in the lowest amount of resolution are projected to allow for the fastest transfer of the most representative picture.

From the field of plastic surgery, imaging has been used over the past fifty years for means of documentation, assessment of operative results, peer-communication and educational purposes. A standard is set for the capture, storage and projection of these images. In the academic world, standardization is necessary to obtain reproducible and valid results. For clinical work, it is important to ensure consistency in patient care at all levels. The advent of digital imaging and the wide availability of affordable data storage devices have made things easier for the consumer. Although wound images may not be as closely scrutinized compared to cosmetic plastic surgery, some sort of standardization, at least within the same program would resolve some of the issues in image quality and projection issues currently faced by telewound care programs. A recommendation for creating consistent digital images in wound care is shown in Table 1 [4].

The importance of standardization is to allow for reliable comparison and reproducibility over time and distance by people of different training levels. These images can be used by everyone involved. At times however, it may be difficult to apply these standards. For example, obtaining professional quality images from rural homes or from a patient with a large, clean granulating wound awaiting a split-thickness skin graft would be impractical or unnecessary. Taking certain views at specific distances in a non-ambulatory patient with a sacral decubitus ulcer would be almost impossible. However, we should try our best to reach these standards within reason and with the available resources so that we can obtain accurate image representations of patients, reproduce them for clinical and educational programs and for objective interpretation of results for academic purposes. When digital technology improves even further, and becomes even more acceptable and affordable, then achieving these standards would be easier.

2.2. Store and Forward Programs

Store-and-forward programs are based on the concept of transmitting digital images, accompanied by text via electronic mail, or through a web-based program.

Using one of the earliest digital cameras (with a resolution of 756×504 pixels/in^2), Wirthlin, in 1988, was able to show the feasibility of digital imaging for the purposes

Table 1. Recommended methods for remote wound assessment using digital images

Type of view	Recommendations	Purpose	Comments
General	Use natural light Adjust the camera white balance manually Use a plain background	To reproduce wound colors accurately	The plain background helps the observer to focus attention on the relevant field
Global view	Include adjacent joints	To show the anatomical situation of the wound	
Regional view	Include adjoining tissues	To assess the skin around the wound	
Dressing view	View after the dressing has been opened	To assess exudate	
Measurement view with centimeter scale	Use two scales, one parallel to the main axis of the wound and the other perpendicular to it Use the camera (axis) perpendicular to the wound	To assess the wound size	The centimeter scale must not hide the edges of the wound The use of two scales instead of one is useful because image distortion is reduced. This improves inter-rater reliability
View centered on the wound	Use the camera's "macro" mode Ensure the camera (axis) is perpendicular to the wound Obtain images before any topical application to the wound	To assess the wound edges and wound bed	In case of large wound size of difficulty in showing the complete wound, it can be useful to have lateral views of the wound as well In case of heavy exudates, a view after cleaning may be necessary It is helpful to obtain images using a probe in the presence of undermining of edges or underlying cavities.

Adapted from Debray M, Couturier P, Greuillet F, et al. A preliminary study of the feasibility of wound telecare for the elderly. J Telemed Telecare. 2001;7:353-8.

of remote wound care [5]. Using the imaging guidelines of Galdino [3], Murphy has taken standardization a step further by introducing the concept of a wound data tool. If accompanied by trained participants, a wound data tool using digital imagery has the ability to provide remote assessment and be equivalent to actual physical examination of the wound [6]. The concept of accompanying digital images with objective data such as wound characteristics, laboratory values, nutritional status, and important aspects of current medical problems is not new. It allows for organized objective data to be used as points of reference over time in patient follow-up, and a standardized system for patient referral and peer communication, across distances. Many programs have used it with success, in the follow up of chronic and post surgical wounds.

As mentioned earlier, most reported programs using store-and-forward technology in telewound care, being pilot projects, lack the numbers and statistical power. They have however, been able to show potential in clinical use by demonstrating good correlation between actual physical examination and digital images. Some of the experiences in the military using this technology have already shown its feasibility in clinical care [7].

2.3. Web-Based Wound Monitoring Programs

The existence of a web-based wound-monitoring program is essential to provide organized data in a chronological and reliable fashion to all its users without the barriers of time and location. Rather than transmitting patient information to a certain individual via email, this system will allow for a wider use and accessibility of the information to achieve more a comprehensive care. Digital images, together with information from a wound data form and treatment recommendations can be transmitted into a website either from a skilled nursing facility or from home visiting nurses (as in the case of the Home Telehealth Consultation System (HTCS) for leg wounds) [8]. To be viewed by a wound "specialist" for evaluation. The advantages of this is multifold as it allows for objective wound monitoring over time, maximizes the convenience of both the patient and care providers, and allows for a larger number of patients to be seen by a specialist over a shorter time period. In this way, the utilization of current resources is maximized. At the same token, various objective assessments of the patient, such as nutritional status, wound images, evolution graphs, rehabilitation data, laboratory results and treatment plans can easily be accessed for a more comprehensive approach by team members from different specialties involved in the care of the patient. Web-based wound care programs can also be an excellent educational tool for students and patients alike.

2.4. Example of a Web-Based Wound Care System

A novel web-based wound care system using standardized guidelines for imaging and data collection has been initiated by researchers and plastic surgeons at the Department of Veteran Affairs (VA) Center for Practice Management and Outcomes Research and the University of Michigan, Ann Arbor, MI [9]. This program targeted patients at home or in long-term care facilities who did not have immediate access to specialized care. Several data tools including visit assessments, nutritional data, diagnoses, and clinical details are submitted to the wound assessment website.

Additional data that can be obtained using various web-based links include the *visit assessments link* which projects enlarged images of wounds; reviews current wound treatment and mobility data. Nursing notes including relevant laboratory and medication data, patient comments or difficulties with image capture, and physicians assessments according to AHCPR guidelines, and all treatment orders that are emailed directly to the on-site health care provider can also be obtained, Using the *diet/nutrition summary link*, the patients nutritional status can obtained. All other relevant clinical diagnose, nursing notes and laboratory data can be found using the *diagnoses summary and clinical detail link*.

This model shows significant promise for the use of store-and-forward technology in wound monitoring of patients, both at home and in skilled nursing facilities. The introduction of electronic health records will only complement the development and progress of these programs.

2.5. Televideo Programs

The power of telepresence is one of the main reasons why patients and care providers love the technology and concept of televideo programs. Success has been achieved in the field of dermatology where the reliability of teleconferencing using televideo for diagnosis and treatment plans has been shown [10]. The management accuracy of teledermatology programs are between 72–90%. One of the largest trials, The Northern Ireland arms of the UK multicentre teledermatology trial has concurred with previous studies that physician preferences, rather than technological reasons play a significant role in management differences [11]. This proves that the current technology available is sufficient to support its use in clinical work. Several wound care programs using televideo have been described. Most were performed using existing video equipment in established telemedicine programs for other medical specialties. The use of low-bandwidth technology has shown to suffice for this purpose. One of the biggest proven benefits of televideo use is in the home setting. It allows live interaction of the patient and the provider without the need of a third party and is a more personalized way of patient care without the need of additional personnel for collection of data, capture of images etc, as is the case of store-and-forward programs.

Both store-and-forward programs and televideo can play a tremendous role in wound care via telemedicine. Several pilot programs have been described across various disciplines.

2.6. Wound Programs

2.6.1. Pressure Sores in Spinal Cord Injured Patients

There are approximately 10,000 new spinal cord injury victims each year, in the United States [12]. The influence of managed care systems has resulted in shortened inpatient rehabilitation center stays. The average stay has decreased from seventy-five to thirty-five days over a twelve year period [13]. The importance of this is that patients and their families now have a much shorter time to adjust psychologically to the devastating diagnosis, learn necessary self care skills, and to integrate important nutritional and therapeutic knowledge into their daily lives. This shift to community and home-based care has resulted in the rise of secondary complications in these patients [14].

Pressure ulcers are the most common but potentially the most preventable complication in chronically debilitated and hospitalized patients. The statistics are quite astounding, about three to four percent (3–4%) of all acute care patients and forty to fifty percent (40–50%) of nursing home patients develop a pressure ulcer. Up to eighty-five percent (85%) of SCI patients develop ulcers at some point in their lives, with twenty-five to thirty percent (25–30%) of young, spinal cord injured patients developing one in the first five years [15,16]. They also become the most difficult complication to manage in this group of patients and the biggest hindrance to continued physical rehabilitation. Complications associated with the development of pressure ulcers include contractures, scarring and resultant deformities, and infectious issues including osteomyelitis leading to loss of limbs, and sepsis, which carries a fifty percent (50%) mortality [17].

The management of pressure ulcers is also a huge drain on health care resources. The annual cost of treatment is estimated to be $8.5 billion a year, averaging $82,000 per person, which does not take into account the tremendous psychological and social pain of patient and their families [18]. This is an excellent example where preventive care and early intervention can make a significant difference in patient outcome and health care dollars.

A response to this problem must include a comprehensive, experienced and multidisciplinary team approach to address the clinical, social, psychological and preventive issues of these patients.

2.6.2. Telerehabilitation in Spinal Cord Injured Patients: Pressure Ulcer Management

"Telerehabilitation" is that team approach aimed at providing comprehensive care via telemedicine. Specialists, in the form of an internist, registered nurse, a physical therapist, nutritionist, psychologist and a recreational therapist form the team [19].

The clinical practice guidelines published by the Agency for Health Care Policy and Research (AHCPR) recommends a minimum of weekly wound assessments in this patient group, where early diagnosis is crucial to avoid potentially life-threatening complications [20].

To achieve this goal, a New York based program has videophones distributed to patients where they interact with the team on a weekly basis. Wound imaging, dietary and physical therapy issues can be discussed with instantaneous feedback and formulation of a treatment plan [19]. Digital images of pressure ulcers have also been incorpo-

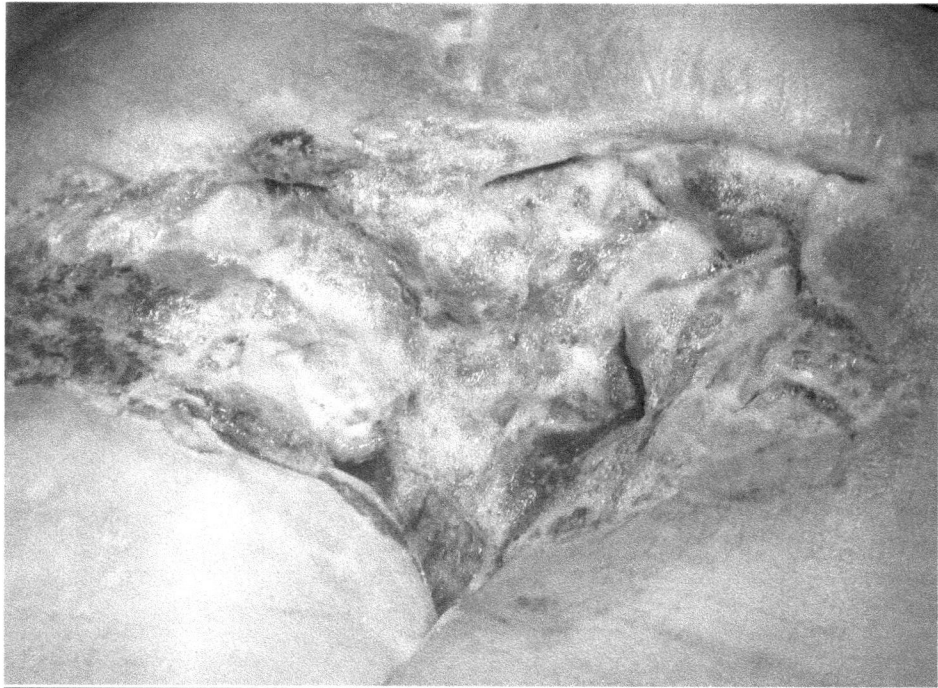

Figure 1. The lack of comprehensive expert care in spinal cord injured patients could result in disastrous results: a large sacral ulcer with exposed bladder, rectal mucosa and an impossible wound to close.

rated into electronic patient medical records as an effort towards monitoring wound progress at a VA setting [21]. The results of a pilot project using the Picasso Still-imaged Videophone (AT&T), across land or mobile telephone lines in Atlanta, Georgia have been encouraging [22]. Although only a small number of patients were enrolled, they were able to show the feasibility of using telerehabilitation to replace regularly scheduled outpatient wound care clinic appointments in pressure sore patients. As with other video-based systems, technical issues related to imaging needed to be fine-tuned, but satisfaction from the patient's standpoint was overwhelming. Many preferred it to regular clinic visits citing comfort in their own environment, elimination of transportation issues and costs and the ability to achieve "specialized" care in their own home as reasons.

The use of telemedicine as a tool for the referral of these patients for further evaluation and higher level of care in teleconsulting and distance care has also been promising [23].

2.6.3. Vascular Ulcers

Vascular patients with chronic ulcers are another group of patients where wound management frequently consumes most of outpatient care. Outpatient monitoring of these wounds are crucial to speed wound healing, and to prevent the complications that could result in limb loss, or additional surgical procedures, requiring in-patient hospitalization. This is currently achieved by frequent office visits to the vascular surgeon's office and home health care visits.

About forty to fifty percent (40–50%) of patients who undergo lower extremity re-vascularization have a non-healing ulcer that may take several months of healing time [24]. In addition, because of the nature of this disease process, twenty to thirty percent (20–30%) of patients undergoing a surgical procedure will develop a wound complication that will lengthen their hospital stay and require prolonged outpatient wound care. Initial work in telewound care in this field started as early as 1988, where a store and forward-based program for remote wound care was created. The results showed potential: there was a high concordance rate between the onsite surgeon and the remote surgeon: 60–83% compared to 64–85% amongst onsite surgeons in relation to wound descriptors. A similar high concordance rate in regards to wound management decisions was also seen [5].

More recently, a pilot project in the UK, using a universal Mobile Telecommunication System, or 3G videophone accompanied by a wound database for home telewound care was tested [25]. This limited study suggests possibilities for the provision of coordinated wound care of vascular patients in the home setting.

2.6.4. Burns

Burn patients require the longest and closest follow-up care amongst all chronic wounds. A typical post-traumatic burn wound frequently consists of regular outpatient visits that may require months or years of dedicated follow-up care [26]. Some of the services being continually performed at outpatient burn centers such as assessments of wounds for healing, follow-up of contractures, monitoring of hypertrophic scar maturation, psychological, social and vocational training, and fitting of compression garments can potentially be done via telemedicine. Since dedicated burn centers are far and between in many countries including the United States, providing such care across telecommunication lines would make sense.

There are several reasons why this concept has been slow to catch on. The first is based on the nature of these evaluations, most of which require the incorporation of live televideo at this time. The fact that comprehensive burn care stretches across several disciplines would imply that long communication times using televideo which can be extremely costly are limiting its widespread use at this time. In addition, before telemedicine can be used for the more technical aspects of burn care such as garment fitting, and in clinical decision-making in regards to scar contractures and maturation (which frequently involves palpation of the wound), sufficient experience in the more basic aspects of burn care and in the technicalities of telemedicine to the users in this field needs to be in place. A study using televideo for follow-up of burn patients across six states in the US, has shown cost effectiveness from the patients' standpoint in terms of time and transport savings but not for the providers of care [26]. This proves that more cost effective methods to incorporate the use of telemedicine using televideo in burn care still needs to be developed.

A two-pronged approach to this problem can be utilized using a store-and forward program, in addition to televideo. Standardization in the imaging of acute burn wounds using compression technology have been initiated to facilitate high transfer speeds of quality images necessary for clinical diagnosis [27]. This will allow for the assessment of wound depth and the ability to estimate wound severity, which will be extremely useful for the set up of a possible store-and-forward program for acute burn center triage and for teleconsulting purposes.

2.6.5. Other Wounds

One of the greatest utilization of telewound care programs is its use in the care of postoperative surgical patients with wound problems. The use of telemedicine program for the treatment of diabetic ulcers has been described [25], but its use in routine postoperative management of problem wounds have largely been under-utilized (or under-reported).

The large number of patients that would benefit from this service would include any postoperative patient with a wound complication. This would stretch across all surgical specialties, and include patients at home, outpatient centers, sub-acute hospitals and nursing homes alike. Home telehealth programs would play a significant role in this aspect of wound care. Patients living in rural and difficult-to-reach areas of the country would benefit tremendously if travel time including its costs were avoided if a simple "wound check" could be performed via telemedicine from a center close to their homes, or through a simple internet based program. Wound care for surgically created wounds such as stomas and fistulas can also be provided by this manner.

Another field that can be incorporated to a telewound care program are patients being treated at a hyperbaric oxygen center for their complicated wounds. Often times, hyperbaric chambers are located at a distance from the wound specialist. During the duration of treatment, wound monitoring can be performed with immediate feedback and treatment plans curtailed to wound progress made without the need of travel.

For teleconsulting purposes, the triage of complex wounds through the use of store-and-forward systems or televideo can facilitate optimal care in a quicker and efficient manner [23]. Life-threatening wounds can be treated quickly to prevent long-term morbidity and mortality. On the other hand, the frequent "wasted trip" to specialized care centers which involves long travel times and poses an inconvenience to all involved, can be eliminated.

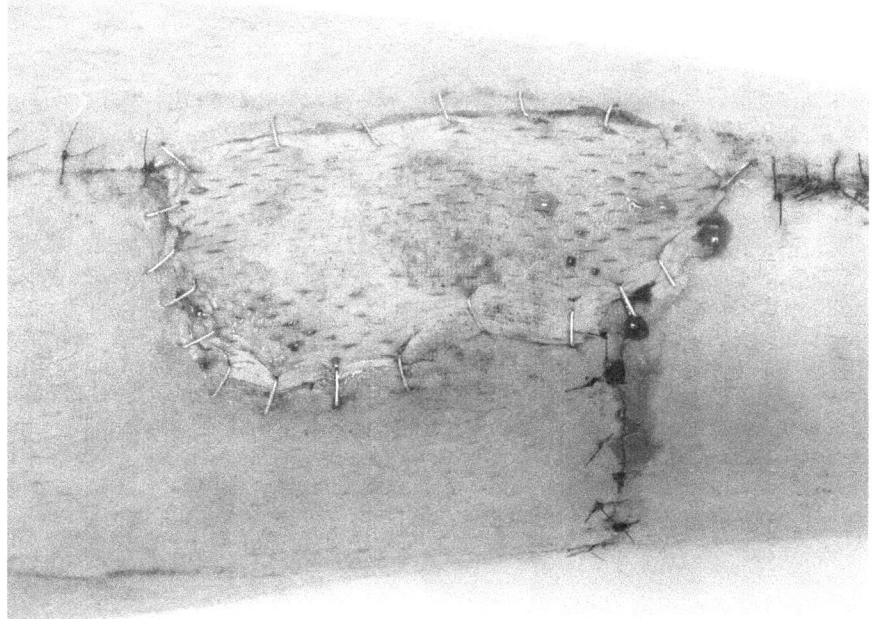

(a) complete graft take requiring no additional therapy

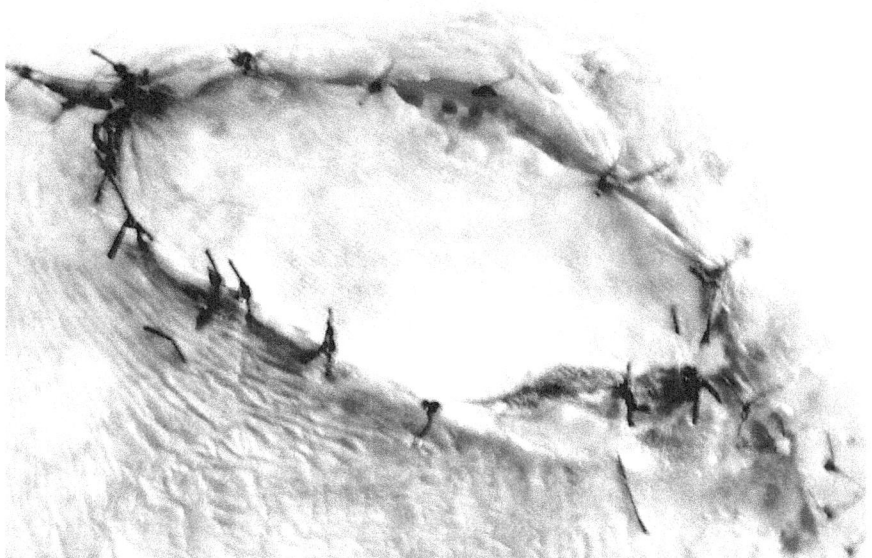

(b) failed skin graft requiring removal and placement of new skin graft

Figure 2. Postoperative skin grafts can be assessed using telemedicine.

Finally the impact of telemedicine in wound care does not stop at the patient level. The frequent interaction with wound care specialists is a welcoming vice especially for the rural health care worker. The educational benefits obtained at all levels of care are tremendous. This will eventually lead to more cost-effective, and improved distribution of quality medical care to patients.

The way I see it, this is a field that relies heavily on the expertise of a "trained eye" in wound care. It is also a specialty in which one has somewhat a luxury of time whereby immediate intervention is not necessary to significantly affect patient outcomes. Much emotional, physical and financial gains can be achieved by all involved, if we can eliminate the need for unnecessary travel, and provide a comprehensive method of care so that patients can obtained the highest level of care in their respective communities where their social support lies. If necessary, these patients can also be triaged to specialized centers of care for their acute problems and then back to their local communities for continued care. We have the resources of telecommunication using phone lines, the web and televideo and the ability to transfer high quality images in a reasonable amount of time. When more programs are in existence, there will be a tremendous amount of education and information transfer between urban and rural communities leading to a more interactive, complete and global health care system.

3. Barriers and Issues at Hand

Why then is telemedicine not used for wound care all across health care centers of the world? Across the country, wound care programs are being cut–down in size or have ceased operation due to the lack of monetary and physical resources to care for these patients. As a result, millions of health care dollars are instead being spent to care for the complications caused by the lack of continual care of these chronic wounds, which are mostly potentially preventable in the first place with adequate specialized care. If there was such a technology that could help provide for these patients and potentially save on time, money and convenience to all involved and ultimately improve overall patient outcome, why is there such a scarcity of its use?

First and foremost, the biggest barrier towards the widespread implementation of telewound care programs is reflected upon all telemedicine services in general. One of the main reasons limiting the widespread use of this technology is due to the fact that reimbursement patterns of telemedicine services including the practice of medicine across state and national borders have not been thoroughly worked out as of yet, although several encouraging legislative outcomes have been made in this regard [28,29]. Privacy laws including patient concerns about being "broadcasted" via the Internet and to unknown individuals are legitimate concerns. The transfer of patient data and images also require the use of Health Insurance Portability and Accountability Act (HIPAA) regulated programs, which are not widely available at this time.

In wound care specifically, these barriers are exacerbated due to the lack of substantial objective data and the small number of telewound programs currently in existence. Most of them are proprietary programs resulting in the lack of standardization amongst programs and software companies. At this point in time, there is no evidence-based data in existence to direct wound care practices. As a result, most current wound care practices in the community and in non-specialized centers are based on reimbursement patterns, which is largely non-operative care. It has been previously shown that improved patient outcomes occur as a result of specialized and directed wound care provided by experts in the field. A more integrated program encompassing aspects of wound care management practices between local communities and specialized centers need to be in place to significantly change the current state of wound care practice. This, to me, would be the biggest contribution that telemedicine can bring to the current practice of wound care. Telewound care can hope to rely on the more 'established' telemedicine services to work in its favor in terms of the recognition and the changing of such reimbursements laws.

Equally important is the inherent lack of knowledge in wound care management amongst health care providers. Despite the prevalence of this problem, currently most physicians undergo training through medical school and residency programs without much exposure to wound care. This has resulted in a very select group of physicians caring for these patients, plastic surgeons and general surgeons in particular. Wound care, which should be considered basic level patient care has become a post-graduate level training specialty.

Another important issue is the lack of familiarity with the technology and reluctance of current health care providers to incorporate it into their daily clinical practice. This change is often a slow process that requires significant time, effort and patience to relearn a new way of practice. The initial reluctance to accept new technology is the first step in this process. As with any new operating system, ensuring a reliable system by providing proper training, technical support and follow-up programs to its users are critical for its expansion. Along these lines, the current pool of wound care providers are far too few to meet the demand, both in the hospital and outpatient setting through home health care programs. Taking time off to relearn a new system and technology may prove to be disastrous to patient care during that time period. However, this becomes a Catch -22 situation, which requires innovation, desire, good organization and utilization of resources to overcome. In addition, the more rural communities and countries are dealt with the issues of lesser experience and receptivity towards modern technology and its capabilities, inadequate reliable access to telecomunication lines, and the lack of adequate resources for program setup and technical support. Most patients are capable of participating and operating home systems if they overcome the initial reluctance to try it. This has been demonstrated in the Virtual Assisted Living Umbrella for the Elderly (VALUE) program where patients and their care-providers were successful in operating home health systems [30].

4. Future

The practice of medicine has changed significantly compared to ancient times as a result of rising and newer technologies. The advent of the roentgengram has evolved into state-of-the-art CT scanners, and MRI technology allowing the human eye to visualize a three-dimensional body part without having to physically enter a body cavity.

Many hospital systems in the United States have switched to computer based systems and electronic data entry ranging from electronic medical records to patient monitoring systems, order entry and imaging files. The VA system is an excellent example where a patient's medical record can be viewed at any time or at any VA health care system across the country.

The wider availability of the Internet, telecommunication lines either via satellite, and GSM mobile services have brought the world closer. Information can now be transferred from one individual to another in a without the barrier of distance. The expansion of wireless technology via Bluetooth, 3G phone services, WiMax services across cities and the potential future of nanotechnology, will allow the potential of telemedicine to be realized in the health care industry. The members of the medical community must embrace technology and use it to our advantage to care for our patients. There is no reason not to fully utilize this potential.

Wound care consultations, can be provided by images of the actual wound together with a wound data tool or patient history over telecommunication lines. This will ensure proper triage of patients and decrease the cost of patient or physician travel. Adequate and reliable followup can be made either at home or in long term care facilities either via televideo or by a store-and-forward program so that care providers can constantly be in touch with wound care specialists without the need for travel. This will allow greater utilization of resources, by freeing up in-hospital beds for acute care patients, decreasing outpatient visits to clinics, overcoming the current shortage of wound care nurses and home health service personnel, and decrease health care expenditure to care for wound complications, and ultimately decrease patient morbidity, and mortality.

This will close the gap between rural and urban health care systems and between developed and developing countries, provide closer relationships and education opportunities, and allow for a more improved and cost effective health care management structure through proper triage of these patients.

5. Conclusion

It is an exciting time to be involved in this rapidly evolving and expanding field. As patient care is shifted towards the outpatient setting, this has led to the expansion of home health systems and skilled nursing facilities. There has also been a slow, but positive response in terms of improved reimbursement plans and passing of laws supporting the use of telemedicine.

In wound care, due to the prevalence and chronicity of the problem, there is much potential for its growth in response to current health care patterns. We are still far away from achieving a "perfect" wound care program. However, with the forward explosion in telecommunications and an open mind, things can change. The current pilot programs should serve as a stepping towards achieving improved wound care systems that would serve to counteract the rising problems currently faced by health care systems: increasing numbers of chronically ill, rural, elderly and debilitated patients requiring long-term wound care in the era of escalating health care costs.

Modern technology is on our side. With the availability of newer technology such as 3G mobile phones, Bluetooth, improved telecommunication systems and nanotechnology, one can only dare to predict what will unfold in the upcoming years ahead.

However, when successful telewound care programs becomes widely accepted and practiced, in every home and in every physician's office we have to remember not to loose sight of one of the most important aspects of humanity: the sense of compassion of a healer. We cannot allow ourselves to be lost in the forest of our own technology, neither to be controlled by it. The comfort, the sense of touch and social interaction amongst human beings should not be lost at the expense of technology. We should incorporate the technology of telemedicine into our current patient care methods to improve patient outcomes, not replace it.

References

[1] Wheeler T. Strategies for delivering telehomecare profiles. Telemed Today 1998;6:37-40.
[2] Gardner SE, Frantz RA, Specht JKP, et al. How accurate are chronic wound assessments using interactive video technology? J Gerontol Nurs 2001;27(1):15-20.
[3] Galdino GM, Vogel JE, Vander Kolk CA. Standardizing digital photography: it's not all in the eye of the beholder. Plast Reconstr Surg 2001;108:1334-44.
[4] Debray M, Couturier P, Greuillet F, et al. Apreliminary study of the feasibility of wound telecare for the elderly. J Telemed Telecare 2001;7:353-8.
[5] Wirthlin DJ, Buradagunta S, Edwards RA, et al. Telemedicine in vascular surgery: feasibility of digital imaging for remote management of wounds. J Vasc Surg 1998;27:1089-99.
[6] Murphy RX, Bain MA, Wasser TE, et al. The reliability of digital imaging in the remote assessment of wounds: Defining a standard. Ann Plast Surg 2006;56(4):431-6.
[7] Scerri GV, Vassallo DJ. Initial plastic surgery experience with the first telemedicine links for the British Forces. Br J Plast Surg 1999;52:294-8.
[8] Baer CA, Williams CM, Vickers L, et al. A pilot study of specialized nursing care for home health patients. J Telemed Telecare 2004;10:342-5.
[9] Lowery JC, Hamill JB, Wilkis EG, Clements E. A Web-based telemedicine system for wound assessment. Adv Skin Wound Care 2002;15:165-169.
[10] Phillips CM, Burke WA, Shechter BA, et al. Reliability of dermatology teleconsultations with the use of teleconferencing technology. J Ame Acad Dermatol 1997;37:398-402.
[11] Loane MA, Corbett R, Bloomer SE, et al. Diagnostic accuracy and clinical management by realtime teledermatology. Results from the Northern Ireland arms of the UK teledermatology trial. J Telemed Telecare 1998;4:95-100.
[12] Hingley AT. Spinal cord injuries: science meets challenge. FDA consumer 1993;7-8:17-23.
[13] Pollack SF, Zuger RR, Walsh J. Moving out services for education and support: a model program for individuals with spinal cord injury. SCI Nurs 1992;9:79-82.
[14] National Spinal Cord Injury Statistical Center: Annual report for the model spinal cord injury systems. Birmingham, AL: University of Alabama Birmingham. 1997.
[15] Jones ML, Evans RW. Outcomes in a managed care environment. Topics in Spinal Cord Injury Rehabilitation 1998;3:61-73.
[16] Niazi ZBM, Salzberg CA, Byrne DW, Viehbeck M. Recurrence of initial pressure ulcers in persons with spinal cord injuries. Adv Wound Care 1997;10(3):38-42.
[17] Allman R. Epidemiology of pressure sores in different populations. Decubitus 1989;2(2):30-3.
[18] Kuhn BA, Coulter SJ. Balancing pressure ulcer cost and quality equation. Dermatol Nurs 1993;5:180-5.
[19] Galea M, Tumminia J, Garback L. Telerehabilitation in spinal cord injury persons: A novel approach. Telemed J e-Health 2006;12(2):160-2.
[20] Bergstrom N, Bennett MA, Carlson CE. Treatment of pressure ulcers. Clinical Practice Guideline, No. 15 AHCPR Publication No. 95-0652. Rockville, MD: Agency for Health Care Policy and Research; December 1994.
[21] Fischetti LF, Paguio EC, Alt-White AC. Digitized images of wounds: a nursing practice innovation. Nurs Clin North Am 2000;35(2):541-50.
[22] Vesmarovich S, Walker T, Hauber RP, Temkin A, Burns R. Use of telerehabilitation to manage pressure ulcers in persons with spinal cord injuries. Adv Wound Care 1999;12:264-9.
[23] Halstead LS, Dang T, Elrod M, et al. Teleassessment compared with live assessment of pressure ulcers in a wound clinic: A pilot study. Adv Wound Care 2003;16:91-6.
[24] Johnson JA, Cogbill TH, Strutt PJ, et al. Wound complications after infrainguinal bypass. Arch Surg 1998(123);859-862.
[25] Clemensen J, Larsen SB, Ejskjaer. Telemedicine treatment at home of diabetic foot ulcers. J Telemed Telecare 2005;11(suppl.2):14-6.
[26] Massman NJ, Dodge JD, Fortman KK, Schwartz KJ, Solem LD. Burns follow up: an innovative application of telemedicine. J Telemed Telecare 1999;5(suppl.1):52-4.
[27] Roa L, Gomez-Cia T, Acha B, et al. Digital imaging in remote diagnosis of burns. Burns 1995;617-23.
[28] http://telehealth.hrsa.gov/pubs/reimb.htm.
[29] Puskin, Dena S. (September 30, 2001) "Telemedicine: Follow the Money" Online Journal of Issues in Nursing. Vol. #6 No. #3, Manuscript 1. Available.
[30] Finkelstein SM, Speedie SM, Potthoff S. Home telehealth improves clinical outcomes at lower cost for home healthcare. Telemed J e-Health 12:2 128-136.

Current Principles and Practices of Telemedicine and e-Health
R. Latifi (Ed.)
IOS Press, 2008

Telemedicine for Pathology

Ekaterine KLDIASHVILI
Georgian Telemedicine Union (Association), Tbilisi, Georgia

Abstract. Telemedicine for pathology, this is pathology in which the specimen is digitally transmitted and examined by a pathologist at a distance. In another words, telemedicine for pathology, or simply telepathology, is a branch of telemedicine and pathology that consists in the exchange of pathology images through tele-communication with the purposes of diagnosis, consultation, research and/or education. The use of telepathology is of great importance in management of patients since it allows fast diagnosis and inter-consultations among specialist pathologists located in every part of the world.

Keywords. Pathology, telemedicine, microscope, virtual slide, imaging

Introduction

Telepathology is the practice of pathology at a distance, based on the transmission through telecommunication means of still or stationary images from pathology specimens for their corresponding interpretation and diagnosis. Included in these transmissions is information about the patient, clinical history, identification numbers, laboratory data, statistics, etc. The central aims of telepathology are (1) the possibility to get a second opinion concerning a pathological-anatomical diagnosis from an expert outside of the normal pathologist's working team, and (2) to deliver primary diagnostics to patients who are treated in hospitals without resident pathologists. All diagnosis in pathology are based on images. In principle a telepathology system should include four basic modules operating independently (i) a module for generating the images (capturing or microscope control); (ii) a module for filing images or other information on the server (filing); (iii) a module for functioning of the expert ("expert module"), and (iv) a module (optional) for remotely controlling the microscope, or another "manipulator" (microscope control).

While telepathology has enormous potential for remote diagnosis, education and obtaining a second opinion, especially in support of isolated pathologists and non-specialty pathologists, telepathology, in general, has been limitedly used for the following reasons.

1. It is an expensive and time consuming process.
2. The limited field of view of telepathology images, unlike glass slides directly viewed on a microscope, often makes pathologists feel uncomfortable.
3. There is no widely accepted method to measure the image quality and accuracy of image parameters such as color.

In general, the uses of telepathology are for 1) primary diagnosis, 2) second opinion, 3) education/QA (quality assurance). Each may require a unique telepathology system design. There are several general types of telepathology systems.

a. In static mode (store and forward or live), images (typically only a few) are captured and transmitted for sequential viewing.
b. In dynamic mode, live video images are transmitted and viewed dynamically in real time.
c. Dynamic systems with a robotic microscope allow the remote viewer to control the microscope at the originating site for a more interactive experience.
d. Combining static and dynamic systems produce hybrid systems with even more flexibility.
e. Whole-slide imaging (virtual slide imaging) is the newest development in which the entire slide is digitized, obtaining the need to select individual or sequential images for viewing.

Depending on the requirements and budget, different types of telepathology systems – with different levels of image quality – can be used. Furthermore, as in the more general field of pathology imaging, a variety of human factors, such as the ability to cut and stain a good tissue section, set up the microscope and optimize contrast and focus, tissue area selection etc. are very important for the effectiveness of the system. This makes telepathology systems even more complex to evaluate and standardize. For example, under-staining or over-staining may hide or fail to reveal important structures in the final image. It may also result in color variation, based not on tissue, but rather on variations in the cutting, processing or staining process. Color differences of the same stain by institution or technicians often occur. Usually pathologists are familiar with the color of stains at their own institution, and sometimes each pathologist has a favorite color. For instance, the color of blood cells in one slide is not always the same as in another slide. This can create confusion even when pathologists correspond by means of a conventional postal consultation, so the problem can be even worse with telepathology. Every type of imaging system has its own limitations.

Static image telepathology depends on the ability of the referring pathologist or staff to both form an appropriate image with the microscope and capture a clear image with the camera. Equally important, static system relies on the operator to capture the appropriate area of the slide in question. Using a 20× objective lens and a standard ¾ inch (8.8 × 6.6 mm) CCD, a single field of view is about 0.44 × 0.33 mm or 0.145 square mm. As a typical cover slip has about 12.5 square centimeters of area, a static system samples only a very small proportion of the potential area of tissue section. It is up to referring pathologist to select several areas of interest and capture images with the appropriate magnification. When the pathologist has specific questions for the consultant, or merely wants to confirm the diagnosis using the telepathology system, static image telepathology works very well. However, when the referring pathologist does not have enough confidence in his/her own diagnosis or needs a primary diagnosis to be rendered, the static image telepathology can be risky, because the consultant pathologist has to make diagnosis based entirely on the transmitted images, which were chosen by the referring clinician. The image quality of static images depends on the person who captured them, potentially limiting the ability of the consultant to render an accurate and confident decision. It is important to understand that a "high resolution" image is not necessarily a good quality image, especially if the optical image from the microscope is out of focus or otherwise imperfect. Most images captured by people who are not experienced in telepathology or digital imaging show problems those are related to the use of the microscope, such as problems with focus and color fidelity.

Dynamic image telepathology is limited by many of the factors already listed for static telepathology, in addition to the fact that the dynamic image quality at the receiver site depends on the bandwidth of network used (and the amount of compression required). In practice, most systems using H323 or H320 for dynamic images cannot provide image quality as good as static systems. For this reason, one often uses both static image and dynamic imaging in one system. This works well. However, when robotic microscopes are used, with motorized stages for remote control, the system needs specialized equipment that is not common in pathology practices, and is unfamiliar to pathologists. Consulting pathologists can use non-robotic microscopes for dynamic telepathology, and let the referring site control them so as to focus on areas of interest, but the same problems with static image of area selection remain.

Another factor in both static and dynamic telepathology systems is that current systems are significantly slower than the manual use of a glass slide on a microscope. No matter what kind of system is used, it takes longer for the pathologist to make a diagnosis using telepathology images. However, if the pathologist uses the system as part of a pathology information system, it might in the future reduce the specialist's total time to diagnose and report.

The key functionality of a telepathology system is the ability to allow a local pathologist to send microscope images of a tissue section, along with text to describe the clinical context, to the remote pathology expert. In the USA and Europe, pathology imaging and telepathology are moving to the use of WSI, and pathologists are able to look at the virtual slide through the Internet from anywhere in the world. However, in the case of developing nations, popular telepathology is still based on email (sender captures static images and sends them as email attachments, with a brief case description) due to limited network bandwidth and technical support.

1. Current Developments: Evidence Based Practice

Telepathology has left its childhood. Its technical development is mature, and its use for primary (frozen section) and secondary (expert consultation) diagnosis has been expanded to a great amount. Those who would attempt to define standards or guidelines for telepathology need to have a clear understanding of the wide scope of image "quality" or "resolution" necessary for imaging to be useful in pathology. One of the best ways of describing these requirements is to examine the way a typical surgical pathologist uses his/her microscope. In examining some cases, the pathologist will not use the microscope at all, making a diagnosis instead on the gross visual examination. In other cases, the pathologist will use a 4× objective lens (with an optical resolution of ~5 microns), while in other cases a 20× lens (optical resolution of ~1 micron) or 40× lens (optical resolution of ~0.5 micron) is used. As a further option, there are very powerful oil-immersion lenses and, beyond that, electron microscopy. The choice of optics is up to the pathologist, and his or her judgment as to what is required for the case at hand. The same argument can be applied to other factors that have an effect on image quality, such as contrast, tissue staining and tissue processing. Imaging guidelines in pathology need to take into account the fact that it is up to the pathologist to determine if the specimen or image is of sufficient quality to render a diagnosis.

Remote diagnosis in pathology is based on color images captured through a camera. Normally cameras are digital cameras capturing the analogue signal by sampling it. Digital sampling can be done through CCD chip (Charge Couple Devices Chip) or

CMOS (Complementary Metal Oxide Semiconductors used as image sensors). The second ones are simpler but suffer a lower signal/noise ratio. Having cameras a non-linear response if compared to human perception of brightness, this should be corrected (gamma correction). This effect on the image is inverted by the gamma correction of the display systems, so obtaining a final effect of adequate visual perception.

As for dynamic ranges 8 bits (i.e. 256 grey levels) are sufficient for color pathology images. The high resolution cameras available on the market directly record digital images with very high spatial resolution. The two main consequences of this are:

1. That the recorded image at a low microscopic power can support digital zooming simulating higher power microscopic views;
2. The image is not affected by the gamma correction of the camera-systems and is therefore comparable to a digital radiography.

The compression techniques include the color reduction further than the usual data reduction ones. The color reduction can be obtained through the following techniques:

1. YUV encoding, usually based on color sampling reduction of 8/4/4 bits information acquisition.
2. Reduction of color palette to 256 colors (8 bits).
3. Median cut color quantization. It is a color quantization technique that optimizes the representation of the original color in the final palette. This technique produces median cuts of colors on RGB to reach 256 colors (8 bits). Therefore the most frequent colors have greater range of color hues then less frequent ones.
4. Dithering. It is another technique, normally coupled with technique 3 and aims to expand the available color palette by juxtaposing pixels of different colors. This creates the illusion of additional color by usual blending.

Telepathology which is the diagnostic work of pathologist at a distance has been developed to routine application within the last ten years. It can be classified in relation to application, technical solutions, or performance conditions. Diagnostic pathology performance distinguishes primary diagnosis (for example, frozen section statement) from secondary diagnosis (for example, expert consultation) and quality assurance (diagnostic accuracy, continuous education and training). Applications comprise (a) frozen section service; (b) expert consultations; (c) remote control measurements; and (d) education and training. The technical solutions distinguish active (remote control, live imaging) systems from passive (conventional microscope handling, static imaging), and the performance systems with interactive (online, live imaging) use from those with passive (offline, static imaging) practice. Intra-operative frozen section service is mainly performed with remote control systems; whereas expert consultations and education/training are commonly based upon Internet connections with static imaging in an offline mode. The image quality, transfer rates, and screen resolution of active and passive telepathology systems are sufficient for an additional or primary judgment of histological slides and cytological smears. From the technical point of view, remote control telepathology requires a fast transfer and at least near online judgment of images, i.e., image acquisition, transfer and presentation can be considered one performance function. Thus, image size, line transfer rate and screen resolution defines the practicability of the system. In expert consultation, the pixel resolution of images and natural color presentation are the main factors for diagnostic support, whereas the line transfer rate is of minor importance. These conditions define the technical compartments, especially size and resolution of camera and screen. The performance of commercially available systems has reached a high quality standard. Pathologists can be trained in a short time and use the systems in a routine manner.

Several telepathology systems have been implemented in large institutes of pathology which serve for frozen section diagnosis in small hospitals located in the local area. In contrast, expert consultation is mainly performed with international connections. There is a remarkable increase of expert consultations by telepathology according to the experiences the Armed Force Institute of Pathology or the Department of Pathology, Thoraxklinik, Heidelberg. In expansion of these experiences, a "globalization" of telepathology can be expected. Telepathology can be used to shrink the period necessary for final diagnosis by request for diagnostic assistance to colleagues working in appropriate related time zones. Telepathology is, therefore, not a substitute of conventional diagnostic procedures but a real environment in the world of pathology.

The morphologic diagnosis of tumor specimens with precise tumor typing, staging, and grading remains the basis of almost all cancer treatments. Thus, in each tumor case, a histologic diagnosis of the highest quality should be the physician's priority. In approximately 10–20% of tumor cases, diagnostic uncertainly remains to some degree, requiring a second opinion in determining the biologic behavior, the histogenesis, the grade of dedifferentiation, or any other parameter. Facilitating the communication between pathologists and the exchange of cases, telepathology gains more and more importance.

The Internet offers a widely available, inexpensive possibility for telepathology consultations. It allows the transfer of image and text files through electronic mail (email) or file transfer protocols (FTP), using a variety of microcomputer platforms. The Internet and relatively inexpensive "virtual microscopy" tools offer a novel technology for telepathology consultations.

A new concept for telemicroscopy has recently been introduced using the Internet and conventional web browser, with java support for microscope remote control as well as image transfer and discussion (http://amba.charite.de/telemic/). The system has two major components: the telemicroscopy server, which is a computer with Internet access connected to the automatic microscope, and the telemicroscopy client, who remotely operates the microscope. This simplified telemicroscopy system allows any Internet user to become a consultant for telepathology without the acquisition of specialized hardware or software. For the inquirer seeking advice, however, this solution is still very expensive, since it requires a fully automated microscope. The system that can be used for conventional microscopes is top actual. In such case a video camera mounted on a microscope with a photo tube is connected to the frame grabber of a personal computer. Java-based telemicroscopy software transforms the computer into an Internet server, which automatically distributes new microscope images, after manual operations, to all connected clients. Any Internet user can access the web page of the server to become a telemicroscopy client. Telemicroscopyy offers new perspectives for telepathology and it is envisaged that many pathologists and scientists will use this facility to connect their personal microscopes to the Internet, forming a network for teleconsultation. Hopefully, this development will promote communication between pathologists and may thus increase the quality of diagnosis.

Recent advances in microcomputers and high resolution digital video cameras provide pathologists the opportunity to combine precision optics with digital imaging technology and develop new educational and research tools. Didactic presentations on the topic of anatomic pathology in front of a live audience have been largely dependent on the use of standard 2×2 inch projection slides of selected still images from the topic at hand. Because of the highly visual nature of the specialty of anatomic pathology, this method has had some serious limitations. With the advent of digital imaging techniques and the availability of new electronic software for the projection of images, new possibilities have become available for didactic presentations in anatomic pathology in front of large, live audience. To provide a seamless transition between the two presentation formats, the personal computer-based PowerPoint slides should be hyperlinked to a browser-based virtual microscope viewer. The presenter, with the use of a mouse, will be able to "move" the image of the scanned slide on the screen, to transition seamlessly among various magnifications, and to rapidly select from the whole-mount scanned slide among any areas of interest pertinent to the topic. Thus, the visual experience obtained by the audience simulated that of viewing a glass slide at a multi-headed microscope during a glass slide tutorial. Because this most closely approximates the experience of reviewing glass slides under the microscope for practicing pathologists, the educational experience of the presentation is greatly enhanced by the use of this technique. Also, this method permits making this type of presentation available to a much larger group of individuals in a live audience.

Another evidence based practice in telepathology is the automated whole-slide imaging (WSI), a new technology that has brought the possibility of standardization in pathology nearer. WSI involves digitizing of entire slides (so there is no issue of sub-sampling), the imaging process being automated (eliminating the need to force specific parameters and eliminating human factors in image capture). However, since the technology is still developing, it will take another few years before it becomes clinically available and a useful system.

2. Barriers and Issues at Hand

The probability of an incorrect handling of a relevant medical data, still dangerously high, mainly is due to:

- Environmental factors – Many medical organizations are not fully able to face every disease, e.g., in a peripheral hospital only the most frequent pathologies for that geographical area are treated.
- Instinctive factors – The decision making of a physician is usually mainly based on the limited number of cases in her/his experience and/or on a static medical knowledge available from databases of main published slides. This factor is very variable between different specialists and general practitioners.
- Emotional factors – Medical decisions are often influenced by the opinions and the decisions that have been taken by the physicians that already have examined the same patient.

As a consequence the probability of a serious error occurrence could be high and the probability of its recognition and correction very low. This frequently causes a repetition of exams in the same time or in different medical units and it slows down the diagnostic process (resources waste) and the proper treatment. So, proper actions for improving the working procedures have to be taken.

Correct medical information management and transmission is a key point, hence the introduction of telepathology can be relevant. There are several diagnostic discrepancies due to sampling error; those are a serious problem in telepathology. For microscopic views the problem can be faced through: (i) a robotics microscopic system allowing remote control of microscope; (ii) by sending low power images with marks of flags where the higher power images will be taken. Virtual slides or complete specimen digitization can be obtained in 2 ways: a. visualizing all fields at high power; b. capturing low power images through a high resolution camera that will allow thereafter a digital zooming.

The difficulty of image standardization in telepathology is that so many factors can influence image quality. The following system components are required for a general pathology imaging station.

1. Microscope: these vary widely according to type of microscope, magnification, type of objective lens, condenser, aperture, filters and light voltage. Each user can change or chose each item every time he/she uses it.
2. Optical coupler: this connects the microscope and camera, and it is an art to choose the right one.
3. Camera: there are analog and digital types, with a variety of parameters such as CCD size, sampling interval, dynamic range, and color characteristics.
4. Computer and software: sizes of RAM and VRAM and CPU speed change the speed of controlling these huge images and the number of colors to display. Image acquisition and manipulation software directly influence image quality.
5. Display: each display has different characteristics (e.g. spatial resolution, maximum luminance) and the user can change the brightness and contrast, affecting perceived image quality. It is also important to properly calibrate the displays.
6. Compression/image format: since the images are so large, it is often necessary to compress the images. With respect to image quality and diagnostic accuracy, issues such as acceptable compression ratio and whether the compression should be lossless or lossy are important.

There are so many pathology imaging systems that can be built with many possible combinations because there are many choices for each component of the system. Each component presents a variety of options to the user; and each user can pick any version of each component. Furthermore, the same system with the same components, when operated by users of different levels of skill and knowledge, can result in different image quality levels. Telepathology performance, and in particular its bandwidth requirements are high and rather asymmetric (there are more often needs for retrieval than for entry or update a medical data).

The discussion about medical image standards commonly includes the discussion of required image resolution, the number of colors, monitor resolution, compression ratio, format etc. As mentioned above, pathology imaging has a wide range of requirements, and is subject to significant human factors and non-imaging-related parameters that make a single standard for pathology imaging problematic. Defining a required "pixel resolution" is meaningless if the optical focus or staining quality is not defined, and even if these parameters could be defined, the image type and quality required for some aspects of pathology is radically different from that required for others. One could decide on a file format for file transfer, but this would not address some of the more basic issues in pathology imaging.

The important concepts for pathology imaging standards to consider are:

1. Systems should be able to share image files.
2. The standards should allow the transmission of information on baseline colors and recommended display parameters.
3. The images should be useful to the pathologist, not necessarily better or worse than direct examination of a slide under the microscope.
4. A mechanism to evaluate image quality objectively should be present.
5. A mechanism to adjust and correct minor errors of tissue processing should be developed.
6. A public organization should support pathologists in the development of standards.

To move pathology imaging into a space where standards can be effectively applied there are two main areas of attack. One involves formal training of pathologists in imaging and image-related activities. This may take form of a web-based formal training process in diagnostic imaging (e.g. continuing education courses). The second area is the development of technical mechanisms to remove human factor issues in the image capture process. The goals are to correct (or at least identify) differences between systems and materials, to develop technical protocols for evaluating and/or grading image quality objectively, and finally, to deploy color standardization technology.

To avoid human factors, automated, whole-slide imaging (WSI) robots and/or imaging microscopes may provide a solution. However, these systems have not yet achieved clinical product status, and are limited to groups that are able to afford them. Also, it takes time and training for pathologists to interpret WSI in an optimal way. However, it is clear that such systems will become more widespread in the next several years. Imaging microscopes (robotic microscopes with built-in cameras and robotic stages) can potentially remove problems related to the human factor, such as variations between users in terms of microscope focus, filter and brightness settings. By having these parameters software-controlled, these systems can help achieve areas of image quality standardization. Automated whole-slide imaging robots capture a complete glass slide (preferable fast enough to be useful for remote diagnosis for frozen sections) without human intervention. With the addition of automated slide loaders and barcodes, along with control slides to monitor resolution and color parameters, these systems can automate the entire image process. Systems to support these quality assurance functions should lead to a major improvement in telepathology imaging, and open the door for extensive quality control and image quality standardization techniques.

Image quality evaluation is another important factor. Currently, the methods used to evaluate image quality are very subjective and vary between individuals and institutions. This subjectivity does not necessarily affect diagnosis by telepathology and/or the imaging system. However, as telepathology systems become more popular and more ubiquitous, it will become necessary to develop more objective image quality assessment methods. Even something as new and untested as the whole-slide imager is making rapid inroads into telepathology, and several commercial systems are available on the market. Each system gives a different visual impression of the images, and different models of the same system give different impressions and image quality. We do not know what level of quality of image we really need for clinical uses, for education or for research purposes, complicating the problem of standardization.

The health care systems, and the education of health care personnel, have to be reorganized to systems that function in a cross-border fashion. Prerequisites for this development shall be a specific emphasis on equity of access, interoperability and standardization of systems and protocols, security and legal aspects. There are technical, legal, organizational, and financial problems to be solved.

Technical problems – Although the technologies needed mostly do exist already today, there are still area-specific technical barriers that have to be overcome. The most prominent barriers are easy-to-use, intuitive, robust and smooth user interfaces and devices. The services must be offered to all users through such interfaces, and all of them have to be implemented in a uniform way. The access to the systems must be smooth and transparent to the users. Otherwise they won't achieve a good acceptance.

Legal problems – The legal barriers that have to be overcome are essentially the general ones applying to the whole telemedicine field. Responsibility, confidentiality, liability and access only to certified professionals are some of the key issues.

Organizational problems – There are serious organizational barriers, however, such as health care at home requiring smooth collaboration of different organizations. This requires a significant redesign of business processes, which is only possible if a change from the enterprise-centric view to a system-wide perspective with the patient/citizen at the centre is achieved. Today the paradigm of service chains in health care, built on telepathology collaboration of service providers linked in a service provision network, is still in its infancy. However, the increasing interest in recent approaches like managed care, disease management, and case management, which are strongly related to this paradigm shift, shows that the necessity of changing the way in which health care systems are organized is more and more recognized and continually becomes transparent. Also country-specific factors, such as the roles of different providers of health and social care services, insurance companies, housing providers, local authorities, and telealarm providers, need to be taken into account when introducing telepathology's possibilities.

Financial problems – The financial barriers largely depend on the different countries' policies. In countries with national health care systems these services will be a part of the overall health care system. In insurance based countries, where services are reimbursed on a fee-for service basis, new codes will have to be established. In countries with market-driven health care systems the prices need to be adapted to market prices driven by the healthcare consumers. At this time there is little evidence on how the broad implementation of such telemedicine and telepathology services will affect the financial situation of health care systems in total, and its participants in particular. The challenge is to create comprehensive systems (networks of services offering the basis for patient-individual service chains) which are financially beneficial for all players.

Other problems – Furthermore, the awareness of the great opportunities that telemedicine and telepathology can help to solve the huge problem of isolated areas has to be promoted in both citizens and politicians. Stakeholders, including health professionals, researchers, public officials, and the lay public, must collaborate on a range of activities. These activities include initiatives to build robust health information system that provides equitable access, development of high-quality, audience-appropriate information and support services for specific health problems, and health-related decisions for all segments of the population, especially for underserved persons, training of health professionals in the science of communication and the use of communication technologies, evaluation of interventions, promotion of a critical understanding and practice of effective health communication both for end-users and for health professionals, and initiatives to gain knowledge about telemedicine consumers' use of and their needs and attitudes with regards to information and communication technologies in health care.

In spite of the potential which telemedicine and telepathology has as mechanism to support health systems, a number of barriers, at various levels, would need to be overcome for health systems to take full advantage of these opportunities. These barriers are not multidimensional constructed, encompassing technical knowledge, economic viability, organizational support and behavior modification. The Telemedicine Alliance, a collaboration between the World Health Organization, the European Space Agency and the International Telecommunications Union studied telemedicine adoption trends through personal interviews with 54 European telecommunications experts, health policy makers, and health care providers (2003). The three most important barriers to telemedicine adoption where identified as: the problem of interoperability (technical, cultural, systematic-financial reimbursement, inter-organizational workflow), acceptance of a "new" health system, and regulatory constraints. This emphasizes that telemedicine and telepathology implementation has to be accomplished by simultaneously horizontal and vertical multisectorial action.

Interoperability is a key change. This is the fragmentation problem – many pieces of information, in many formats, on many platforms, in many stakeholder environments, and in many geographic locations. The data sets are this heterogeneous both physically (stored in different locations) and logically (not organized in the same fashion) accentuating issues of interoperability that are raised by lack of compatibility of systems and equipment. The problem of interoperability is not limited to technical standardization as typically assumed, but encompasses the complex issues of integrating cultural, financial and workflow systems. Ensuring that the 'ways of working' of health systems are interoperable is a major challenge.

Acceptance of telemedicine and telepathology presents a particular challenge. It is important to promote the use of automated tailoring of information access and summaries to accommodate variations in culture, language, literacy, and health-related goals, as well as integrated decision-support systems that can proactively foster best practices. Unfortunately, collection and delivery of the necessary epidemiological and patient data on which such systems must be built are problematic. However, once collected, telemedicine and telepathology can be used for timely transfer of data to central services for planning and management purposes. At the organizational level, revolutionary advances in medicine and technology as a whole during the past few decades have resulted in shifts in the boundaries between hospitals, primary health care, and community care. In the future, telemedicine and telepathology is likely to add to this by changing the way in which health services are provided, from clinical messaging (advice, results and referrals), to distributed electronic health records, increased connectivity between health services, patient appliances to assist self-management, and the use of technology to improve communication. These changes need to be sensitive to acceptance concerns related to changing established medical traditions, professional autonomy and loss of control.

Liability in connection with standards of care and medical malpractice, responsibility for security and confidentiality of patient-specific information are major legal changes. Owing to the computerized communications involved in telepathology, determining where transactions occurred, which laws apply and which courts have jurisdiction will be problematic. At the policy level, challenges include professional standards of providing care and licensing of care givers, and regulation of medical devices and telepathology application software. Telepathology is currently unregulated, unlike all other aspects of the telemedicine. This field also raises or accentuates ethical, legal and policy issues. Confidentiality of information, protecting the privacy of patients and safeguarding the integrity of information will present significant challenges with increasing use of telepathology. There will also be gender issues to be addressed and model guidelines will be needed to resolve the problems brought on by cultural differences among countries engaged in telepathology activities.

3. Suggested Solutions to Overcome Barriers

Interconnectivity comprises a lot more than merely devising and installing the technological infrastructure so as to be able to communicate and spread medical/pathology data through defined secured channels from one point on the earth to another. Interconnectivity is responsible for several aspects of telepathology service delivery when installing and running it:

- Technical aspects
- Organizational aspects
- Psychological aspects
- Social and socio-cultural aspects
- Financial aspects
- Political aspects
- Security aspects.

With the availability of electronic patient record systems which try to integrate not merely both the stationary and the ambulatory medical/pathology workflow of diagnostics and treatment, but deliver real-time medical patient data in a ubiquitous fashion to hold these data available at any time and any location, the basis for a global data exchange in the field of medicine/pathology is given. The main stakes today comprise HL7 (HL7 2004) and information servers, CDA (CDA 2004), SCIPHOX (SCIPHOX 2004), and many other existing and to become documentation standards. More and more, the availability and performance of terrestrial communication lines becomes continually better: back from analogue telephone line to digital ISDN and nowadays xDSL lines. Whereas these communication line types are financially affordable usually for private and small business applications and services, such lines of even better quality (e.g. optical fiber) are today too expensive to compete adequately for a substantial market share in medicine/pathology.

The necessary forms of organization within hospitals and the medical practices are only partially compatible to each other. As of yet, there are no general recommendations as how to organize services which have to deal with a more through electronification of medicine/pathology. This, however, is independent of the underlying communicating technology used.

Many staff members in a medical setting – irrelevant of their hierarchical position – are still reluctant to use computer-based help in their daily routine work. It has clearly been shown that for pathologists, the "option to possess a gadget" to handle medical instructions is interesting, but this interest soon enough looses intensity after a very short period of time.

The Internet can be seen as the main background, which will ensure the implementation of many tasks in telepathology. There are a few examples of telepathology that utilize the Internet as their mode of communication. The list is not intended to be comprehensive, but illustrative of the range of telepathology activities occurring globally. The Armed Force Institute of Pathology are long-standing players in this field, providing second-opinion consultation via simple store-and-forward but also utilizing the BLISS system for slide digitization. The John Hopkins University Department of Pathology and University of Maryland Department of Computer Science have a complex virtual microscope project which use Java applets as the primary interface. The University of Pittsburgh Medical Center offers web-based consultation services via store-and-forward telepathology. They also have the facility for robotic telepathology consultation. The UICC (Union Internationale Contre le Cancer) established a Telepathology Consultation Center at the Institute of Pathology of the Charité, Humboldt-University, Berlin, Germany. The purpose of this site is to offer store-and-forward telepathology consultation services at an international level. A similar web-based service exists in Tromso, Norway, although not in English. Intra-operative frozen section consultation is also undertaken in Berlin using their Java-applet controlled robotic microscope.

In conclusion, the Internet represents a major confirmation conduit and the means by which telepathology practice can become truly global. Telepathology can only benefit by the developments which will continue to occur in this area.

4. Future

The most important and perspective application of telepathology is education of health care professionals at a distance, so called distance education (eLearning). It may be defined as the application of communication technologies to acquire new knowledge or skills across the whole range of areas which will affect health care professionals, and enrich their experience in rendering the best possible care to patients through out the process of medical care. Distance education has the abilities to apply new concepts, and ideas in which the learner becomes an owner of that knowledge, without any respect to distance. As such, telemedicine overall, and in particular telepathology education, is significant part of health care revolution, since the event of modern medicine. Telepathology education process as a culture, uses for the most part, distance education as the medium of dissemination of advanced information, and while it is an important aspect of today's education process, this medium should not be distracting, and the principles of learning and education should be unchanged. The addition of technology should not substitute for failed pedagogical process, but technology should allow that educational process, and the message to be disseminated, and tailored to individual groups and professionals, by retraining along some of the educational principles of traditional education. Telepathology education centres on these principal issues:

- Distance learning
- Continuous Medical Education (CME) for pathologists
- Advanced telepathology professionals education in the changing environment
- Patient's education in pathology related issues in the information age.

While distance learning benefits are not challenged by most, it is difficult to estimate the impact on education overall. Nonetheless, is becoming more and more prevalent around the world. In a survey of Internet found more than 3,000 programs and 1,100 accredited institutions using distance learning in 1,400 fields of studies, represented by over 50,000 courses. The impact of distance learning should be measured by the content of the curriculum which should be based on the process, perception, product and the mode of delivery. As such distance learning and distance education process should be scrutinized just as traditional curriculum has been in the past and continue to be so. The only "change" should really be the medium of dissemination. Not the content per se, not the overall approach, and certainly not the end product, which is the education of the students, health professional and, the patients themselves. The differences between classical teaching and learning, and new and modern form of teaching as well as learning is substantial in this new era. Instead of confined classroom teaching and learning, the entire universe has become a workplace, a learning environment, anywhere, anytime, 24 hours a day. This creates a sense of shared knowledge and virtual networking alliances. The demand for distance learning stems from the common sense of its applicability, but it requires the same standards of production, and evaluation of such programs.

The main reasons to implement distance learning in health education are:

- Health care professional, in the information age, will acquire new skills and new knowledge without major disruption of their work.
- The need to reduce the cost of obtaining such education on new information (travel expenses, lodging, registration fees on venues like clinical conferences, congresses, and other forms of meetings).
- Need for better convergence of information age health care professional on communication and computing technologies.

CME is an important aspect of health care professionals in order for them to maintain the acquired knowledge, and to gain new information, which will make possible:

- To offer the best possible care to their patients implementing current standards of care.
- To satisfy governmental, institutional and scientific and clinical societies requirements for licensing, membership, and good standing in societies, associations and other organized forms of health care professionals.
- To ensure that, they are set up to speed with current medical practices.

Distance learning and advances in technologies allows health care professionals to participate in CME programs without disrupting their daily routine work to participate in the traditional meetings. Furthermore, it allows and ensures consistency throughout the educational process among peers, institutions and countries.

Education of health providers is a major issue in the current environment, as there is a great need for advancing the education process of all health care professionals. The report of the Institute of Medicine in 2001 states that clinical education simply has not kept pace with or has been responsive enough to shifting patient demographics and desires, changing health system expectations, evolving practice requirements and staffing arrangements, new information, focus on improving quality and new technologies. As such, healthcare providers have not been prepared adequately in either academic or continuing education venues to address these major changes in patient population. Health care providers are more and more asked to work on inter-disciplinary teams, often supporting patients with chronic conditions, although they may lack the training and education that is based on a team-based approach. Based on multiple reports and analysis, the twenty first century health care provider, and system, should ensure that all health care professionals be educated to deliver patient-centred care as members of an inter-disciplinary team, emphasizing evidence-based practice, quality proven approaches and informatics.

The proper techniques and methods of disseminating the existing knowledge and evidence-based medicine education programs and processes from renowned institutions and universities to countries around the world is a matter of some debate. What is not a matter of debate at all anymore, is the fact that, this dissemination of knowledge and expertise should be a priority of those who posses the knowledge and skills to disseminate it. Such initiatives should come as an international concerted action and collaboration of telepathology in order to facilitate the implementation of telemedicine/telepathology networks around the world.

The implementation of telepathology education as an expression of needs and demands from the public and health care providers is based on a growing concern for medical errors, advances of patient-centred health care systems; need to improve cost-benefit ratios and rationalizations of health care.

The entire aspect of needs and demands as pertained to telepathology education process needs to be centred in described issues of distance learning, advanced telepathology professionals education in the changing environment, CME for medical professionals, and patient's education in pathology related issues in the information age, and change. Furthermore, it should be taken in mind, the core competencies needed for health care professionals that have been created and required common vision across the topics. These competencies are:

- Patient centred care
- Work on inter-disciplinary teams
- Employ evidenced-based practices
- Apply quality improvement techniques, and
- Utilize informatics.

While all five these competencies are extremely important, the utilization of informatics as an important element of telepathology can effectively:

- Reduce the medical errors.
- Helps manage the knowledge and information, and support the decisions making process based on evidence based practice guidelines.
- Ensures better communication between health care providers and patient.
- Advance the goals of redesigning the health care systems.

As a result, the core competencies help implement new evidence-based pathology protocols and support the notion that, every citizen of the world need to receive the best possible existing care.

The implementation of telepathology education process remains one of the most important issues among current health challenges, that are staggering and numerous, as illustrated by numerous studies:

- Only in the USA each year 98,000 people die from medical errors, more than those who die from motor vehicle crashes, breast cancer, or AIDS.
- Other challenges include the lack of the "best system," poor accommodation of patients' needs, inability to assimilate the increasingly complex scientific advances, failure to address the growing consumerism among the patients.
- Health care provider's workforce shortage and discontent.

These are important issues that have led to medical errors, poor quality of care, and dissatisfaction among patients and health care providers. In this environment of technological advances, information technology and evidence based medicine has the potential for transformation of health care. The integration of more recent advances and visions with goals of the institutions, nations and more broadly of the world is the main challenge, however.

The use of well defined education programs for health care providers will be the cornerstone of the new revolution of the "e-era". Current specific challenges in implementing telepathology education and other revolutionary advances for health care professions educations are:

- Lack of funding, lack of faculty and faculty development programs.
- Lack of coordination and integration of accreditation, licensing, and certification process at the governmental and institutional level.
- Lack of application existing evidence based medicine.
- Shortage of visionary leaders and champions.
- Crowded curricula of pathology education for health care professional, often with irrelevant courses.
- Insufficient channels to share the information on the best practices, among medical professionals, governments and institutions.

Telemedicine in pathology training could supplement greatly pathology education of pathologists in developing countries for example, without the expenses of moving those pathologists from one country to the other for supplemental education. Eventually, pathology education could be advanced to pathology telementoring which could assist in the provision of pathology care to underserved areas and potentially facilitate the teaching of advanced pathology skills worldwide. Although there are still multiple logistical, technical and legal barriers to the widespread application of telepathology mentoring and telepresence pathology great progress has been achieved in this complex field.

Telepathology education is a very important element of overall progress in the telepathology. In order to be able to advance this, as an accepted culture and part of the daily practice of health care professionals, there are many initiatives that need to be taken, or existing one to be supported. Few issues that need resolved in order for telepathology education to prosper and be accepted are:

- "Product" acceptance by traditional medical educators, scholars, and legislators.
- Changing the old style of education to the new one and thus breaking the "traditional" classroom pathology teaching and learning methods.
- Lack of capability and availability of technology in most of the world for disseminating the knowledge, or in other words lack of communications.
- Language and cultural diversity.
- Socio-economic and political status of the countries in need for telepathology education.
- Legislative policies and championships for new information age.

While technological means for broadcasting and transmission of the telepathology education programs and clinical data is becoming abundant around the world, there is a great part of the planet that is not covered by Internet and will not have the ability to overcome the digital divide for decades to come. This should be our chance to advance the cause, and the issue, of infrastructure and perhaps a vision in some cases.

5. Conclusion

Perspectives and strategies for telemedicine for pathology, telepathology, are currently evolving, as emerging operative requirements would allow self-sustainable large scale exploitation while recent technological developments are available to support integrated and cost-effective solutions to such requirements. However, as far as we know few telepathology services have proceeded to large scale exploitation, even after successful technological demonstration phases. Main exploitation drawbacks, problems and deficiencies have been:

1. Partial solutions approach instead of integrated total approach to health care assistance needs.
2. Lack of economical drive and consequently no self-sustainability for large scale exploitation.
3. Insufficient H24 (24 hours/day 365 days/year) medical and social operators support.
4. Insufficient networking approach for medical operators and scientific/clinical structures.

Telemedicine and telepathology is the most important for the ensuring the safe medical care. It is well known, that the first contact with patients needing medical help is the contact with the local primary care health center. Second opinions from specialists are often required in primary care health centers. An efficient and appropriate strategy of medical care can be worked out at the initial steps of patient's contact with health care. Such an approach can avoid unnecessary hospitalization, and will be a substantial contribution to the reduction of health costs.

Telepathology has the potential for offering the worldwide medical community the following qualitative and quantitative improvements:

1. Distance consultations, diagnosis and advice for treatment.
2. Opening up new ways for education and training. Improvement in qualification of national specialists and health technicians, by opening up international medical databases.
3. Overall improvement of service by regional centralization of resources (specialists, hardware and software packages).
4. Effectiveness and efficiency in a management of actions related to reduction of waiting times for consultations, and introduction of medical information systems.

Telepathology is able to reduce health care costs in the following ways:

For the patient:

1. Cutting down on the journeys to major health care centers or for specialist consultations.
2. Reduction of length of stays, and therefore cost of hospitalization, since the patient can be treated and checked at a distance.

For providers of health care services:

1. Reduction of operating costs through centralization and optimization of resources (expertise, laboratories, equipment and etc.).

2. Reduction in travel cost and time for specialists visiting other hospitals and centers for consulting.
3. Reduction in costs for training and updating, improvement of specialists' qualifications through distance learning and access to medical databases.

Telepathology by comparison with the usual pathology service introduces added value and a positive impact at social, economic and cultural levels. As a result, telepathology is initiating to have an important influence on many aspects of pathology service in countries with low and middle income. When implemented well telemedicine for pathology may allow these countries to leapfrog over their developed neighbors in successful health care delivery.

References

[1] International Telecommunication Union. Making Better Access to Healthcare Services, 2005.
[2] Dzenowagis J. Global E-Health Strategy Draft for Consultation. Geneva, World Health Organization, 2004.
EU. E-Health Ministerial Declaration, 22 May 2003, made at 2003 e-Health Ministerial Conference. http://europa.eu.int/information_society/eeurope/ehealth/conference/2003/doc/min_dec_may_03.pdf. May 2003.
[4] Beolchi L. Telemedicine Glossary (5th Edition), 2003.
[5] Menabde N. Country Work is Paramount. Eur J Public Health, 13(3):28, 2003.
[6] Lareng L. Telemedicine in Europe. European Journal of Internal Medicine, n.13, pp.1-13, 2002.
[7] Della Mea V., Cortolezzis D., Beltrami C.A. The Economics of Telepathology – A Case Study. J of Telemedicine and Telecare, 6 suppli 1: S168-9, 2000.
[8] Furness P., Rashbass J. The Virtual Double-Headed Microscope: Telepathology for All? Histopathology, 36(2):182-3, 2000.
[9] Kekki P. Communications and Distance Learning: More Towards than Action. Towards Unity for Health – Coordinating Changes in Health Services and Health Professions, Practice and Education, WHO/EIP/OSD/NL/A/2002.2/2000(2), 30-31.
[10] Kwankam Y. E-Health Department of Knowledge Management and Sharing (KMS). World Health Organization, 2000.
[11] Leong F.J.W-M. Telepathology and the World Wide Web – Internet resources applicable for telepathology. XXIII International Congress of The International Academy of Pathology and 14th World Congress of Academic and Environmental Pathology, 2000.
[12] Moura A., Del Giglio A. Education via Internet. Rev. Assoc. Med. Bras., vol.46, no.1, p.47-51, 2000.
[13] Rosenberg M. E-learning, Strategies for Delivering Knowledge in the Digital Age. McGraw Hill, 2000.
[14] Tsuchihashi Y., Okada Y., Ogushi Y., Mazaki T., Tsutsumi Y., Sawai T. The Current Status of Medicolegal Issues Surrounding Telepathology and Telecytology in Japan. J of Telemedicine and Telecare, 6 Suppl 1: S143-5, 2000.
[15] Baskerville R. and Lee A. Distinctions Among Different Types of Generalizing in Information Systems Research. In New IT Technologies in Organizational Processes: Field Studies and Theoretical Reflections on the Future of Work. New York: Kluwer Academic Publishers, 1999.
[16] Haux R., Swinkels W., Lun K.C. Health and Medical Informatics Education: Transformation of Healthcare through Innovative Use of Information Technology for 21 Century. Int. J. Med Informatics, 1998.
[17] Hasman A., Albert A., Wainwright P., Klar R., Sosa M. Education and Training in Health Informatics in Europe. State of Art – Guidelines-Applications. Amsterdam, IOS Press, 1995.
[18] Hooper S. Cooperative Learning and Computer-Based Instruction. 1998.
[19] Mason R. Globalising Education. Trends and Applications. Routledge, London. 1998.
[20] Cimino J.J. Beyond the Superhighway: Exploiting the Internet with Medical Informatics. J. Am Med Inform Assoc, 4(4):279-284, 1997.

Current Principles and Practices of Telemedicine and e-Health
R. Latifi (Ed.)
IOS Press, 2008
© *2008 R. Latifi. All rights reserved.*

Tele-Dermatology in Australia

Jim MUIR and Lex LUCAS
Australian College of Rural and Remote Medicine

Abstract. Australia is a large country with a small and scattered population. Specialist dermatology services are concentrated in the capital cities and larger urban centers on the coast. This has meant access to these services for Australians in rural and remote areas has been limited to those able to travel the often long distances to their nearest dermatologist. Due to a considerable shortage of dermatologists, waiting times to see one are more than six months.

The challenge was to provide a dermatology service that overcame these twin obstacles of distance and demand. Telecommunication infrastructure in Australia is good and most towns have at least one general practitioner. More than 75% of all general practices are equipped with computers and have broadband internet access.

Dermatology is a specialty with few life threatening disorders. However short delays in diagnosis and management of a skin condition rarely have any serious impact on a patient's long-term health. At the same time many skin problems are distressing, and difficult to diagnose and treat. Many skin conditions last for considerable periods of time and patients need ongoing care. Due to the highly visual nature of the specialty, most skin conditions can be diagnosed from an image especially if there is some history available. This often requires a trained specialist. Paradoxically, any needed investigations such as skin biopsy or blood tests can be performed by any qualified doctor. Dermatological treatments can be instituted and monitored by these same practitioners without any specialist training. These factors make tele-medicine an ideal solution to the problems of isolation from and excess demand for specialist dermatological services.

In 2004 the Australian College of Rural and Remote Medicine (ACRRM) in a joint initiative with Queensland Divisions of General Practice (QDGP) set up Tele-Derm with funding from the Commonwealth Department of Health and Ageing under the Medical Specialist Outreach Assistance Program (MSOAP).

Tele-Derm was set up as an online consultation service combined with a central portal for online dermatology education, resources, links, discussions and professional development activities. It was set up with the belief that a teledermatology service must offer ongoing education as well as a specific case consultation service. If the remote doctor does not have the skills to perform required procedures such as biopsy and excision then the patient will still need to travel.

The common misconception about tele-dermatology is that this form of consultation is not as good as a face-to-face one with a dermatologist. But, in the majority of cases it is [1]. In any event Tele-Derm is not trying to provide a service that is necessarily better then the traditional mode of delivery. It wishes to provide a service where none currently exists. To this end, Tele-Derm provides teleconsultation and online education in dermatology to doctors Australia wide.

Keywords. Australia, dermatology, Tele-derma, online education, rural medicine

1. Introduction

1.1. Platform

Tele-Derm is an online dermatology service hosted on the Australian College of Rural and Remote Medicine's (ACRRM) Rural and Remote Medical Education Online (RRMEO) platform. The site is located at www.rrmeo.com.

RRMEO is an online platform designed to assist ACRRM members to:

1. locate relevant educational experiences using an online searchable database
2. record all their educational experiences toward fellowship, vocational registration and other credentialing using a unique online learning planner
3. engage in online education using the RRMEO's integrated learning management system.

Tele-Derm is just one of the interactive online communities available on the RRMEO platform.

1.2. Australia

The Australian Bureau of Statistics (2004) estimates Australia has a current population of more than 20 million people. They are dispersed over a land mass the size of continental Europe. However, 84% of this population is contained within the most densely populated 1% of the continent. 14% of the population lives in rural areas. This rural population includes people living on private rural properties, in very small communities, and bounded localities (population clusters of 200 to 999 people) [2].

Australia, like many other countries has a shortage of doctors particularly specialists. At the same time the Australian population is affluent and well educated by world standards and expects ready access to medical care.

Australia has 22,000 General Practitioners (GPs) and 300 Dermatologists, with the majority working in capital cities and major metropolitan areas.

With a warm climate, Australians enjoy an outdoor lifestyle and spend a lot of time in the sun. Skin disease accounts for up to 15% of all GP consultations. Patient waiting times for a traditional face-to-face consultation with a Dermatologist are often up to 6 months. With the vast majority of Dermatologists practicing in the state capitals, rural patients are traditionally required to travel many hours by road or air to see a Dermatologist.

The challenge Tele-Derm faced was to overcome these obstacles to dermatological care without compromising the quality of the advice received.

Dermatology is a highly visual specialty. Although the conditions seen are often distressing, they are rarely life threatening. Most can be diagnosed from a digital photograph or at least the possible diagnoses can be narrowed down. Most investigations and treatments can be readily performed by any GP.

Australia has a more than adequate telecommunications networks allowing rapid transmission of information and images across the nation.

All these factors mean that dermatology is the perfect specialty for tele-medicine.

Tele-Derm National was designed with the needs of a rural doctor in mind. The aim was to provide ready access to specialist dermatological advice. Coupled with this, the site seeks to impart the skills needed to diagnose and manage skin disease to the doctors using it.

1.3. Set-Up

In 2004, the Australian College of Rural and Remote Medicine (ACRRM), in a joint initiative with Queensland Divisions of General Practice (QDGP), secured funding for Tele-Derm via the Commonwealth Department of Health and Ageing under the Medical Specialist Outreach Assistance Program (MSOAP).

At this time, a leading Australian Dermatologist, Dr. Jim Muir, was contracted to moderate, and supply educational content, for the site.

Due to initial funding and medical indemnity issues, Tele-Derm began largely as a Queensland project, with only Queensland Doctors being able to submit cases for advice. Success of the project (and a desire to roll the project out nationally) led to Dr. Muir being registered in every state, and Tele-Derm was subsequently launched nationally by Australia's Federal Minister for Health, Dr. Tony Abbott MLA, in the first few months of 2005.

2. Current Developments

2.1. Submitting Cases

The heart of Tele-Derm is the online consultation service.

A doctor seeking advice on the diagnosis and management of a patient is only required to submit clinical details and, if needed, a digital photograph. For medico-legal reasons doctors must accept a disclaimer stating that Tele-Derm only provides advice not treatment, that an online consultation may not be as good as a face-to-face one with a dermatologist and that their patient has agreed to them using the service. To protect the privacy of the patient, no identifying details are sent other then their age and sex.

Minimal computer skills are needed to use the service. An internet connection, the ability to type a text message, and to attach an image, is all that is required.

Tele-Derm uses a store and forward system for online consultation. This allows the Dermatologist to be separated in time, as well as space, from the requesting doctor. Most cases are responded to within 24 hours. Tele-Derm cannot formally make any assessment of how accurate its tele-dermatological diagnoses are. This is because there is no ability for these patients to be seen face-to-face.

However, extrapolating from other studies (see Table 1) there has been shown to be an interobserver reliability between teledermatology and traditional consultation of up to 90%. This would suggest that a teledermatology consultation is very effective. Informal feedback from Tele-Derm's referring practitioners also suggests that the majority of cases submitted have been able to be managed without recourse to face-to-face consultation with a Dermatologist. Teledermatolgy has been demonstrated to produce similar management plans to traditional consultations for medical therapy. When dealing with skin malignancy there is less concordance between online and traditional consultation [14]. Therefore Tele-Derm does not provide a diagnostic service for pigmented skin lesions. This is primarily due to medico-legal concerns at this stage. Advice on management of diagnosed skin malignancy is provided.

Studies have shown that the use of videoconferencing can increase interobserver reliability in teledermatology [14]. However, videoconferencing was not incorporated

Table 1. [3] Interobserver diagnostic reliability between clinic-based dermatologists and teledermatologists using store and forward technology – point estimate data reported as simple proportion agreement

Reference	Complete Agreement	Partial Agreement
Kvedar [4]	0.61–0.64	0.67–0.70
Zelickson [5]	0.88	–
Lyon [6]	0.89	–
High [7]	0.64–0.77	0.81–0.89
Whited [8]	0.41–0.55	0.79–0.95
Taylor [9]	0.44–0.51	0.57–0.61
Lim [10]	0.73–0.85	0.83–0.89
Eminovic [11]	0.41	0.51
Du Moulin [12]	0.54	0.63
Mahendran [13]	0.44–0.48	0.64–0.65

Complete Agreement – considers the single most likely diagnosis.

Partial Agreement – considers both the single most likely diagnosis and differential diagnoses or comparable diagnoses.

1 History of presenting complaint.
2 Past Medical History, including history of atopy, asthma, hay fever etc.
3 Past Skin History, including rashes, skin cancers etc.
4 Drug History, including over the counter, prescribed and "alternative" therapies, topical, systemic and inhaled. If female are they on the OCP.
5 Cigarette and Alcohol use.
6 Allergies.
7 Family History of skin disease, auto-immune disease, diabetes etc.
8 Age, sex, occupation, hobbies etc. If female, pre or post menopausal, pregnant etc.
9 A detailed description of the rash. A detailed outline of treatment attempted and its outcome.
10 Results of any investigations to date.
11 Anything else they feel may be of use.
12 Digital photos showing distribution and a close up.

Figure 1. Proforma for Tele-Derm case submission.

into the Tele-Derm model because of impracticalities. Organising a time when the tele-dermatologist, referring doctor, and perhaps the patient, can be available for simultaneous videoconferencing is always very difficult. This is made more so by the fact that Australia has three different time zones. To overcome this, a detailed proforma was developed, to be completed by the referring doctor requesting a detailed history to enhance diagnostic ability (Fig. 1).

Below is a typical case as originally presented from the flying doctor in Mt Isa, a two hour plane flight from the nearest Dermatologist. This is followed by advice offered on Tele-Derm and subsequent follow through to final diagnosis.

Remote Doctor (05/12/2005 16:17):

Another case for you from the Isa. This 42 yo man presented with this rash after 1 week of mild URTI symptoms. It was mildly itchy and seem to be worsened by sunlight. It came on over about 36 hours and seemed to affect only his limbs.

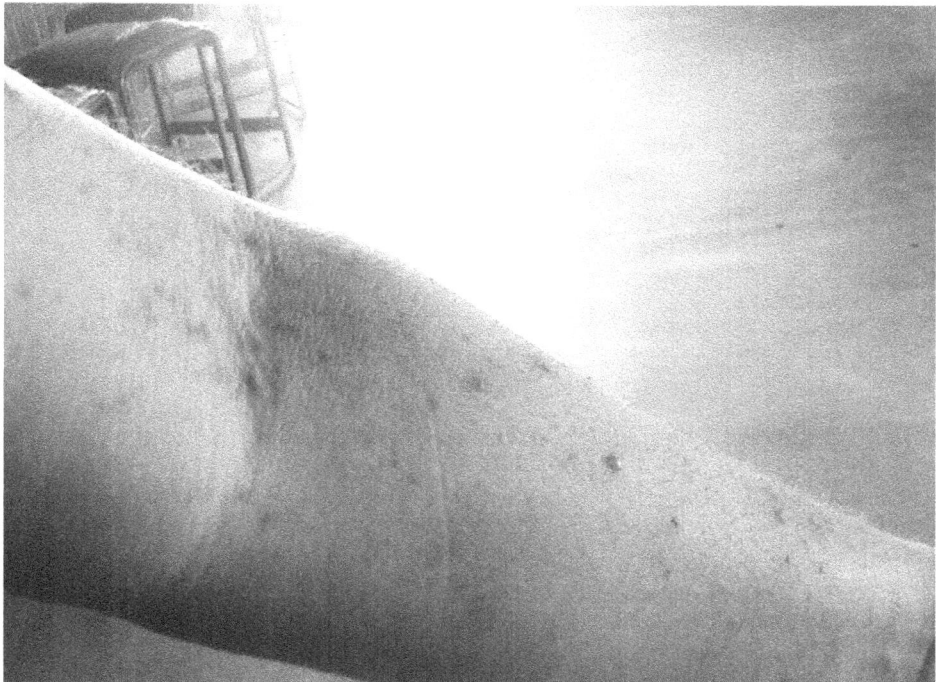

Tele-Dermatologist (05/12/2005 17:31):

In some areas looks purpuric/petechial in others seems to be vesicular. I would consider the following:

1. Queensland tick typhus. This usually has mild malaise/fever/adenopathy followed by rash after 1–12 days. Rash can be maculopapular, purpuric or vesicular. Ask re tick bite, look for the 'tache noir' which is a black eschar with surrounding erythema and seen in 70%. This is at site of tick bite. Regional draining nodes may be inflamed.

2. Drug eruption. Ask re antibiotics/NSAIDs given for URTI.

3. Vasculitis although is a bit widespread. Will be purpuric of course and usually maximal lower leg. Can be vesicular.

4. If he was ill I would worry re meningococcal.

Suggest:

1. Examine etc for above.

2. Biopsy for histol and send some off for culture. Biopsy an acute lesion from the upper limb.

3. Take blood for FBE/renal liver function. Take blood for culture and serology. There is specific serology for Qld tick Typhus available. Check urine for blood. Check coag profile.

4. See if you can beat a history of tick bite etc out of him. Doxycycline is supposed to help if no contraindications.

Remote Doctor (06/12/2005 17:03):

Bloods showed a CRP 9 and ESR 35 with WCC 11 normal renal and liver function. Hep B/C negative.
ANCA negative.
ANA speckled pattern 130 titre.
Anti DS DNA positive 2 titre.
Complement mildy raised.
Biopsy showed lymphocytic vasculitis.
No preceding drug exposure before rash.

Any ideas about follow up? His rash resolved within 10 days and he is asymptomatic.

Tele-Dermatologist (06/12/2006 20:46):

Have you ordered the serology for Tick typhus?? Can be done on blood for ANA. Still likely diagnosis.
I would repeat ANA etc in a while, if still up get rheumatology opinion.
Ask the pathologist if histol consistent with tick typhus, probably is.
Would expect rash to go spontaneously with this but not if he has lupus etc.

Remote Doctor (07/12/2005 09:13):

I have ordered the typhus serology on old blood today and the patient is coming for a remote clinic review next week when we can repeat the ANA and typhus serology on fresh blood.
Interestingly we asked a rheumatologist about the case and without seeing the images of the rash he told us the diagnosis was most likely urticarial vasculitis secondary to a viral URTI!!!? He dismissed the ANA and anti DS DNA results and said if the patient is getting better then not to bother with any followup.
I will let you know about the serology results. No one in the Mount Isa RFDS operations has ever diagnosed or suspected a case of typhus in our region so it will be a first if you are right.

Remote Doctor (16/12/2005 10:45):

Well you've done it again.
The patient's serology for spotted fever was reactive!
He must have had a relatively mild infection as a recent case report in the MJA from SA reports four cases of spotted fever all having to be hospitalised and treated with doxycycline (MJA 2005;182(5):231-234).

With the aid of clinical images this vasculitic eruption was diagnosed as Queensland tick typhus and appropriate management instituted without the patient having to leave home.

Tele-Derm is a service that can be used while awaiting a 'normal' visit to the Dermatologist, and is not intended as a substitute for a traditional specialist consultation. It provides a 24 hour turn around between submission of a request for advice and response. Biopsy performed by the local doctor will provide some confirmation of the teledermatology diagnosis in many cases. The response to treatment for an inflammatory skin condition, for example, can be assessed by the patient and referring doctor and the patient can seek a face-to-face consultation with a dermatologist if still required. In this, so far rare instance, the patient has not been disadvantaged in any way.

Another benefit of teledermatology is that it is a valuable educational tool for the referring doctor. The practitioner is intimately involved in the diagnosis and management of their patient. They have to provide a detailed history, take representative images, perform any diagnostic tests required and pass on the teledermatologists advice to their patient. From this comes a greater understanding of the patients condition than can be achieved through the more passive referral to a distant Dermatologist.

2.2. Online Education

Rather then reproduce what is available in text books, a case based approach to dermatology teaching has been employed. There are currently more than three hundred cases on Tele-Derm.

Each case presents the user with a clinical problem and asks them a series of questions. The user has to work their way through each case with the aim of being shown how to diagnose and manage the clinical problem. Detailed and specific answers, relevant to the case seen, are available. The online cases explore clinical assessment, relevant history and investigation and finally management. There are 'after images' to show response to treatment.

At the conclusion of each case there is a short multiple choice question which, once completed, earns participants professional development points which are automatically recorded in their RRMEO electronic Learning Planner.

To enable users to find information on a specific condition, all cases are indexed in alphabetical order by 'condition'. This allows a doctor, examining a patient with a specific condition, and wanting further information, to be able to select that condition from the index, to take them directly to that case. In this way they can get instantaneous advice on a condition seen in their practice.

Each week all Tele-Derm subscribers receive a 'Case of the week' in their e-mail. Subscribers are invited to log-in to RRMEO and share their suggested answer via online discussion forums. This is like a 'grand rounds' session with online peer discussion about a specific case. Detailed answers for the case are posted at the end of each week.

To keep subscribers up to date, interesting articles from the latest journals are reviewed and posted in discussion forums on Tele-Derm. Users are invited to comment on the reviews or to add their own.

Educational online tutorials in basic surgical skills are also available. Topics currently include: Cryotherapy; Curettage; Drug Eruptions; Skin Biopsy; Punch Biopsy; Shave Biopsy; Biopsy of a Difficult Site; Skin Check; Skin Tags; Second Intention Healing; Marini Suture; Pulley Suture and Acne Typical Treatment Regimes.

These tutorials are designed with medical students in mind and go into exact detail of how they are performed, from marking the site, through anaesthesia to applying a dressing.

Streaming video footage demonstrating excision and suture techniques, curettage, biopsy and even skin examination is also available.

Specific online tutorials in the use of topical 5 flurouracil cream, acne and drug eruption management, links to other useful sites and even histopathology is available on the site.

3. Barriers (and Suggested Solutions) to Issues at Hand

In a recent independent study of the Tele-Derm project [15] it was found that 45 doctors from around Australia submitted a total of 103 cases to Tele-Derm over a period of 11 months during 2005. A clinical response was provided by the teledermatologist within one working day for the majority (96%) of cases. All referring physicians agreed that the teledermatology consultations had helped with the management of their patients and that they would recommend Tele-Derm to another colleague and use Tele-Derm again in the future for teleconsultations. Seventy percent of users who had not yet submitted a case to Tele-Derm, reported they would consider using Tele-Derm in the future for consultations. Although most users saw no significant barriers to using Tele-Derm, the two most common negative aspects quoted were the increase in workload, and the process being too time consuming (Fig. 2).

Anecdotal evidence indicates that each Tele-Derm submission adds 20 minutes of extra time to a consultation. This is the time it takes to photograph the patient, document the history and upload the photograph to the Tele-Derm site. Currently this is an unchargable 20 minutes of time.

The other issue is funding the specialist to provide the service. While there is current government funding for the Tele-Derm service – this is not guaranteed ongoing funding. At the moment a fee for service model for specialist remuneration is not feasible.

What are the negative aspects of using Tele-Derm

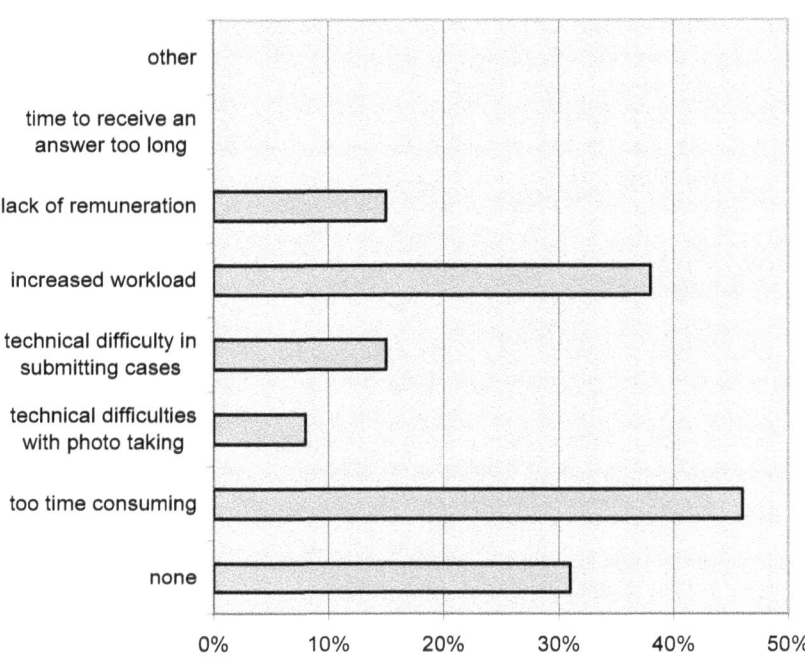

Figure 2. Referring doctors' views on the negative aspects of using Tele-Derm.

Australia needs to find a way to allow greater exploitation of telemedicine as an option for diagnosis and treatment. Clearly there are enormous potential savings to be made in travel and waiting times, but no incentives for specialists to provide the service, or for doctors to use them.

4. Future

It is hoped that the future will see increased use of the Tele-Derm service (and other services like it).

It is anticipated that some form of funding model will become available to allow such services to be set-up and used in a sustainable way.

References

[1] Tele-Dermatology in the Highlands of Scotland, J Telemed Telecare, 1996;2 supp 1:7-9.
[2] The Australian Bureau of Statistics. (2004). *AusStats* [Online]. Available: http://www.abs.gov.au/
     Ausstats/abs@.nsf/95553f4ed9b60a374a2568030012e707/282E34EA888D4ECCCA256E7D0000263E
     ?opendocument [Accessed 10 October 2006].
[3] Whited JD. Summary of the Status of Teledermatology Research. Teledermatology Special Interest
     Group, American Telemedicine Association 2006.

[4] Kvedar JC, Edwards RA, Menn ER, Mofid M, Gonzalez E, Dover J, et al. The substitution of digital images for dermatologic physical examination. Arch Dermatol 1997;133:161-7.

[5] Zelickson BD, Homan L. Teledermatology in the nursing home. Arch Dermatol 1997;133:171-4.

[6] Lyon CC, Harrison PV. A portable digital imaging system in dermatology: diagnostic and educational applications. J Telemed Telecare 1997;3(S1):81-3.

[7] High WA, Houston MS, Calobrisi SD, Drage LA, McEvoy MT. Assessment of the accuracy of low-cost store-and-forward teledermatology consultation. J Am Acad Dermatol 2000;42:776-83.

[8] Whited JD, Hall RP, Simel DL, Foy ME, Stechuchak KS, Drugge RJ, et al. Reliability and accuracy of dermatologists' clinic-based and digital image consultations. J Am Acad Dermatol 1999;41:693-702.

[9] Taylor P, Goldsmith P, Murray K, Harris D, Barkley A. Evaluating a telemedicine system to assist in the management of teledermatology referrals. Br J Dermatol 2001;144:328-33.

[10] Lim AC, Egerton IB, See A, Shumack SP. Accuracy and reliability of store and forward teledermatology: preliminary results from the St. George Teledermatology Project. Australas J Dermatol 2001; 42:247-51.

[11] Eminovic N, Witkamp L, Ravelli ACJ, Bos JD, van der Akker TW, Bouseam MT, et al. Potential effect of patient-assisted teledermatology on outpatient referral rates. J Telemed Telecare 2003;9:321-327.

[12] Du Moulin MFMT, Bullens-Goessens YIJM, Henquet CJM, Brunenberg DEM, de Bruyn-Geraerds, Winkens RAG, et al. The reliability of diagnosis using store and forward teledermatology. J Telemed Telecare 2003;9:249-252.

[13] Mahendran R, Goodfield MJD, Sheehan-Dare RA. An evaluation of the role of a store-and-forward teledermatology system in skin cancer diagnosis and management. Clin Exp Dermatol 2005;30: 209-214.

[14] Baba M, Seckin D, Kapdagli S. A comparison of teledermatology using store and forward methodology alone, and in combination with Web camera videoconferencing. J Telemed Telecare 2005;11:354-360.

[15] Lee, EY, Muir J. The Tele-Derm National Store and Forward Teledermatology Service: A Review of Submitted Cases and Quality Assessment by User Satisfaction.

Telemedicine in Oncology: European Perspective

Markus MOHR, MD
Tumor Centre, University Hospital of Regensburg, Germany

Abstract. Telemedicine in oncology or teleoncology integrates many so far well-known telemedicine elements such as teleconsultation, telesupport, telesurgery and telerobotics, teleeducation, and many others and is integral part of many disciplines such as internal medicine, surgery, dermatology, but also dentistry and psychooncology/psychiatry. Changes in ICT, new developments in oncology, the need to think and work interdisciplinarily, geographic and economic challenges as well as the transgression of sectoral boundaries as elements of modern teleoncology. Whereas the northern parts of Europe show a well-developed telemedicine infrastructure with a growing tendency to incorporate teleoncology for documentation, data analysis and quality assurance, in more southern countries this process is still underway and often marked by project status. Modern technology using xDSL and other terrestrial network lines but also satellite connectivity is at hand to cover a wide variety of telemedicine applications and services from which teleoncology benefits. More and more specifically designed software applications can be used to assess the medical workflow of an oncological patient and determine a life-long oncological electronic patient record. The trend, however, goes to the systemic integration of single applications and services into clinical information systems with a telemedicine approach. Although past evaluations of telemedicine applications and services have shown very positive results, only the right financial funding determines their survival and wide-spread usability in daily routine medical use. Formerly identifiable barriers for this use nowadays can be overcome more easily.

Keywords. Telemedicine, Oncology, Interdisciplinary, Developments, Europe, Technical Issues

Introduction

The search for international literature specifically for the terms of "telemedicine in oncology" or "teleoncology" throughout the last ten to 15 years is very scarce and primarily follows a general telemedicine consideration. Very often, telemedicine in oncology is part of other disciplines such as telemedicine in pathology, in surgery, in internal medicine, etc. Telemedicine in oncology can be seen as a discipline with a heterogeneous group of both applications and services combining patient-based ongoing medical documentation of oncological diagnostic, primary therapeutic, and follow-up data, the integration of most recent assured oncological knowledge, the process of therapy-centered discussion within oncological expert rounds for primary and secondary opinion over geographical and financial boundaries in order to assess a proper way of delivery of medical care for oncological patients. All of the current activities are concentrated around changes in information and communication technology (ICT), development of oncology in terms of diagnostics and treatment in different medical disciplines especially over the past ten years. This new approach includes interdisciplinary within expert rounds, geographic and economic considerations and thus creating eHealth in oncology, as an expression of multidisciplinary approach in oncological science. Thus, the historic meaning of telemedicine has given way to a far more modern understanding of what telemedicine in oncology implies nowadays such as ongoing documentation of the patient's oncological history from first diagnosis over a follow-up until the end of treatment, documented discussion of (diagnostic and) therapeutic procedures within interdisciplinary expert rounds, and evaluation and analysis of patient findings and oncological data for quality assurance and benchmarking.

1. Issues at Hand

1.1. Changes in ICT

Whereas in the late nineties of the last millennium video conferences were the most outstanding instruments for communicating medical findings over distances, nowadays many software applications can handle the encrypted and secure transport of medical data irrespective of their underlying formats (text, audio, video, etc.).

1.2. Developments in Oncology

The inclusion of many new insights from scientific fields such as molecular medicine, functional and descriptive genomics, pathology of cancer development into modern oncology has led to much more refined diagnostic procedures. In consequence, oncological grading and staging has both been unified and standardized for the majority of malign diseases so that the process of deciding which therapy shall be delivered has been facilitated and follow-up can be attached to defined criteria which include the chance of early detection of relapses or metastases.

1.3. Medical Disciplines

Some malign diseases such as breast and colon cancer, but also melanoma and leukemias bear the potential to quickly worsen the patient's medical condition without prior warning. Others develop slowly and more in a chronic fashion. Wherever medical intervention requires fast and consensus-derived decisions for the further delivery of medical care, telemedicine procedures has been agreeably found the right instrument to be applied. Examples are not merely documentation or second opinion, but the global availability of DICOM sequences with a defined user-authorized access, robotic aids in oncological surgery such as endoscopy, telediagnosis by medical colleagues thousands of miles away, and telesurgical procedures especially in oncology.

1.4. Interdisciplinary

Worldwide, medical specialization more and more leads to the formation of cancer competence centers and organ centers. They all have their respective need to continually document and to discuss the delivery of medical care. Therefore, telemedicine in these scenarios has to take care of interdisciplinary expert rounds in the therapeutic decision making process.

1.5. Geography and Economy

Geographical conditions, especially limitations for easy traveling (e. g. mountains, deserts, war-ravaged countries, remote locations), and lack of physicians can be overcome by telemedicine, even more so for oncological conditions. For patients in a bad medical shape, among which are often individuals with malign diseases in a progressive state, telemedicine consultations can be of essential quality. Hence, Stalfors et al. (2005) describe that through multidisciplinary team (MDT) meetings used for establishing diagnosis for TNM classification and for treatment in head and neck tumour patients in the western region of Sweden it was possible to save costs compared with face-to-face consultations (FTF) [1].

1.6. eHealth in Oncology

The term telemedicine has been supplemented by the notion eHealth within the last decade. Whereas telemedicine a priori describes the delivery of medical care through distances not to be overcome easily otherwise according to the original WHO definition [2], eHealth implies many modern medical services in terms of broadening the original definition (cf. [3]). Some aspects are the transgression of sectoral boundaries (clinics, medical institutions, general practitioners, etc.), the fortification of ongoing digital documentation as a post-paradigm change phenomenon (widespread ICT facilities within the routine of medical documentation), and the integration of many formerly separated functionalities and procedures in the context of the delivery, but also the administration of medical care.

In trying to combine all these factors into one coherent definition, it becomes clear that the original definitions of telemedicine have to be accepted as historic and are still valid. But they have to be supplemented by a wide differentiation of the various aspects mentioned so as to overlook the entire field.

2. Current Status of Oncological Documentation in Europe

In most states of the European Union, oncological documentation in cancer registries is determined not to be central, but to be carried out in geographical areas or provinces.

In the UK, for example, there are two cancer registries in Scotland and Wales with regional competence, whereas England per se has more than nine cooperating cancer registries.

Originally centrally organized, in the mid-eighties of the last century there has been a regional differentiation of cancer registries in Sweden. Norway nowadays tries to combine cancer registry-like institutions in one large southern and one northern institution for geographical reasons. Cancer registries were begun in most Scandinavian countries during the 1950's, and reporting became obligatory during the 1960's. The informants who submit data on cancer cases include all hospitals, physicians, pathological, cytological and hematological laboratories and also dentists. Furthermore, the Cause of Death Registry contains information on dates and causes of all deaths according to the ICD. Official statistics on the death rates are available since the early 1900's in Scandinavian countries. In Austria, oncological documentation is organized on the level of the ten provinces each of which has one cancer registry. Up to now, a complete documentation has been available only from Tyrol. The Netherlands have one single cancer registry founded in 1989. They derive their data from all in all nine comprehensive cancer centers with disjunctive catchments areas containing five to 20 clinics each.

France, Italy, and Spain, however, do not have a common oncological documentation all over their respective countries. In France, there are some population-based registries in geographic areas (provinces and departments). Furthermore, there are specialized registries for gynaecologic, haematologic, and gastrointestinal malignancies.

And finally, in Germany there is a range of 43 cancer registries up to now (political changes imply a reduction in number to be expected). Each of these registries has different internal and external functions such as epidemiological and clinical documentation, populations-based statistics, regional comparability of oncological data, and many more. Regulated by law in 1994, oncological documentation is mandatory for all physicians involved in the phases of diagnostics, treatment, and follow-up.

Most important, the attempt to manage the comparability of data of regional cancer registries for a German-wide description of the cancer situation is the declared aim of both epidemiological and clinical cancer registries. Whereas epidemiological registries primarily care for the detection and documentation of incidences, prevalence, and other statistical measures, the task of clinical registries implies a principally life-long patient follow-up with exact data analysis for clinical quality management.

In conclusion, even more than ten years after the first introduction of practical telemedicine instruments one still sees the pre-eminence of Scandinavian countries concerning the telemedicine practicability on a country-wide scenario. Germany, Austria, and Switzerland have developed national regimes of cancer registries (epidemiological and clinical) to handle and evaluate the vast amount of oncological data. Most important for all these countries, however, remains the evaluation of oncological data for the sake of quality assurance and especially the consequence of optimizing diagnostic and therapeutic procedures for cancer patients. Other European countries are underway to build similar models as the ones mentioned.

3. Modern Telemedicine Uses, Applications, and Services in Oncology

Olver [4] recently has well described the range of telemedicine applications in oncology that range from real-time videoconferencing for primary and secondary opinion gathering through both generalists and specialists in a geographically circumscriptive area [5,6] to the gathering of second opinion through international experts [7] and CT-based remote 3D radiation oncology treatment planning [8,9].

He also contrasts ISDN as cost-effective telecommunication lines to formerly used analog (telephone) lines. However, most recent developments in low pricing for xDSL technology (speeds up to 25 Mbit/sec in downlink mode) will lead or already leads to its wide-spread use and will be supplemented by even faster technologies (E1, ATM, SDSL etc.) within a narrow period of time. This holds true, on the other hand only for such countries in which these technologies are available. The situation is completely different in countries with economy in deficit: The affordability of telemedicine equipment is directly proportional to the readiness of well faring countries to sponsor such poor economical environments for the good of telemedicine consultation.

4. Technical Issues

Technical aspects in telemedicine more and more incorporate not only terrestrial data transfers, but imply an intensified use of satellite communication where geographically applicable (and necessary) [cf. Introduction] and financially affordable. Excellent examples with international applicability are the Satellite-based networks for DELTASS (Disaster Emergency Logistic Telemedicine Advanced Satellite Systems) [10], MEDASHIP (Medical Assistance for Ships) [11], and EMISPHER (Euro-Mediterranean Internet Satellite Platform for Health, Medical Education and Research) [12], where oncology more and more comes into the focus of attention.

Transfer facilities on the one side have to be supplemented by suitable documentation systems on the other. Here, mostly country-wide solutions without any option to "internationalize" them are in wide-spread use.

A very good example of an integrative tumor documentation system, however, is the German multilingual software OncoLutions® [13]. OncoLutions® offers a large variety of features that include oncological life-long electronic patient record (patient- and secondarily case-based, all malign entities can be comprised) in a client-server and a web-based flavor and selective data extractions (clear names, pseudonyms, anonyms) and transport processes (email, ftp etc.) for various data analysis institutions in various formats. Overall this integrates hospital physicians, general practitioners, pathological institutes, tumor centers, and other medical establishments through principally the same graphical user interface (second telemedicine component) and thus provides interdisciplinary expert discussions in a forum-like user interface (third telemedicine component) in a bidirectional mode of delivery of medical data to the tumor centre in charge (fourth telemedicine component). Furthermore, OncoLutions® integrates data analysis and anonymized benchmarking among the data providers (fifth telemedicine component) as well as videoconference-like user interface for second opinion consultations (sixth telemedicine component).

More and more, individual telemedicine applications are integrated into the larger clinical information systems (CIS). This process reduces the often highly complicated media breach through interfaces (e.g. HL7) which must be established and configured. One internationally used CIS with a general telemedicine approach is SOARIAN® Integrated Care from SIEMENS [14], others will follow. As this process is continually ongoing, the literature does not yet report global results.

When it comes to evaluation of telemedicine applications and services in oncology, one has to focus on the individual points of view of the patient, the physician, the technician, but also to consider financial and political aspects. There are many publications to this topic, but all of them focus on historic telemedicine scenarios which have lost their actuality as of today [15–21]. In conclusion, they describe well the individual benefit both patients and physicians are able to derive from telemedicine applications and services. However, often enough the economic premise for a project has run out after a number of years so that there is also a report of many promising approaches and beginnings to have ended without their integration into routine daily medical use [22–26]. Much work still has to be done to fortify continuous funding for this.

5. Conclusion

Whereas telemedicine applications and services used to be rather informal and unstandardized in the past, nowadays these procedures largely are standardized and both workflow- and process-oriented. Thus, the integration into daily hospital routine use is facilitated at least on a technical level. In combination with many economic aspects such as value chain orientation, just in time aspects and many others, but also the growing acceptance of digital documentation in general prepares the way for teleoncology within hospitals and specialized general practitioners' offices. As for a vision, teleoncology as well as all other telemedicine and eHealth disciplines shall be integral instruments for a standardized and logical workflow of delivery of medical care in every patient.

References

[1] Stalfors J, Bjorholt I, Westin T: A cost analysis of participation via personal attendance versus telemedicine at a head and neck oncology multidisciplinary team meeting. J Telemed Telecare 11 (2005): 4, 205–210.
[2] WHO 1998. Telehealth and Telemedicine will henceforth be part of the strategy for Health for All. Press Release 23, December 1997. World Health Organization, Geneva, 1997–1998.
[3] Dario C, Dunbar A, Feliciani F, Garcia-Barbero M, Giovanetti S, Graschew G, Güell A, Horsch A, Jenssen M, Kleinebreil L, Latifi R, Lleo MM, Mancini P, Mohr MTJ, Ortiz García P, Pedersen S, Pérez-Sastre JM, Rey A: Opportunities and Challenges of eHealth and Telemedicine via Satellite. Eur. J. Med. Res. 10 (Suppl. 1): 1–52 (2004).
[4] Olver I: Telemedicine in Oncology. In: Burg G (ed.): Telemedicine and Teledermatology. Curr Probl Dermatol. Basel, Karger, 2003; 32: pp. 121–126.
[5] Olver IN, Selva-Nayagam S: Evaluation of a telemedicine link between Darwin and Adelaide to facilitate cancer management. Telemed J 2000; 6: pp. 213–218.
[6] Dootlittle GC, Allen A: Practising oncology via telemedicine. J Telemed Telecare 1997; 3: pp. 63–70.
[7] Vorozhtcov G, ChissovV, Danilov A, Kazinov V, Sokolov V, Frank G: Perfect DiViSy technology for video network in medicine (Moscow Information Network for Teleoncology). In: Nerlich M, Kretschmer R (eds.): The Impact of Telemedicine on Health Care Management. Moscow, IOS Press, 1999, pp. 119–125.
[8] Stitt J: A system of teleoncology at the University of Wisconsin Hospital and Clinics and Regional Oncology Affiliate Institutions. Wisc Med J 1998; 97: pp. 38–42.
[9] Purkable TL, Bauer JJ: A telementored transrectal ultrasound-guided prostate biopsy. Stud Health Technol Inform 1999; 62: pp. 275–277.
[10] Graschew G, Roelofs TA, Rakowsky S, Schlag PM: Disaster Emergency Logistic Telemedicine Advanced Satellite Systems – DELTASS.1st Arab I.T. MED, 1st Pan Arab Congress on I.T. in Medicine in collaboration with 1st World Congress of I.T. in Medicine, Cairo, Egypt, 12.–14.03.2003. Proceedings, pp. 17–18.
[11] Graschew G, Roelofs TA, Rakowsky S, Schlag PM: Satellite-based Networks for MEDASHIP and EMISPHER. Tromsoe Telemedicine Conference, Tromsø, Norway, September 15–17, 2003. Proceedings, p. 36.
[12] Graschew G, Roelofs TA, Rakowsky S, Schlag PM: Real time Telemedicine and the EMISPHER-Project. 1st Arab I.T. MED, 1st Pan Arab Congress on I.T. in Medicine in collaboration with 1st World Congress of I.T. in Medicine, Cairo, Egypt, 12.–14.03.2003. Proceedings, pp. 5–6.
[13] Mohr M, Klinkhammer-Schalke M: Electronic medical report for tumor documentation: A new software and service implementation combining different intrahospital and general practitioners' systems for the Tumor Center Regensburg, Germany. TTeC 2004 – Tromsø Telemedicine and eHealth Conference, Tromsø, 2004 (presentation and poster).
[14] Bocionek S, Brandt S, Cseh J, Haskell B, Rucker D, Thomas D: Built for Success: The new Clinical and Financial IT Solution from Health Services. electromedica 2001; 69: pp. 76–81.
[15] Lipsedge M, Summerfiled AB, Ball C, Watson JP: Digitised video and the care of outpatients with cancer. Eur J Cancer 1990; 26: pp. 1025–1026.
[16] Yellowlees PM, Kennedy C: Telemedicine; here to stay. Med J Aust 1997; 166: pp. 262–265.

[17] Allen A, Hayes J: Patient satisfaction with teleoncology. A pilot study. Telemed J 1995; 1: pp. 41–46.

[18] Kunkler IH, Rafferty P, Hill D, Henry M, Foreman D: A pilot study of teleoncology in Scotland. J Telemed Telecare 1997; 4: pp. 113–119.

[19] Mair F, Whitten P, May C, Doolittle GC: Patients' perceptions of a telemedicine speciality clinic. J Telemed Telecare 2000; 6: pp. 36–40.

[20] Allen A, Hayes J, Sadasivan R, Williamson SK, Wittman C: A pilot study of the physician acceptance of teleoncology. J Telemed Telecare 1995; 1: pp. 34–37.

[21] Hicks LL, Boles KE, Hudson ST, Koenig S, Madsen R, Kling B, Tracy J, Mitchell J, Webb W: An evaluation of satisfaction with telemedicine among health-care professionals. J Telemed Telecare 2000; 6: pp. 209–215.

[22] Olver IN: Telemedicine: Prospects and realities. Med Today 2001; 1: pp. 81–83.

[23] Hakansson S, Gavelin C: What do we really know about the cost-effectiveness of telemedicine? J Telemed Telecare 2000; 6 (suppl. 1): pp. 33–36.

[24] Whitten P, Kingsley C, Grigsby J: Results of a meta-analysis of cost-benefit research: Is this a question worth asking? J Telemed Telecare 2000; 6 (suppl. 1): pp. 4–6.

[25] Doolittle GC, Harmon A, Williams A, Allen A, Boysen Cd, Wittman C, Mair F, Carlson E: A cost analysis of a teleoncology practice. J Telemed Telecare 1997; 3 (suppl. 1): pp. 20–22.

[26] Mair FS, Haycox A, May C, Williams T: A review of telemedicine cost-effectiveness studies. J Telemed Telecare 2000; 6 (suppl. 1): pp. 38–40.

V. The Internet and Medicine

Current Principles and Practices of Telemedicine and e-Health
R. Latifi (Ed.)
IOS Press, 2008

The Authority and Utility of Internet Information

Ronald C. MERRELL, MD, Stephen W. CONE, MD and Azhar RAFIQ, MD
Medical Informatics and Technology Applications Consortium,
Virginia Commonwealth University, Richmond, VA

Abstract. Internet use for health information by both practitioners and consumers continues to expand geometrically. The impact of Internet on practice, access and health decisions is considerable and will probably grow to the predominant mode of health information delivery in the coming years. As the growth of this unregulated global bulletin board continues, how do we assure the quality of the information retrieved by professionals and patients? What are the indicators of quality? How should we measure impact? How do authoritative sources get the attention and who should decide? What should practitioners recommend? What should medical teachers advise trainees? This review of Internet content, access and application considers the history, patterns of use, evaluation studies and specialty examples. A few authoritative sources are recommended and that recommendation is justified. Changes in health care delivery must take best advantage of the Internet with least disruption to the important principles of practice and patient relationships. The health community needs effective interaction with medicine's inevitable partner, the Internet.

Keywords. Internet, information technology, evidence based medicine, peer reviewed data, internet services, e-health, telehealth

Introduction

The Internet is such a dynamic and rapidly evolving phenomenon that it seems impossible for traditional human information systems such as libraries, in person consultation, pedagogical instruction, and peer reviewed print media to keep pace. The current situation of unregulated information on the Internet, unedited sources and commercial motives that keep the Internet more or less free of charge cannot assure coherent, accurate and accessible information. There is no authority responsible for accuracy and appropriate application of Internet information, medical or otherwise. A blog is a personal rather than authoritative communication; more like graffiti than truth inscribed for all time on stone! What is the history of the Internet? How did we get here?

The ARPANET in 1969 connected Leonard Kleinrock at UCLA to Douglas Engelbart at the Stanford Research Institute. Standard protocol (Transmission Control Protocol/Internet Protocol – TCP/IP) for communication and registration was introduced by Robert Kahn, Vincent Cerf, et al., in 1983 and a play toy of science was quickly recognized as a very useful tool for communication, relying upon the power of shared computing. ARPANET was transferred to the National Science Foundation in 1990 to become a vehicle for imagination, connecting select universities. By January 1992, the monthly net traffic exceeded 12 billion packets or a trillion bytes with a further doubling of volume by November of that year. The utility of the Internet at that

Table 1. History of the Internet

Year	Event
1963	Hypertext language introduced
1969	ARPANET connected UCLA to Stanford Research Institute
1983	Standard protocol (TCP/IP) becomes core Internet protocol
1990	National Science Foundation acquires ARPANET
1991	Gore Bill creates the National Research & Education Network or Internet
1993	MOSAIC browser introduced
1995	World Wide Web Consortium established at MIT

time was for information exchange. The use of the Internet as a tool for information storage and retrieval became a reality with the MOSAIC browser introduced by Andreessen and Bina in 1993. Hypertext for language management had already been introduced into computing by Ted Nelson in 1963. The global spread of the almost mythical Internet cloud was realized with the Tim Berners-Lee server and the World Wide Web Consortium was established at MIT in 1995 (Table 1). The Internet or world wide web is a huge, nebulous domain of shared computers and digital information encircling the globe with immense power to inform and share. Proper access to the Internet can eliminate forever the tyranny of single source propaganda and the errors of anecdotal evidence. Although much of the information in this paragraph is pretty much common knowledge in the Internet community, the facts were checked at a web site, of course [1,2].

So obtain an Internet Service Provider and an IP address and prepare to leap into cyberspace! Share the knowledge of the planet accumulated for all time through a network of servers. Share your thoughts, explore the thoughts of others, search cyberspace with engines and participate in the greatest exchange of human mental activity ever imagined in history. There are over one billion Internet users in a world with only 6 billion people. The penetration varies from less than 3% in Africa to 36% in Europe and 68% in North America [3] (Table 2). It is certain these numbers will grow by the time this book is published. Perhaps the only things the world population consumes with greater regularity than the Internet are oxygen, water and essential nutrients. The Internet is pervasive, economically aggressive, almost free to the user and available in many languages.

Medicine quickly realized the utility of the Internet, bringing forth what would be known as "telemedicine," "telehealth" and "e-health." While early efforts in Russia [4] and remote regions [5] were often troubled by Internet interference and dropped messages, the frustrations were more than matched by the promise of cheap long distance interaction and experimentation continued. By the late 1990's every major medical center and medical association had a web site. The National Library of Medicine put its MEDLINE archive on the web with PubMed in 1997. From a meager start, the number of searches reached 80 million per month in early 2006 [6]. The subject "Internet" summons 27,452 references on PubMed [7]. A recent estimate claims that nearly 5% of all Internet searches in the world relate to accessing medical information. Most medical school curricula in the US are web based and most medical journals are now online

Table 2. World Internet usage and population statistics

World Regions	Population (2006 Est.)	Population % of World	Internet Usage, Latest Data	% Population (Penetration)	Usage % of World	Usage Growth 2000–2006
Africa	915,210,928	14.1%	**32,765,700**	3.6%	3.0%	625.8%
Asia	3,667,774,066	56.4%	**394,872,213**	10.8%	36.4%	245.5%
Europe	807,289,020	12.4%	**308,712,903**	38.2%	28.4%	193.7%
Middle East	190,084,161	2.9%	**19,028,400**	10.0%	1.8%	479.3%
North America	331,473,276	5.1%	**229,138,706**	69.1%	21.1%	112.0%
Latin America/Caribbean	553,908,632	8.5%	**83,368,209**	15.1%	7.7%	361.4%
Oceania/Australia	33,956,977	0.5%	**18,364,772**	54.1%	1.7%	141.0%
WORLD TOTAL	6,499,697,060	100.0%	**1,086,250,903**	16.7%	100.0%	200.9%

with web-based manuscript management. There are entirely paperless Internet journals and new medical libraries around the world are likely to use the HINARI program of the WHO to access some 2000 journals with full text at very low prices [8]. Internet virtual libraries are saving libraries in the developing world, where the average number of print subscriptions had fallen below ten as the rapidly rising costs of print media became prohibitive, from grievous isolation.

Lest this report be entirely laudatory, there are some very serious problems with Internet information. No one ever expected the telephone to stay pure without annoyance calls, false advertising, seedy solicitations, and foul mouthed anonymity. The television is not a gleaming cultural achievement of the 20th century. Indeed, the Internet covers the entire spectrum of human expression from pornography to theology, artistic literature to science, matters arcane and banal. Just because something is found on the Internet, there is no guarantee of truth, innocence of intent or full attribution. Without any control, the Internet may be used to post outrageous claims from scam healers, unscientific claims in the alternative medicine realm, commercial bias for a drug product, unsupported claims for a debatable surgical procedure, personal aggrandizement by an author touting a poorly executed clinical trial or simultaneous blaring of conflicting claims from legitimate information sources without anyone explaining the subtleties to the Internet reader. At the same time the Internet provides the very latest in evidence based medicine, science that will change the course of our species and advice that could save uncounted lives if applied properly.

1. Current Developments

With a standard search engine such as Google™, the order of the citations is based upon frequency of prior access. Some engines use some degree of commercial priority in the order of presentation. The references are not in any way sorted by accuracy and the search process simply cannot review the content. Among the debris, rare flowers bloom but they may be hard to find. Actually, even highly respected databases like CINAHL®, MEDLINE, Cochrane, etc., do not certify the reliability of citations. Medical readers are taught to differentiate a randomized controlled trial from a case report but the general public is not trained. The medical reader relies upon the peer review process, the prestige of a particular journal and the citation index or publication impact factor. However, the lay searcher is not so well equipped. Numerous evaluations have found problems in Internet material. A study of the general population in the UK by Larner in Liverpool revealed that almost 40% of searchers reached inappropriate information based upon their searches. This was in a population with 40% Internet access at home. Older patients were even less likely to be successful in finding accurate information. However, the author kindly pointed out that no harm seems to have come to any patient getting the wrong information [9]. Information for eating disorders was very much lacking in quality in another study of two popular search engines [10]. In a paper by Bernstam, the quality of health information was assessed with PubMed and five search engines to find any Internet quality studies. Of 273 distinct quality instruments applied, only 80 (29%) made the evaluation obvious. Only seven had entirely objective criteria and, of these, only one had criteria with proper interobserver kappa scores [11].

Evaluation of web material is far from reassuring. A 2004 paper found that consumer use of search engines was impaired by spelling and the use of general search engines without good qualifiers. The users also tended to fatigue after the first page of entries and did not pursue further [12]. Bernstam published another study in 2005 that questioned the usability of quality measures for material found on line. That paper was somewhat more optimistic, finding that inter-rater agreement could be improved with greater precision of the terms of study [13]. Health search engines can be improved. A study by Gaudinat, et al., examined a specialized health search engine and found advantages. However, the new engine was informative only 65% of the time compared to 59% for general purpose search engines. It was reliable 72% of the time compared to 41% for the standards [14]. It is hard to be reassured by 65% and 72% if a life depends upon the information retrieved.

For practitioners the situation can also be less than desirable. Shaneyfelt, et al., looked at evaluation of education in evidence based practice. Of 357 articles searched, 115 were excluded with only 104 unique instruments identified in those remaining. Acquiring evidence and appraising evidence were the matters most commonly evaluated and the users were medical students and postgraduate trainees. Only newer instruments looked at applying the information to patient care. At least one type of validity tool was used in 53% of the instruments applied in the study but three or more validity tools were utilized in only 10%. They concluded that although there are instruments for testing the validity of evidence based medicine they are not used with sufficient frequency [15]. Therefore, many publications of evidence based practice may not be the critical sources trainees and practitioners need and should expect.

For patients the situation is quite difficult in terms of authoritative sources. The lay person is not trained to understand the hierarchy of authority in study design and outcome analysis. There have been efforts at certifying sites. The HON code was introduced in 1996 with eight principles of practice for web sites offering medical information. Although disclosure and attribution figure strongly here, there is still no referee to assure accuracy of the material. In fact, the HON voluntary subscription by web publishers has not been very extensive [16]. Still the code is a good start and perhaps the best effort to date to assure ethical information [17]. The American Commission for Health Care began offering accreditation for web sites publishing health information in 2001 and, within the first year, 21 companies had successfully obtained certification; while, in the next 6 months an additional 12 web sites were certified. Please compare this to the thousands and thousands of web sites offering health information. It is clear that the impact has been limited. The European Commission has a code of practice that would be very sound if more widely implemented [18].

Medical organizations of high integrity and credibility are likely to sponsor web sites of implicitly higher quality. In this regard the US government offers the National Health Information Center with its Health Information Resource Database [19]. This site will access such impeccable sites as the American Cancer Society, various professional societies also devoted to cancer care, and prestigious treatment sites such as the MD Anderson Cancer Center in Houston. The Ontario Medical Association and the Ontario Ministry of Health and Long Term Care have developed a Guidelines Advisory Committee to address these issues [20]. However, the number of medical conditions for which resources have been evaluated is limited and the evaluators may not be altogether familiar with the expert community. The National Library of Medicine, in general, will lead patients to credible sites but maintains a distance that does not allow discrimination among information sources. The AMA and its journals are accessible to patients and offers an abundance of information [21] as does the World Health Organization [22]. These are sound sources that, unlike the standard search engines, may limit links to those considered authoritative. Senior web surfers number about 10 million in the US. They tend to spend little time on the searches and may become confused rather than informed [23].

Specialty organizations have every motivation to assure the quality of information for patients and accountability among its specialists. However, studies of web information for a given specialty strongly indicate the need for concerted and urgent effort by the specialty society or other body. In a study of web sites for cosmetic surgery Parikh found that of 200 sites, 115 failed to reach an acceptable standard of information. In fact, only 14 sites met the expected criteria in all areas [24]. In a study of sites about liver transplantation, the first 50 sites in a search were assumed the ones most likely used by a lay searcher. Four search engines led to a total of over two million sites! Examining the first 50 of the four engines, 200 sites were studied but of these only 58 sites were not repeated and therefore unique. On a standardized information score, the sites from the US were at about half the optimal and international sites were about half that of US and European sites [25]. In a study of web based information on psychological trauma, the top 20 hits from Google™, AllTheWeb, and Yahoo were tabulated for three synonyms and 94 unique sites were found. Of these, seventy-two were actually pertinent and were studied for content, design, disclosure and ease of access. Of these 42% had patently inaccurate information, while 82% did not indicate a source and in 41% a mental health professional had not been involved in preparing content [26]. Murphy, et al., studied web information on vasectomy using six search engines and the top 25 sites in each were scored. The study was conducted over a four year period to better understand the dynamic of information. In fact, there was no improvement over the time period and the engines continued to direct the searcher to irrelevant sites. They conclude that the Internet "cannot be recommended" for health information! [27] Similarly grim findings are published for pediatric orthopedics [28], nutrition [29] and scoliosis [30]. The latter study did find a superiority with academic sites over commercial but even academic sites did not score terribly well.

Despite the condemnation of so much web information by scientific sources there is no way to turn back the public from this source. In the September 12, 2006, New York Times, Deborah Franklin offers a very fine report on the use of the Internet for support from other patients [31]. The professional societies in medicine, surgery and in general are improving monthly and seem to recognize increasingly the responsibly to better serve the public with high quality and accessible information. Patients will never again rely solely on their doctor for the ultimate truths about their condition and its treatment. The Internet has become the idea forum for finding a protocol or treatment even before seeing the first consultant who is confronted by patient research. It seems certain that the Internet has become the second opinion of choice for many US patients. Patients routinely arrive with printouts about the doctor they are visiting and the treatment they have chosen. This matter of Internet use by patients is irreversible but the process can be improved by standards and professionalism.

2. Conclusions and Recommendations

At the moment the Internet is a highly suspect information source for health workers and patients. It is also clear that users will rely upon the source with all its flaws and that from time to time someone is going to get hurt by acting upon very bad advice. That may be a patient whose physician consults the Internet or a patient who consults the Internet and pursues erroneous advice. If health workers and patients are going to use the web no matter it seems futile to complain too stridently. Rather it is an ethical responsibility to remedy the situation. The following recommendations are offered.

1. Every health worker should have access to the Internet.
2. Every health worker should have training in evaluating e-health information as critically as any other publication. The assessment skills can be taught in medical school and in continuing medical education for older practitioners.
3. Every practitioner should be familiar with what is available on the web in his or her area of specialty and should be able to recommend sites. The recommendation would probably start with the appropriate professional society and every member of such groups should know what is being put on the web to represent the highest standards for the discipline.
4. Every specialty society should take the time and evaluate its own electronic health content to assure that the information is timely, pleasantly presented and an accurate reflection of the image of the specialty. In addition, the societies should use the expertise of the membership to assure the accuracy of the content.
5. Governmental sources should be certain that their information has had what amounts to peer-review and is updated with sufficient frequency to assure accuracy.
6. Every treatment facility and research organization should put on the web information that is accurate, timely and has been carefully reviewed for content.
7. Some of the international standards for quality should be applied to all e-health web sites and the additional assertion of truth in the content should be the responsibility of the organization and its specialized members.
8. It seems advisable for every practitioner to be accessible by the web. The web site could be used to answer questions about credentials, practice hours, information for referral and appointments with practice emphasis. Educational materials could be downloaded from the site and hyperlinks could lead to web sites known for quality and usefulness. Annotation of the hyperlink and suggestions on use would be desirable.
9. It would be advisable to ask patients about the quality and utility of the Internet access provided by the practice. This should be an element of patient satisfaction surveillance. Patients will also tell practitioners how to make their

electronic information better. Such an approach to patient communication is badly needed and has been adopted by many practitioners.

10. Finally, the consumer, the patient, the public should be educated in secondary school and beyond through community action to be prudent gatherers of information on the Internet and careful evaluators of content. The public must not lose confidence that medicine will always apply truth and human understanding to patient issues and will always behave with high ethical standards.

Acknowledgements

We would like to thank Ms. Chasity Roberts for her editorial work with this chapter.

References

[1]   Living Internet website http://www.livinginternet.com/. Last accessed September 22, 2006.
[2]   Internet Society website. http://www.isoc.org/internet/history/. Last accessed September 22, 2006.
[3]   Internet World Stats website. http://www.internetworldstats.com/stats.htm. Last accessed September 22, 2006.
[4]   Angood PB, Doarn CR, Holaday L, Nicogossian AE, Merrell RC: The Spacebridge to Russia Project: Internet-Based Telemedicine. Telemed J; Winter 4(4):305-311, 1998.
[5]   Williams DR, Bashushur RL, Pool SL, Doarn CR, Merrell RC, Logan JS: NASA Strategic Planning Workshop Proceedings – A Strategic Vision for Telemedicine and Medical Informatics in Space Flight. Telemed J E Health; 6(4):441-448, 2000.
[6]   National Center for Biotechnology Information website. http://www.ncbi.nlm.nih.gov/About/tools/ restable_stat_pubmed.html. Last accessed September 22, 2006.
[7]   US National Library of Medicine PubMed website. www.pubmed.gov. Last accessed September 22, 2006.
[8]   WHO Health InterNetwork Access to Research Initiative (HINARI) website. http://www.who.int/ hinari/en/. Last accessed September 22, 2006.
[9]   Larner AJ: Searching the Internet for medical information: frequency over time and by age and gender in an outpatient population in the UK. J Telemed Telecare. 12(4):186-188, 2006.
[10] Muphy R, Frost S, Webster P: An evaluation of web-based information. Int J Eat Disord. 35(2):145-54, 2004.
[11] Bernstam EV, Shelton DM, Walji M: Instruments to assess the quality of health information on the World Wide Web: What can our patients actually use? Int J Med Inform. 74(1):13-19, 2005.
[12] Morahan-Martin JM: How internet users find, evaluate and use online health information: a cross-cultural review. Cyberpsychol Behav. 7(5):497-510, 2004.
[13] Bernstam EV, Sagaram S, Walji M: Usability of quality measures for online health information: Can commonly used technical quality criteria be reliably assessed? Int J Med Info. 74(7-8):675-83, 2005.
[14] Gaudinat A, Ruch P, Joubert M, Uziel P: Health search engine with e-document analysis for reliable search results. Int J Med Inform. 75(1):73-85, 2006.
[15] Shaneyfelt T, Baum KD, Bell D, Feldstein D: Instruments for evaluating education in evidence-based practice: a systematic review. JAMA. 296(9):1116-27, 2006.
[16] Consumer Informatics: Applications and Strategies in Cyber Health Care. Rosemary Nelson and Mario Ball (eds.) Springer-Verlag New York, 2004.
[17] Wilson P: How to find the good and avoid the bad or ugly: a short guide to tools for rating quality of health information on the internet. BMJ. 324(7337):598-602, 2002.
[18] Watson R: European Commission to publish a code of practice for websites. BMJ. 324(7337):567, 2002.
[19] National Health Information Center, U.S. Department of Health and Human Services, Health Information Resource Database website. http://www.health.gov/NHIC/. Last accessed September 22, 2006.
[20] Guidelines Advisory Committee webpage. www.gacguidelines.ca. Last accessed September 24, 2006.
[21] American Medical Association webpage. http://www.ama-assn.org/. Last accessed September 22, 2006.
[22] World Health Organization webpage. http://www.who.int/en/. Last accessed September 22, 2006.

[23]   Moore GA: On-line communities: helping "senior surfers" find health information on the web. J Geron-
       tol News. 31(11)42-48, 2005.
[24]   Parikh AR, Kok K, Redern B: A portal to validated websites on cosmetic surgery: the design of an ar-
       chetype. Ann Plast Surg. 57(3):350-352, 2006.
[25]   Hanif F, Sivaprakasam R, Butler A: Information about liver transplantation on the World Wide Web.
       Med Inform Internet Med. 31(3):153-160, 2006.
[26]   Bremner JD, Quinn J, Quinn W, Veledar E: Surfing the Net for medical information about psychologi-
       cal trauma. Med Inform Internet Med. 31(3):227-36, 2006.
[27]   Murphy JO, Sweeney KJ, O'Mahony JC: Surgical informatics on the Internet: any improvement? Sur-
       geon. 1(3):177-9, 2003.
[28]   Aslam N, Bowyer D, Wainwright A: Evaluation of Internet use by paediatric orthopaedic outpatients
       and the quality of information available. J Pediatr Orthop B. 14(2):129-133, 2005.
[29]   Sutherland LA, Wildemuth B, Campbell MK: Unraveling the web: an evaluation of the content quality,
       usability and readability of nutrition web sites. J Nutr Educ Behav. 37(6):300-305, 2005.
[30]   Mathur S, Shanti N, Brkaric M: Surfing for scoliosis: the quality of information available on the Inter-
       net. Spine. 30(23):2695-2700, 2005.
[31]   Deborah Franklin. Support for Patients, Just a Mouse Click Away. New York Times, September 12,
       2006. http://www.nytimes.com/2006/09/12/health/12cons.html?ex=1160539200&en=7fcbcdaf3043a20
       9&ei=5070. Last accessed October 9, 2006.

VI. New Frontiers of Telemedicine

Current Principles and Practices of Telemedicine and e-Health
R. Latifi (Ed.)
IOS Press, 2008

Telepresence and Telemedicine in Trauma and Emergency

Rifat LATIFI, MD, FACS
Professor of Clinical Surgery
Trauma, Surgical Critical Care and Emergency General Surgery
Department of Surgery, The University of Arizona, Tucson, Arizona, USA

Abstract. Telemedicine for trauma and emergency management is emerging as new frontier and is evolving as an integral part trauma care of modern trauma practice. This chapter will review the current applications and future endeavors of telemedicine and telepresence to trauma and emergency care as the new frontiers of telemedicine application.

Keywords. Telemedicine, trauma, teletrauma, telepresence, emergency management, wireless technologies

Introduction

Trauma requires fast, definitive and precise care as well as major resources and continuous expertise; otherwise the consequences may be enormous for the individual patient, family and society as a whole. The major trauma centers and trauma specialists around the world are concentrated mainly in urban settings. Subsequently, most of the population of the USA, and the world for that matter, is not covered by specialized trauma systems. Although only 23–25% of the population in the USA lives in rural America, 56.9% of deaths caused by motor vehicle crashes (MVC) occur in this population [1]. Furthermore, only 15 states in the USA have state wide 911 or enhanced 911 systems. As a result, rural patients are at greater risk of traumatic death than their urban counterparts [2]. In fact, patients involved in motor vehicle crashes in rural America have twice the rate of mortality when compared with those in an urban setting with the same injury severity score [1–7].

Each day, more than 600 people die or sustain long-term disability from traumatic injuries in the United States. Up to 40% of the deaths could be prevented if access to a well organized system of trauma care was uniform throughout the country [2]. Residents of Loving county Texas (population 240 in 1990), are almost 600 times more likely to die following an automobile crash than residents of downtown Manhattan [5]. Although it is not entirely clear why there is such a discrepancy in trauma care between rural and urban America, a few factors have been identified by many authors [2–5]. First, emergency room personnel in low volume trauma care "centers" often have limited experience with major traumas, which may lead to management errors and departures from the standard of care. In addition, many rural emergency rooms are not adequately staffed with properly trained personnel, and there are limits to the ability to provide continuing medical education (CME) to ER personnel and emergency medical service (EMS) providers in the rural setting [6]. Another reason for poor outcomes for rural trauma patients is the lack of access to immediate subspecialty care (trauma surgeons, neurosurgeons, orthopedic, vascular or cardiac surgeons) in remote locations.

One of the most important challenges, therefore, arises to develop means to reduce the major discrepancy between urban and rural trauma care. Advances in technology including telemedicine and telepresence applications may be the solution as the mean to reduce and/or eliminate the gap in trauma care between rural and urban areas, but the implications of telemedicine may be far beyond the simple video-teleconference.

The patient population for a Level I trauma center consists largely of patients who have been transferred from rural communities for definitive tertiary trauma care. In most current systems, the decision to transfer a patient to a trauma center is based on a phone call from the referring rural physician to the emergency room physician or trauma surgeon. Based on the experience of many trauma centers, a large number of patients transferred to trauma centers could be adequately cared for in the rural or community hospital with the help or "telepresence" of a trauma surgeon in these remote hospitals from a central location. In order to accomplish this goal, small emergency rooms or other centers in rural areas need to have access to major trauma centers and trauma surgeons 24 hours a day, seven days a week with modern technology. This "telepresence" undoubtedly will have a major impact in major trauma centers that will evaluate and eventually manage most critically ill patients who need specialized and definitive trauma care.

Current Telemedicine and Telepresence Programs

Wireless Mobile Telemedicine and Telepresence in Prehospital Assessment and Intervention: Tucson ER-Link Project

The City of Tucson and the University of Arizona Medical Center in Tucson, Arizona are have implemented the concept of digitized emergency services with seamless integration of multiple video processing and wireless communication. This concept will improve the quality of emergency medical services and it is hoped that early intervention will increase the survival of most critically ill patients.

The City of Tucson Emergency Room Link or "ER-Link Tucson" project allows physicians to be virtually present at the scene and/or in the ambulance, while the patient is being transported to the hospital emergency room. This program will provide emergency dispatchers and responders a view of the incident scene(s) in order for them to optimally assign emergency first responders and other necessary resources for incident management. The project allows video and audio teleconferencing capabilities between the University Medical Center and all of the City of Tucson Fire Department Advanced Life Support (ALS) Ambulances. The system ensures near-constant two-way audio-video and medical data transmissions between the attending paramedic in the ambulance and the trauma and emergency room medical personnel. The communications is envisioned to be via regional traffic control and city communications infrastructure and wireless technology. The telepresence at the scene of event is made possible from cameras mounted externally to the emergency vehicle. These cameras, in conjunction with the existing highway cameras, operating along the freeway or at intersections, provides command and control video to the regional E-911 centers and emergency department. These images are intended to facilitate the dispatch and management of emergency resources for incident command, accident management and medical triage/mechanical assessment of the scene for the trauma team.

This project funded by the Federal Department of Transportation makes Tucson one of the first cities in the nation to use combinations of traffic control and communications infrastructure to relay "real-time" accident video to the E-911 center and patient information to the trauma/emergency room physicians. The system's goals are to get advanced trauma level medical assistance to the citizens of Tucson and surrounding communities when time is critical and when they need help the most. A secondary goal is to clear an accident scene sooner and reduce the potential for secondary collisions, which further enhance the public's safety by not tying up additional emergency services and congesting our transportation system. In addition, Tucson's program fits well into the goals and objectives of Homeland Security by expanding the communications capabilities of the emergency service providers and regional trauma center(s). "ER-Link Tucson" can help assist hospitals and public health agencies and upgrade communications and other emergency medical technologies to quickly identify victim's needs and formulate appropriate responses.

The goal of the first phases of Tucson's ER-Link is the development of a successful technological implementation of a mobile telemedicine communications system in the city using current traffic control and communications equipment. Once the technology is proven, the inclusion of more private partners, air and land emergency transporters, rural fire districts and Indian Nation fire departments will become more feasible. The combination of the skills of the fire paramedic and the remote trauma specialist is expected to expand the level of care to injured patients when time is the most critical.

Interhospital Telemedicine and Telepresence: The Southern Arizona Tele Trauma Program

The creation of the Southern Arizona TeleTrauma Program (SATT), at the University of Arizonahas been completed and is functionalThis will include rural towns which lie along the Arizona-Mexico border, including the towns of Douglas, Bisbee, Benson, Sierra Vista, Nogales, and other small towns and communities. Teletrauma consultations is provided through existing T1 lines of the Arizona Telemedicine Program (ATP). The trauma surgeon will have video and audio access to events unfolding in trauma and emergency rooms throughout the "border belt" as well as other rural communities.

Discussion

The first attempt to simulate the use of telemedicine in trauma resuscitation was recorded in 1978 by Dr. R. Adams Cowley, who staged a disaster exercise at Friendship Airport in an aged DC-6 aircraft [3]. He transmitted real-time images of burn victims via satellite transmission to San Antonio's Burn Unit and other medical centers around the Washington DC area. This was accomplished with an old and cumbersome technology, yet it is the first successful attempt to use technology and telemedicine in trauma care. Since then, numerous efforts have been made to resuscitate trauma patients from a distance.

Rogers et al. [4,6] reported their use of a tele-trauma service in rural Vermont, where 68% of the population lives in rural areas. Their initial experience with 41 tele-trauma consultations was very encouraging. Ninety-five percent of the injuries were caused from blunt trauma, primarily MVC (49%), pedestrians/bicyclist struck by vehicles (10%) and injuries caused by all terrain vehicles (7%). Thirty one of 41 patients that were seen via the tele-trauma system were transferred to the tertiary care center. In 59% of the cases transfer was recommended immediately, due to the critical condition of the patient; 41% of transfers were accomplished by helicopter. While in three cases, tele-trauma consultation was considered life saving, the most common recommendations from the tele-trauma consultant were regarding patient disposition. For example, in 15% of cases the trauma surgeon recommended keeping the patient at the referring facility. Other recommendations included suggestions for diagnostics such as obtaining or foregoing a CT scan, as well as recommendations for additional therapeutics (placement of an NG tube, or a chest tube, transfusion of blood, etc.).

Other investigators have also reported various techniques to establish trauma tele-consultations in rural settings [8–10]. In a study of 40 orthopedic trauma cases, radiographic images were photographed by a digital camera and transmitted via dedicated T1 based network to a consulting hub, where two orthopedic and two radiologists reviewed the cases [8]. This and other reported studies have demonstrated that a simple digital camera can be used effectively in many cases, as long as the proper region of interest on the x-ray has been photographed and transmitted to the consultant [8,9].

Lambrecht et al. also demonstrated the effectiveness of telemedicine technology in the evaluation and treatment of extremity and pelvic injuries [10]. The most important element in this report was that 68 of 100 patients referred for tele-consultation remained in the rural community hospital. This certainly has major implications on the cost of transferring of these patients to major medical centers, increased utilization of local health care facilities and other social and financial issues of treating these patients away from their families.

Clinical Accuracy of Telemedicine in Trauma Care

The clinical accuracy of telemedicine in evaluating trauma patients has been assessed. When telemedicine was used for minor trauma consultation and compared with face-to-face consultations in two hundred patients, skin color changes were accurately defined in 97%, the presence of swelling or deformity in 98%, diminished joint movement in 95%, presence of tenderness in 97%, weight bearing and gait 99%, and radiological diagnosis was made correctly in 98% of cases [11]. The severity of injury was overestimated in one and underestimated in five cases, but the final diagnosis was correct in all but two cases. Similarly, other authors have shown that remote evaluation of trauma patients using telemedicine is accurate and feasible [13]. In a two-phase project using ATLS-based evaluation tools, it was found that accurate clinical data could be recorded, tasks delegated, and therapeutic measures advised and applied using telemedicine. This application of telemedicine can make expert trauma care available to patients in hospitals and emergency rooms without advanced trauma systems, and potentially reduce costs, prevent unnecessary transfers, and promote early transfer when indicated.

Health Care Providers Satisfaction

Patient and healthcare provider's satisfaction with telemedicine is a major issue that has been examined in the past, and continues to be an important element. Multiple studies have demonstrated that patients' satisfaction has been one of the positive elements of telemedicine. When 52 patients with brain injury were interviewed via high quality teleconferencing these patients were very satisfied and wanted to repeat their sessions more than patients interviewed in person, especially those in the assessment phase of their disease [11].

In order to fully implement remote trauma resuscitation, the remote trauma surgeons and referring health care providers must feel comfortable and confident in their ability to supervise and mange trauma resuscitation in the remote site from a central location. When the level of satisfaction with teletrauma [4,7] was analyzed, eighty-three percent of referring doctors and 61% of the trauma surgeons thought that the consultation improved patient care. In addition, 67% of all the physicians involved in tele-trauma care, thought that the consultation could not have been performed as well by telephone. This study demonstrated the effective use of telemedicine for consultation, expert opinion, and to determine the need for transfer of the patient to the major trauma center and as such has been successfully implemented in a rural setting [4], where both patients and the referring doctor benefited greatly from the expert at a distance. Senior trauma experts located centrally have used ATLS protocol to supervise trauma scenarios performed by a physician at a remote site [15] and recorded the degree of confidence in the supervision of the tasks on a five point predetermined Likert scale (1 – poor; 2 – unsure; 3 – satisfactory; 4 – sure; 5 – certain). Fifteen trauma scenarios were evaluated on three points: the primary survey, resuscitation and secondary survey. The average score was between 3 and four for the assessment of the primary survey and resuscitation phase.

Telemedicine in Follow-Up and Wound Care in Trauma Patients

Telemedicine is also being applied to the follow-up care of trauma patients. In Kentucky, 22 telemedicine-based follow-up assessments of trauma patients were performed with the assistance of a nurse, an electronic stethoscope and a close-up imaging instrument [16]. The average duration of the video-teleconference appointment was 14 minutes. Both patient and physician satisfaction were high, significantly decreased travel distances and time were observed. In a follow-up survey, all patients involved strongly agreed with the statement "Telemedicine makes it easier to get medical care" [16]. Telemedicine tools have also been applied to the field of wound care management. In one study, bedside wound examination of 38 wounds in 24 vascular surgery patients was done by onsite surgeons and was compared with viewing digital images of those wounds by remote surgeons [12]. Agreements regarding wound description (the presence of edema, erythema, cellulitis, necrosis, gangrene, ischemia, and granulation), management issues (such as the presence of problem wound healing, need for emergent evaluation, antibiotics and hospitalization) were analyzed and compared between onsite and remote surgeons. Agreement between onsite and remote surgeons matched for wound description and wound management. Sensitivity of remote diagnosis ranged from of 78% for gangrene to 98% for identification of problem wound healing respectively, whereas specificity ranged from 27% for erythema to 100% for ischemia. The agreement was influenced by the wound type (p < 0.01), but not by the certainty of diagnosis or level of training (p > 0.01). This combination of telemedicine and digital photography may prove to be very useful for outpatient wound care in complex vascular surgery and in trauma patients in their post operative care.

Conclusion

Telemedicine will become a major tool in trauma care and trauma education. Trauma resuscitation can be performed successfully and safely using telemedicine principles, when guided by and under direct supervision of a trauma surgeon. Furthermore, major trauma centers can render direct help in primary resuscitation of trauma victims to small hospitals without trauma specialists, potentially reduce cost, prevent unnecessary transfers, and promote early transfer when indicated to Level I trauma centers. There a need for investment in technology and creation of substantial networks and for creativity among trauma surgeons, emergency medicine physicians and other healthcare workers providing care to trauma and injured patients.

References

[1]   Congressional Office of Technology Assessment. Rural Emergency Medical Services. Special Reports US, Washington, DC, 1989. Publication OTA-H-445.
[2]   Voelker R. Access to trauma care. JAMA 2000; 284.
[3]   Maull K. The friendship airport disaster exercise: pioneering effort in trauma telemedicine. Eur Jour Med Research 2002; 7 (supplement) 48.
[4]   Ricci MA, Caputo M, Amour J et al. Telemedicine Reduces Discrepancies in Rural Trauma Care. Telemed Journ & e-Health 2003; 9(1):3-11.
[5]   Baker SP, Whitfield RA, O'Neil B. Geographic variations in mortality from motor vehicle crashes. N Eng J Med 1987; 316:1384-87.
[6]   Flowe KM, Cunningham PRG, Foil MB. Rural trauma. Surg Annu 1995; 27:29-39.
[7]   Rogers F, Ricci M, Shackford S, Caputo L, Sartorelli K, Dwell J, and Day S. The use of telemedicine for real-time video consultation between trauma center and community hospital in a rural setting improves early trauma care. Preliminary results. J Trauma 2001.
[8]   Rogers FB, Shackford SR, Osler TM et al. Rural trauma: the challenge for the next decade. J Trauma 1999; 47:801-21.
[9]   Krupinski E, Gonzales M, Gonzales C and Weinstein RS. Evaluation of digital camera for acquiring radiographic images for telemedicine applications. Telemed J E Health 2000; 6(3):297-302.
[10] Carr P, Cooper I, Beninfield SJ, and Mars M. A simple telemedicine system using a digital camera. J Telemed Telecare 2000; 6(4):233-6.
[11] Lambrecht CJ. Telemedicine in trauma care: Description of 100 trauma teleconsults. Telemed J 1997; 3(4):265-8.
[12] Tachakra S, Lynch M, Newsom R et al. A comparison of telemedicine with face-to faces consultations for trauma management. J Telemed Telecare 2000; 5(Suppl 1):S178-81.
[13] Wirthlin DJ, Buradagunta S, Edwards RA, Brewster DC et al. Telemedicine in vascular surgery: feasibility of digital imaging for remote management of wounds. J Vasc Surg 1998; 27(6):1089-99.
[14] Aucar J, Granchi T, Liscum K et al. Is regionalization of trauma care using telemedicine feasible and desirable? Am J Surg 2000; 180(6):535-39.
[15] Schopp LH, Johnston BR, Merveille OC. Multidimensional Telecare strategies for rural residents with brain injury. J Telemed Telecare 2000; 6(Supp 1):S146-49.
[16] Tachakra S, Jaye P, Bak J, Hayes J, Sivakumar A. Supervising trauma support by telemedicine. J Telemed Telecare 2000; 6(Suppl 1):S7-11.
[17] Boulanger B, Kearney P, Ochoa J, Tsuei B and Snads F. Telemedicine: a solution to the follow-up of rural trauma patients? J Am Coll Surg 2001; 192(4):447-452.

Current Principles and Practices of Telemedicine and e-Health
R. Latifi (Ed.)
IOS Press, 2008

Appendix

Author Information:

Sandra J. Beinar
Associate Director, Administration
Arizona
Telemedicine Program
1501 N. Campbell Avenue
PO Box 245105
Tucson, AZ 85724-5105

Gail Barker, MBA, PhD
Co-Director, Maricopa
Arizona Telemedicine Program
550 Van Buren, Room 1372
Phoenix, AZ 85004

Charles R. Doarn, MBA
Deputy Director
Advanced Center for Telemedicine and
Surgical Innovation
Executive Director
Center for Surgical Innovation
Associate Professor of Surgery and
Biomedical Engineering
Editor-in-Chief, Telemedicine and
e-Health Journal
Department of Surgery
University of Cincinnati
231 Albert Sabin Way, MSB 2463A
ML 0558
Cincinnati, OH 45267-0558
Voice: (513) 558-6148
Fax: (513) 558-7061
Cell: (513) 403-9604
E-mail: charles.doarn@uc.edu
Web: http://surgery.uc.edu/csi.html

Brett Harnett
Assistant Professor, Research
University of Cincinnati Medical Center
231 Albert B. Sabin Way
Cincinnati, OH 45267
E-mail: brett.harnett@uc.edu

Michael Holcomb
Associate Director, Network Architecture
Arizona Telemedicine Program
1501 N Campbell Avenue
PO Box 245105, Tucson, AZ 85724-5105

Dr. Anastasia N. Kastania
Department of Informatics
Athens University of Economics
and Business
Patission 76 Str
Athens 10434, Greece

Stephen W. Cone, MD
Medical Informatics and Technology
Applications Consortium
Virginia Commonwealth University
Richmond, VA

Prof. K. Ganapathy
Head, Apollo Telemedicine Foundation
Secretary, Asian Australasian Society of
Neurological Surgery
President, Neurological Society
of India. 2006
Fax/Tel. No.: 91 44 28295447
Web: http://kganapathy.com

Robert H. Groves, Jr., MD, FCCP
System Medical Director Critical Care
Banner Health
Medical Director iCare, Intensive Care
Banner Health
2145 W. Southern Ave
Mesa, AZ 85202

Georgi Graschew
Surgical Research Unit OP 2000
Robert-Roessle-Klinik and
Max-Delbrueck-Centrum
Charité – University Medicine Berlin
Lindenberger Weg 80, D-13125 Berlin
Germany

Barry W. Holcomb, Jr., MD, FCCP
Senior Intensivist iCare, Intensive Care
Banner Health
2145 W. Southern Ave
Mesa, AZ 85202

Eka Kldiashvili, PhD
Executive Director
Georgian Telemedicine Union
(Association)
75 Kostava str., 0171 Tbilisi, Georgia
E-mail: kldiashvili@georgia.
telepathology.org
Web: http://georgia.telepathology.org

Elizabeth A. Krupinski, PhD
Research Professor Dept. Radiology
Research
University of Arizona
1609 N. Warren Bldg 211 Rm 112
Tucson, AZ 85724520
krupinski@radiology.arizona.edu

Jim Muir and Lex Lucas
Australian College of Rural and Remote
Medicine

Rifat Latifi, MD, FACS
Professor of Surgery
Interim Chief, Section of Trauma &
Critical Care
Director of International Affairs
University of Arizona Telemedicine
Program
1501 N. Campbell Ave., PO Box 245063
Tucson, AZ 85724-5063

Ana Maria Lopez, MD, MPH
Medical Director, Arizona Telemedicine
Program
1501 N Campbell Avenue, PO Box
245024, Tucson, AZ 85724-5024

Cheri A. Ong, MD
Department of Plastic Surgery
Vanderbilt University
D4207 Medical Center North
Nashville, TN 37232-2345
E-mail: cheri.ong@vanderbilt.edu

Marshall (Mark) Smith, MD, PhD
FACOG
Medical Director of Telemedicine
WT-1 1111 East McDowell Rd
Banner Good Samaritan Medical Center
Banner Health
Phoenix, Arizona

Theo A. Roelofs, Stefan Rakowsky
and Peter M. Schlag
Surgical Research Unit OP 2000
Robert-Roessle-Klinik and
Max-Delbrueck-Centrum
Charité – University Medicine Berlin
Lindenberger Weg 80, D-13125 Berlin
Germany

Deborah Theodoros, PhD
Associate Professor and Head
Division of Speech Pathology
School of Health and Rehabilitation
Sciences
Phone: 07 3365 2806
Mobile: 0411 090 681
E-mail: d.theodoros@uq.edu.au

Ronald Merrell, MD
1101 E Marshall St
Sanger Hall 8017
PO Box 980480
Richmond, VA 23298-0480
Phone: 804-827-1031
Fax: 804-827-1029
E-mail: rmerrell@mcvh-vcu.edu

Richard A. McNeely
Co-Director, Arizona Telemedicine
Program, Arizona Telemedicine Program
1501 N Campbell Avenue
PO Box 245032, Tucson, AZ 85724-5032

Azhar Rafiq, MD
Medical Informatics
and Technology Applications Consortium
Virginia Commonwealth University
Richmond, VA

Keith Shelman, MD
Information Systems Services

University Medical Center
1501 North Campbell Avenue
PO Box 245173
Tucson AZ, 85724-5173
Phone: 520-694-4766
Fax: 520-694-4764
E-mail: kshelman@umcaz.edu

Trevor Russell
Division of Speech Pathology
Division of Physiotherapy
School of Health and Rehabilitation
Sciences
The University of Queensland
Brisbane, Australia

Laurence S. Wilson
CSIRO ICT Centre, Sydney, Australia

Ronald S. Weinstein, MD
Director
Arizona Telemedicine Program
1501 N Campbell Avenue
PO Box 245105, Tucson, AZ 85724-5105

Subject Index

‒irrent Principles and Practices of Telemedicine and e-Health
k. —atifi (Ed.)
IOS —ress, 2008
© 2(8 R. Latifi. All rights reserved.

Author Index